www.harcourt-international.com

Bringing you products from all Harcourt Health Sciences companies including Baillière Tindall, Churchill Livingstone, Mosby and W.B. Saunders

▶ **Browse** for latest information on new books, journals and electronic products

▶ **Search** for information on over 20 000 published titles with full product information including tables of contents and sample chapters

▶ **Keep up to date** with our extensive publishing programme in your field by registering with eAlert or requesting postal updates

▶ **Secure online ordering** with prompt delivery, as well as full contact details to order by phone, fax or post

▶ **News** of special features and promotions

If you are based in the following countries, please visit the country-specific site to receive full details of product availability and local ordering information

USA: www.harcourthealth.com

Canada: www.harcourtcanada.com

Australia: www.harcourt.com.au

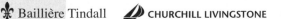 Baillière Tindall  CHURCHILL LIVINGSTONE Mosby 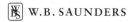 W.B. SAUNDERS

Effective Management of Musculoskeletal Injury

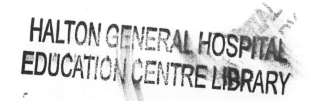

For Churchill Livingstone:

Editorial Director, Health Professions: Mary Law
Project Development Manager: Dinah Thom
Designer: George Ajayi

Effective Management of Musculoskeletal Injury

A Clinical Ergonomics Approach to Prevention, Treatment and Rehabilitation

Andrew Wilson ND DO MNZRO
Registered Osteopath (New Zealand) and Consultant Ergonomist, Tauranga, New Zealand

Foreword by

Jeffrey D. Boyling MSc BPhty GradDipAdvManipTher MAPA MCSP MErgS MMACP MMPA SRP
Director, Jeffrey Boyling Associates, Chartered Physiotherapists and Ergonomists, London, UK

Illustrations by

Colleen Parsons

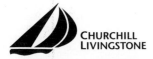
CHURCHILL
LIVINGSTONE

EDINBURGH LONDON NEW YORK PHILADELPHIA ST LOUIS SYDNEY TORONTO 2002

CHURCHILL LIVINGSTONE
An imprint of Harcourt Publishers Limited

© Harcourt Publishers Limited 2002

 is a registered trademark of Harcourt Publishers Limited

The right of Andrew Wilson to be identified as author of this work has been asserted by him in accordance with the Copyright, Designs and Patents Act 1988

First published 2002

ISBN 0 443 06353 2

British Library Cataloguing in Publication Data
A catalogue record for this book is available from the British Library

Library of Congress Cataloging in Publication Data
A catalog record for this book is available from the Library of Congress

Note
Medical knowledge is constantly changing. As new information becomes available, changes in treatment, procedures, equipment and the use of drugs become necessary. The author and publishers have taken care to ensure that the information given in this text is accurate and up to date. However, readers are strongly advised to confirm that the information, especially with regard to drug usage, complies with the latest legislation and standards of practice

The
publisher's
policy is to use
**paper manufactured
from sustainable forests**

Printed in China

Contents

Foreword

Ramazzini (1633–1714) described the relationship between work and ill health in his book *De Morbis Artfactum Diatriba*. Today, ill health caused by work is still an issue and a costly one too. Despite the efforts of researchers worldwide, as well as legislative changes in numerous countries, the toll on the worker does not appear to be lessening. Furthermore, the quantity and quality of occupational health provision varies around the globe, and it varies between employers within countries. If anything, the problems of spinal pain and upper limb disorders in the workplace appear to be on the rise.

By the very nature of the resulting musculoskeletal problems experienced by workers it is no surprise to find that the front-line troops managing these problems are manual therapists such as osteopaths and physiotherapists. Unfortunately, apart from pure clinical books, there are not many texts written by osteopaths or physiotherapists that deal with work-related musculoskeletal ill health. The majority of those written tend to be either edited works or suited for the dedicated therapist working in occupational health.

Taking the ergonomic perspective, those texts dealing with musculoskeletal problems lack the clinical know-how of 'hands on' therapists. The late Stephen Pheasant, a well-respected and distinguished writer on the subject of ergonomics, used the expression 'clinical ergonomics' approximately 10 years ago. The few pages that he wrote gave a foretaste of his thinking. What Andrew Wilson has written in over 250 pages covers three areas, namely the injury process, low back pain and finally the neck, shoulder and upper limb pain. However, what distinguishes this material from previously published work is the blend of the clinical and ergonomic aspects.

Andrew's writing on the injury process in Section 1 draws together numerous strands without overburdening the reader. These strands are essential if the clinical and ergonomic aspects of musculoskeletal injuries are to be effectively managed. Similarly, the problem of low back pain is addressed by means of chapters on epidemiology, risk factors, injury type, the complex low back and management of low back pain. Numerous worthwhile facts are presented along with illustrations for the reader. Helpful tips such as plateau breakers are suggested. The neck and upper limb are also covered with chapters on the various joint complexes as well as on nerve entrapments and multiple tissue disorders. Throughout, a blend of clinical management and the application of ergonomics is fostered.

As an Australian physiotherapist and ergonomist based in the United Kingdom it gives me great pleasure to write the foreword for this text by Andrew Wilson, an osteopath based in New Zealand. The text will appeal to many, from the undergraduate student needing a foundation in the area of clinical ergonomics to the clinician who has seen the error of treating a work-related condition in isolation from the workplace. Those already attempting to blend clinical and ergonomic roles will also find valuable material here. This book will create much interest and therefore the future of the work is assured.

Jeffrey D. Boyling

Acknowledgements

A huge thanks to Colleen Parsons, whose dedication to the illustrations has provided such an important part of this book. Thank you to Dinah Thom and Mary Law of Churchill Livingstone, who persevered with this author despite ever-changing formats, and to Jeffrey Boyling, who provided comments and suggestions at various stages of development.

In the great forest of knowledge, my original contribution is equivalent to a pair of tender buds. A project like this is not possible without access to the research that has gone before it. My thanks to the researchers and writers whose work has contributed to the development of this project. Some researchers do more than just research, they have the ability to expand existing knowledge and provide directions into the future, like a spotlight shining through the dark. Some of the people whose work has provided particular inspiration to me are: Michael Adams, Kim Korr, James Fisk, A. C. Mandal, Stephen Pheasant and Barbara Silverstein. My colleagues, my patients, my clients and my students have all played important roles in the learning process.

Most of all, my love and gratitude to Elspeth, who supports and encourages me. To my children, Emily, Charlotte and Jamie, I promise not to write another book for a long time!

Andrew Wilson

Acknowledgements

Introduction

Clinical ergonomics is the art and science of managing the demands of the environment to enable people to comfortably meet those demands, and to enhance their capacity to meet the challenges of their environments, including the prevention, treatment and rehabilitation of musculoskeletal injury.

The development of an injury suggests an imbalance between a person and his or her environment. The person has been affected by demands that were beyond his or her capacity to endure without developing symptoms. This can be due to an unpredictable event, such as driving into a brick wall at 100 kmph; to a mismatch between the predictable demands of the environment and the capacity of the person to meet these demands on one or more occasions, resulting in tissue failure, such as back injury following repeated lifting; or it can be due to prolonged and cumulative exposure, which causes a progressive reduction in efficiency of action and the ability to recover, such as in the classic overuse injuries.

The main concerns of the clinical ergonomist are to:

- reduce pain and dysfunction
- identify barriers to recovery (ergonomic, psychosocial and personal)
- assess people's ability to function in their environment
- improve people's ability to meet the demands of their environment
- reduce the demands of the environment to suit the individual and the population at risk
- minimize the risk of developing symptoms.

Clinical ergonomics is predominantly focused on the individual, trying to optimize the fit between people, their environment and the myriad of influences: work and domestic, biomechanical, physiological or psychosocial. The clinical ergonomics approach is likely to be alerted by the presence of symptoms and the need to manage these. However, it can be extended to a more systems- or population-based approach to improve the match, and decrease the risks, of different populations and their respective environments.

When people are injured they benefit from therapy, guidance, rehabilitation and education. They need empathy and understanding in a positive, honest and constructive manner. The manual therapy approach aims to minimize the effects of the injury and reduce any musculoskeletal dysfunction that may be exacerbating the symptoms or contributing to the injury. There is now a significant body of research into manual therapy and there is sufficient evidence to suggest that it is probably the most effective modality for dealing with recent injuries, although the evidence is less convincing for more chronic injuries.

Chronic injuries are often complex, and a comprehensive treatment model is required. Early indications from research suggest that progressive exercise designed to strengthen the injured joints and improve their adaptation to the tasks involved has been helpful in reducing disability. Exercise therapy has shown good long-term outcomes with chronic patients but is generally less effective for acute patients.

Psychosocial factors can be important in the development of injury and in the transition from acute to chronic injury. A thorough understanding of these issues and of the practical solutions for dealing with them is an important part of injury management. Anxiety or depression are often associated with injury and these also need to be addressed.

However, even the best efforts of skilled, well-educated, musculoskeletal practitioners, working with well-motivated patients, are often not sufficient to effect a good outcome. If the environment is not conducive to recovery there is an increased likelihood of chronicity. Being a clinician can become frustrating when there is an obvious environmental cause to a patient's symptoms that they find difficult to influence. People are often unaware that the tasks they do every day can contribute to the cause of an injury or can exacerbate an existing injury. Patients are frequently confused by advice or feel powerless to make effective changes. The therapist can play an important role as a catalyst for change. A visit to, or an assessment of, someone's working environment can be vital to understanding a person's injury and effecting the changes that may be crucial to recovery. When I began visiting workplaces I was amazed how closely injuries could be related to a person's at-risk postures or behaviours. On returning to my clinic I was pleasantly surprised to find how I could often predict people's postural faults by their muscle tension patterns – a neck that is flexed too much, or too frequently rotated in one direction; a shoulder that is held in elevation. Musculoskeletal practitioners should beware of confining themselves to the comfort zone of their treatment rooms and of neglecting the environment where the injuries are produced; the most important manipulations are often to the patient's environment.

There is a large body of sound research on ergonomics and its role in the management of injury. This has been for the most part neglected by the musculoskeletal fraternity. The extension of my practice into clinical-based ergonomics has enabled me to provide genuine benefits to many chronic patients who would otherwise prove very difficult to manage and would frequently suffer patient disability (and practitioner burnout).

There is a considerable art involved in healing the sick and providing a positive support role. This has tended to become subsidiary to the current focus on evidence-based medicine (EBM). While not wanting to diminish the importance of developing EBM, it must be placed in context of the practitioner who is faced on a daily basis with managing patients and providing solutions where the evidence is confusing, conflicting or even absent. Even in areas where there is a considerable body of research, different epidemiologists may reach startlingly different conclusions when reviewing the same body of literature. In the absence of scientific consensus, principles and philosophy based on sound homeostatic principles become important. This book attempts to identify practical and clinically based solutions for chronic and overuse injuries and so provide busy practitioners with working tools for their patients. I have attempted to support this with reference to sound research where possible. However, in many areas research is still very much in its infancy and it is difficult to reach consensus on the problems, let alone their solutions.

While research is rarely definitive it is often sufficient to provide some direction, to act as a signpost toward the desired outcome. Practitioners do not have the luxury of waiting for sufficient evidence before proceeding; we are faced with challenges every day where we must do our best under the circumstances available. There is much that we do know, and much that we can extrapolate to provide helpful tools to prevent and manage injury. I have been selective in my use of references. I have chosen references that support the models for injury management developed in Section 1. I have focused on research involving manual medicine, exercise and ergonomics – the approaches that seem to be demonstrating the most success in injury management. I have concentrated on recent research, as this tends to reduce the risk of methodological errors; it is easier to access and it better reflects our modern environment. In this rapidly changing world research can date quite quickly.

I apologize to the researchers who have made valuable contributions to research in these areas that I have not included. It is becoming increasingly difficult to keep up with all areas of research, particularly when the net is cast wide. In most developed countries the amount of time spent off work due to back pain has increased around 600% since the 1970s. The 1980s saw a similar explosive increase in work-related upper limb disorders, which are now similar to low back pain statistics. The 1990s have shown some dropping-off of the rate of claims in these types of injuries but it is open to debate whether this is due to a genuine reduction in symptoms or because of changes in claims management. Why do these injury statistics remain at very high rates? Despite a therapist on every corner, despite widespread dissemination of advanced techniques, despite medical advances in imaging, we are losing the battle against back pain and its attendant morbidity in a spectacular fashion.

In this rapidly changing world, the type of injuries that people get seems to be changing. There has been a trend towards an increasing number of chronic and overuse injuries, in addition to the traumatic injuries traditionally seen. Our traditional models for injury management, such as surgery and medicated pain relief, are often applied inappropriately to this emerging injury trend. The traumatic, pathological and inflammatory causes of injury, and the models of management that have developed from these, have often proved to be blunt tools for the complexity of chronic pain or overuse injury. A different model of injury will be explored and an attempt made to develop a coherent management approach to musculoskeletal injury to take into account the multifactorial nature of modern musculoskeletal problems.

Our lifestyles and workplaces are changing at an extraordinary rate. We are becoming more sedentary, spending more time in sitting postures. Most of us sit for long periods at work, on transport and at leisure. The computer is playing an increasingly important role in our work and home environments. Never before has a new piece of technology become used so much in so many different workplaces in such a short space of time. Computer work involves a change in work patterns that we are not well adapted to:

- a constrained, sitting posture
- long periods of low level isometric contraction
- a large amount of mental processing
- little opportunity for social interaction.

These changes in workstyle have produced subtle changes in our physiological processes, which alter both the risk of injury and the nature of the injury. If we perform less physical work we have reduced muscle tone. If we have less activity we have reduced muscular pumping of our vascular and lymphatic systems. This reduces effective oxygenation of our muscles and reduces the ability to deliver nutrients and remove waste products. Our muscles fatigue more quickly and become more prone to dysfunction and injury.

This book is not the definitive guide – the knowledge is too recent and the research too limited to provide this – but it attempts to develop a framework for understanding injury and for developing solutions. In this ever-changing world there is an increasing need for practitioners to identify emerging problems and predict solutions. The research on which to base this often takes many years and is frequently incomplete. We do not always have time to wait for research.

This book is not a definitive guide on differential diagnosis, or treatment techniques – there are many books that do this very well. Instead, it will provide basic clinical knowledge on the most common injuries relevant to the parameters of the model. Readers are expected to be familiar with anatomy, differential diagnosis and to have some clinical skills. The emphasis will be on identifying practical solutions for the busy clinician, based on the probability of the most common things happening most commonly. This book is only a beginning in a new and rapidly evolving field.

Understanding, and influencing, the environmental factors of the injured patient must be a priority for practitioners. They must see their role as more than treating an injured tissue in the confines of the clinic but as developing a multi-dimensional view of injury that encompasses a wider view of cause, effect and solution.

The types of injuries we get are changing. Our treatment modalities and our injury management must adapt and meet the challenge of these changes. The successful practitioner of the future will be not just a therapist, but also an ergonomist, a teacher, a motivator and a psychologist.

Treat people as if they were what they ought to be and you help them become what they are capable of becoming.

Goethe

New Zealand, 2001   Andrew Wilson

The injury process

1

The type of injury

Not all injuries are the same. How the injury is sustained has a clear bearing on the nature and prognosis of the injury, and on the subsequent management and therapeutic regimen. When patients present with a musculoskeletal injury they can be categorized according to the cause.

TRAUMATIC INJURY

A traumatic injury is caused by a clear precipitating event, where the load on the tissues is greater than their load-bearing capacity, resulting in tissue failure. The injury process is directly associated with the onset of pain and is responsible for subsequent symptoms. This process can be triggered by:

- impact, e.g. a fall or a motor vehicle accident
- an unexpected increase in musculoskeletal load, e.g. a slip while carrying an object
- attempting to carry a load, or series of loads, above the musculoskeletal tolerance.

In these cases there is an acute injury with some type of tissue failure. This type of injury has characteristic symptoms and physical findings related to the injured segment. This may be muscular, ligamentous or articular and diagnosis is reasonably straightforward. Symptoms will usually peak within the first few days and are followed by a healing process that is reasonably predictable. The practitioner's role is to manage the healing process and recovery to best advantage, attempting to reduce pain and morbidity and recover normal function in a realistic time frame. The effectiveness of the healing process will be modified by such factors as the age and condition of the patient, the amount of stress involved and the patient's life and workstyle habits. Most patients with a traumatic injury would be expected to make a full recovery and the practitioner's role is to assist this. The knowledge that the recovery process is likely to produce a resolution of the symptoms, and that the practitioner's role is to facilitate this, makes a traumatic injury more reassuring for the practitioner than some other types of injury (see below).

Minor trauma injury

A minor trauma injury is due to a clear precipitating event, where the event is not of sufficient magnitude to explain the extent of the injury. This may be due to an activity that is performed frequently without causing injury, e.g. doing up a shoelace or reaching to a high shelf; although on this occasion it clearly produced symptoms. The injury may involve acute tissue failure, with a traumatic injury, or it may be more dysfunctional in nature, for example joint strain or muscular/tendon disturbance in the rotator cuff. A minor trauma injury may present complications in recovery as there is an unpredictability about its cause and there may have been precipitating events leading up to the minor trauma that rendered the tissues more susceptible to injury. The practitioner will need to identify and address these issues.

A common example of this type of injury is the minor trauma overuse injury. A man is coping well with a daily exposure just below the threshold level of musculoskeletal tolerance; a relatively minor trauma takes him over this threshold, precipitating symptoms of greater complexity than would be expected by the initial trauma. He would probably respond to treatment but would be prone to relapses due to the on-going high exposure. To gain a more permanent improvement the overuse component of the injury needs to be addressed by reducing the exposure or improving the musculoskeletal tolerance.

INSIDIOUS INJURY

An insidious injury is one in which there is no clear precipitating event. The onset of symptoms may be acute – 'I woke up with it' – or it may be of a longer duration, with symptoms building up to an acute, subacute or even chronic pain pattern, or the symptoms may not peak so rapidly but develop more gradually over a period of time. Usually, the natural healing process is not so active as with a traumatic injury and the insidious injury will either stabilize at a certain level of dysfunction or continue to get worse. In addition to improving the symptoms and facilitating the recovery, the practitioner must be something of a detective, identifying and minimizing the causative events and removing any barriers to recovery. This type of injury may have ongoing exposure to musculoskeletal stressors that will affect the recovery. The more stressors that can be identified and minimized, the greater the powers and extent of recovery.

Patients with an insidious injury will benefit from a much more proactive role by the therapist in the recovery programme. Frequently, the stressors may be unrelated to the direct pain sensation, which makes their identification more of a challenge. 'I wake up with a stiff neck and headache every morning' suggests a failure to recover normal muscle balance during the sleeping hours but does not provide any clues to the stressor that creates the tissue fatigue and strain. Clearly, in these gradual process cases a good case history is paramount.

It seems that, in a changing society, patients with insidious pain onset are occupying a greater proportion of presenting cases. It is difficult to put an exact figure on this, as the reporting of injuries is often biased by the need to describe some precipitating event for insurance claim purposes, or simply by the desire to try and find a simple explanation for a more complex injury. The flow diagram in Figure 1.1 suggests that some type of ongoing exposure may be an important factor for 75% of injuries.

Practitioners may try to explain-away the appearance of symptoms by blaming an old trauma in the patient's history, such as a long-distant motor vehicle accident. While old injuries may affect future tissue tolerance to musculoskeletal exposure, they cannot be regarded as the cause of the new injury, even though the patient

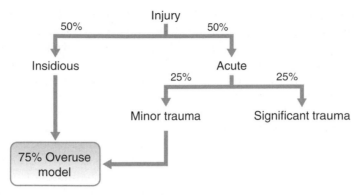

Figure 1.1 A breakdown of presenting patients shows that up to 75% can fit the overuse model (adapted from Pheasant 1994, with permission).

often seems impressed by such assumptions ('He knew I must have had a car accident!').

Young, healthy tissue is less likely than older tissue to suffer from an overuse injury because the tissue tolerance is greater and there has not been the degree of cumulative exposure. Although insidious injuries do occur in young people – note the high incidence of back pain in school-age children – most injuries require a combination of degenerative change and tissue exposure in order to become symptomatic. The tissue exposure to musculoskeletal stressors is the main cause of an overuse injury leading to the typical symptoms of musculoskeletal strain. Many modifying factors can affect the threshold of injury, the ability to recover and the patient's coping mechanisms. These will be covered in subsequent chapters.

It is important to emphasize that an insidious overuse injury cannot occur without musculoskeletal strain greater than the tissue tolerance, and this should be regarded as the principal cause of overuse injuries. These patients will often make some progress during the treatment process. However, if they are returned to the same environment, with a similar level of musculoskeletal stress, they will soon re-present for therapy or start doing the rounds of therapeutic possibilities. Clearly, these patients need to be identified early and more actively managed and educated.

A plot of the progression of symptoms against time clearly shows the different progression of different types of injury and suggests the different management strategies required.

Figure 1.2 shows a typical, acute, traumatic injury profile with a rapid progression and peak of symptoms followed by a gradual recovery period. This process usually occurs without therapeutic intervention and the role of the treatment provider is not as critical as with other types of injury, although their involvement may become more critical if some dysfunction intervenes and the symptoms fail to progress beyond a certain point – this is quite common with spinal injuries.

Figure 1.3 shows the gradual, insidious, cumulative nature of an overuse injury and illustrates the need to reduce musculoskeletal stressors below the threshold level in order to effect recovery. The profile suggests that the injury will continue to progress unless some interventions are made to curtail the injury-producing process.

Figure 1.4 shows a more rapid-onset overuse injury where the stressors are significantly

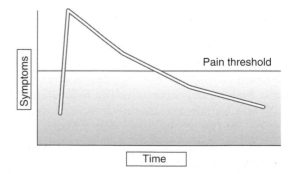

Figure 1.2 An acute injury – a rapid onset of symptoms followed by a gradual and largely predictable recovery process.

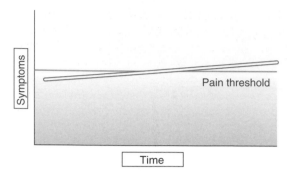

Figure 1.3 An overuse injury – shows a gradual accumulation of musculoskeletal strain where the exposure is greater than the tolerance level.

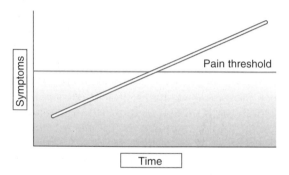

Figure 1.4 A rapid-onset overuse injury – the tissue exposure is much higher than the tissue tolerance, leading to a rapid onset of symptoms. Urgent interventions are required.

greater than the tissue tolerance and the injury process is accelerated, rapidly reaching crisis proportions. It is vital to identify these cases early on, as the symptom progression is rapid and the interventions required to reduce stressors below recovery threshold will be more urgent and of greater significance. Patients will often present in a highly charged, 'ground to a halt' situation and urgent intervention, such as reduction of work hours or change of the type of work, may be required to reduce their exposure until the situation is under control.

These figures illustrate a general process and there are as many variations on these profiles as there are injuries. Although the symptom threshold has been depicted as a constant line for the sake of clarity, this is not normally the case and a number of factors influence the perception of symptoms. The symptom threshold often becomes lowered after an injury, as the tissues become more sensitized as a result of the injury. In overuse injuries there can be a gradual lowering of symptom threshold as the progressively fatigued tissues become less physiologically efficient and more sensitized. Most tissues have a lower threshold of tolerance for repetitive loading than for a single loading, hence the cumulative nature of the injury. This will be explored in more detail in the following chapters.

Figures 1.5 and 1.6 show common variations of the above injury profiles. It is important that the practitioner recognizes these and manages the case accordingly. Figure 1.5 shows an acute-type injury from which the patient seems to recover but where a post-injury sensitivity makes him

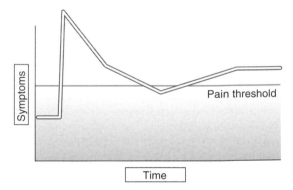

Figure 1.5 A post-traumatic overuse injury – a postinjury sensitivity can follow a traumatic injury. This can render people more sensitive to exposures they were previously adapted to.

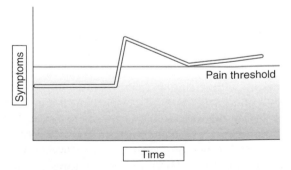

Figure 1.6 A minor trauma overuse injury – a minor trauma creates a symptom picture more complex than the nature of the patient's injury would suggest due to a combination of high musculoskeletal exposure and tissue sensitivity.

more sensitive to an exposure he was previously well-adapted to. Patients develop a subsequent overuse-type injuries when their ongoing exposure is too great for their musculoskeletal systems to tolerate without developing symptoms. This can be quite common in cases of whiplash.

Figure 1.6 illustrates the type of minor trauma injury described on page 4, where a minor trauma can precipitate symptoms greater than the trauma would suggest. The individual's high ongoing exposure (although previously asymptomatic) was precipitated over the symptom threshold by a minor trauma, and here it stubbornly remains, due to a combination of tissue sensitivity and dysfunction. This type of injury is remarkably common and successful management depends on addressing both the ongoing exposure and the trauma-induced symptoms. These scenarios illustrate how the overuse concept of injury causation can contribute to the management of many apparent acute or traumatic injuries.

DEFINING THE INJURY

Terminological variation and confusion are rampant in the area of overuse injuries. The various terms used place different emphases on different facets of the injury. The labels used to describe an injury are very important, but frequently provide misinformation, misunderstanding and often contribute to mismanagement. An injury can be defined by its cause, such as insidious, cumulative or acute – there are a number of different terminologies for this. Identifying the nature of the injury causation is crucial in determining the most efficient management and appropriate treatment procedures. As most definitions of injuries are by causation of the problem rather than anatomical pathology, they must be clarified by a further definition of location. For example, 'Work-related upper limb disorder – common extensor tendonitis' or 'occupational overuse strain – tension neck syndrome'.

Overuse or chronic injuries do not usually exist within neatly defined boundaries. It is normal to have some spread to neighbouring tissues or joints as part of the process of chronicity. Thus, although the symptoms may be predominantly in one region, the practitioner should be aware that other joints or regions are involved to a greater or lesser degree and that the symptom picture may change to reflect this. If the location of pain changes, this is probably due not to a new injury but a different manifestation of the same injury process and should be treated and managed accordingly, rather than as a new acute injury.

Common terms for overuse injuries include:

- Repetitive strain injury (RSI) – this term has good consumer recognition but has fallen out of favour with health professionals. It has come to be associated with a particularly chronic form of neck, shoulder and arm pain, frequently computer related. The term is not particularly accurate or informative and has developed a number of historical and emotional connotations to its use. The injury it commonly describes is not necessarily due to repetitive trauma. This term RSI is tending to be replaced by work-related musculoskeletal disorder (WRMSD).
- Work-related musculoskeletal disorder (WRMSD) – this term makes two statements – that of work-relatedness and that of a disorder. It avoids any categorization of the injury in terms of traumatic or overuse, which avoids some political issues, but it does not provide enough information to develop the appropriate management. WRMSD is often further defined as work-related upper extremity disorder (WRUED) or work-related upper limb disorder (WRULD). The issue of work-relatedness is often very important to determine funding of treatment and lost wages by insurance agencies.
- Occupational overuse strain (OOS) – this term is favoured in Australasia and provides a clear indication of the type of injury as an overuse injury, in addition to its work-related form. This may help with developing management plans. Unfortunately, it sounds unattractive in its contracted form and its use is not without controversy, although this relates to the whole

overuse injury concept and the reluctance of some organizations and their advisors to recognize this type of injury.

● Cumulative trauma disorder (CTD) – this term is favoured in North America. 'Cumulative' neatly describes the gradual injury process involved and 'trauma' suggests that some mechanical stress is involved in the production of the injury. There is no clear distinction between private or work causation, although it is usually used to describe work-related injuries.

● Refractive cervicobrachial disorder – this term is neither accurate nor descriptive, tending to place the emphasis on neurological symptoms.

The above are generic terms for overuse injuries and have all been used in the book, at different times, to keep the text true to the original sources of information. Where possible, the terms 'cumulative' or 'overuse' have been used to describe the process of injury.

Other terms that are commonly used to describe chronic injuries or chronic pain syndromes include:

● Fibromyalgia – this term is used to describe chronic pain that conforms to certain criteria. The criteria usually used are those of the American College of Rheumatology for the classification of fibromyalgia syndrome (Wolfe 1990). These include:

– pain that has been present for over 3 months
– pain on the left and right sides of the body, and both above and below the waist
– pain in at least 11 of 18 tender points on digital palpation, using 4 kg of pressure.

The term 'fibromyalgia' remains somewhat controversial and there are many difficulties in applying these criteria. Interpractitioner reliability of identification and interpretation of tender points is notoriously poor, particularly if an algometer is not used. Asking patients to discriminate between tenderness and pain will lead to individual variation in interpretation, and interpretation may vary on different occasions

with the same subject, depending on the immediate environment and the preceding activities or exposures to stressors.

Assuming that the criteria for establishing a diagnosis for fibromyalgia are satisfied, this means that a person has a 3-month history of pain with multiple trigger points, but does not signify that there is another disease process in existence. Thus, the definition of fibromyalgia would include most chronic injuries where gradual spread of pain sites is a normal and explainable phenomenon as a consequence of injury that has not fully resolved. So the term 'fibromyalgia' provides no useful insight into the cause of the problem, the injury process or the treatment process. It replaces logic with mystique.

Cohen et al (1992) made similar observations: 'Fibromyalgia is no more than another descriptor and contains no pathological insight'. Troup & Videman (1989) go further:

The belief that the diagnosis of a musculoskeletal symptom can be encapsulated in a single word or phrase is no longer defensible. ... It is imperative to search for diagnoses that take full account of all the causative and contributory factors which underlie the condition; diagnoses in which the logical choice of therapeutic management, or prevention is implicit.

The value of using a term to describe a set of findings that have no identifiable cause, no known pathology and provide no clue to patient management is questionable. The difficulty arises when the term is used as a diagnosis, when it is nothing of the sort. Most chronic injuries, whether traumatic or overuse, will fit the criteria if they are given time to develop the secondary symptoms of chronicity. Medical reports that state 'this is not an overuse injury it is fibromyalgia', cloud the real diagnosis and contribute to mismanagement.

● Myofascial pain syndrome or regional pain syndrome – this suggests that the pain originates in the muscles and fascia; that it is not neurological or bony and hence it cannot be diagnosed by X-ray or other objective screening. It is usually used to describe pain and tenderness of a regional nature with palpable taut bands known as trigger points. The trigger point is painful on compression and creates a characteristic referred pain. The concept has been well developed by Travell and Simons (1983, 1992) in *Myofascial pain and dysfunction, the trigger point manual*. It tends to be a definition of palpable findings rather than a diagnosis. By providing a regional description it allows the possibility for neighbouring myofascial tissues to be involved. Although the title makes an important statement that assists with treatment procedures, it is incomplete, as it does not provide information regarding the cause. Most chronic injuries will develop active trigger points and the cause is a little more complicated than this descriptor gives credit for. The trigger point manual provides an excellent treatment rationale for practitioners interested in manual therapy. The trigger point theories and treatment methods fit comfortably into the overuse injury model.

• Reflex sympathetic dystrophy (RSD) – This is a complication arising from trauma, overuse or surgery where the sympathetic nervous system has become significantly involved. It can lead to vasoconstriction – cold, blue or purple limbs, paraesthesia, muscle weakness, atrophy of skin, bone loss and loss of hair. It is often a feature of chronic overuse injuries and the increased sensitivity of the sympathetic nervous system renders it quite difficult to treat. It can be present to a greater or lesser degree in chronic injuries and it is not necessarily progressive.

In an attempt to overcome the hurdle of the myriad of diagnostic terms used for overuse injuries, and their inherent prejudices and belief systems, I have recently become tempted to develop my own terms.

LIFE OVERLOAD ADJUSTMENT DISORDER (LOAD)[1]

This generic term suggests accumulation of musculoskeletal (MS) strain at a greater rate than the individual's recovery capacity, resulting in musculoskeletal symptoms.

The 'life' component suggests the whole of life – not just one compartment such as work or stress. It also suggests a chronological process.

The 'overload' component clearly states a load in excess of the individual recovery mechanisms.

'Adjustment' suggests an individual component to the problem; that there is a difficulty in adapting to the exposure. It suggests that it is not necessarily the exposure that is extreme, but the way it is managed; the individual has not been able to adapt to the load. This helps develop a sense of individual responsibility.

The term 'disorder' reflects the fact that, although there are musculoskeletal symptoms, these may not be in the form of an identifiable pathology.

The acronym LOAD suggests work being performed, a load on the mind or a load being moved, which helps conjure a sense of use of our musculoskeletal system as part of the injury process.

LOAD can be further divided into workLOAD and non-workLOAD. WorkLOAD would be an overuse injury primarily caused by work-related exposure. Non-workLOAD would be an overuse injury primarily caused by non-work exposure. Deciding whether an injury is work-related or otherwise can be very tricky, with a great many financial considerations hinging on the final decision, such as funding for treatment, compensation and employer liability. The decision can be highly charged – employers often refuse to recognize the work-relatedness of an injury and employees are often reluctant to accept any personal responsibility. The decision should be based on relative balance of probability. If a worker who develops an injury is working full-time in an occupation with an identified increased risk ratio for that disorder, then there is a probability that the work is a significant factor. If the worker uses postures or other exposures that have been identified with increased risk of injury, there is an increased probability of work involvement. Longer hours, higher exposure and poor ergonomic or psychosocial environment suggests a greater probability of work-related exposure being the major factor. For example, working over 4 h a day doing word processing at high output levels with few breaks is related to

---

[1] I am indebted to Mary Law, my publisher at Churchill Livingstone, who first coined this term. We were discussing terminology to use for the book and she came up with this elegant acronym.

increased incidence of neck, shoulder and forearm problems.

However, decisions we make about our personal lives can influence how well we cope with work-related exposure. For example, moderate aerobic exercise followed by relaxation and effective sleep will help the word processor operator while a long period of competitive tennis or squash followed by a late night party will significantly handicap effective recovery.

The decision is rarely black and white. With full-time employees in occupations with significant work-related exposure, work must be implicated unless there is a significant source of non-work exposure. The time spent at work and the intensity of the work are factors that must be taken into account. Practitioners who make these kinds of decision must be up-to-date with the international ergonomic literature relating to work-related musculoskeletal exposure.

Non-workLOAD has an emphasis on stressors in the non-work environment. These can have a clear biomechanical cause, such as sport, household work or hobbies, or can be due to constrained postures such as knitting and sewing. There are also people who are disposed toward developing musculoskeletal tension but have no clear history of biomechanical cause. In these cases, the emphasis will be on personal and psychosocial factors. These are the patients who have tended to be given the label 'fibromyalgia'. The label 'non-workLOAD' reflects a management model that does much to help them identify and manage their personal risk factors.

SUMMARY

The causative nature of an injury will have a clear bearing on its prognosis and management. Most injuries occur when a threshold combination of predisposing factors and biomechanical strain has been reached.

The uncomplicated, traumatic injury that readily improves with manual or electrotherapy, with little else required, is a clinical luxury. The emerging pattern of lifestyle where people do less physical work, more mental processing and long periods of sitting followed by short bursts of activity, is producing a much higher incidence of overuse-type injuries characterized by poor posture, muscle imbalance and strain. The management of these types of injury requires a new set of skills from the practitioner, who will have to teach, motivate and counsel the patient in addition to providing the usual treatment methods. Practitioners need to look not just at patients and their physical structures, but also at how they interact with their environment. Some of the most important treatment methods should be aimed at the environment!

This type of approach to patient management can be exciting and challenging for both practitioner and patient, as the pieces of the jigsaw puzzle of pain gradually emerge to form a realistic picture.

2

Developing a management model

This chapter will provide an overview of the injury process, to set the scene for the development of a structural model for injury management. Subsequent chapters will give more detail and referencing to further explore the generalizations made in this chapter. The chapter attempts to categorize the contributory causes of overuse injuries and incorporate them into a structure that allows a clear management plan in an area that is often fraught with misinformation and misunderstanding.

Overuse injuries involve an ongoing exposure to fatigue and strain that exceeds the capacity of the individual's recovery processes. Recovery involves identifying the risk factors and reducing the tissue exposure below the recovery threshold. This is most likely to be successful if as many as possible of the factors that contribute to the exposure are identified and minimized, while at the same time a supportive and cooperative environment is provided. Single interventions in overuse injuries are rarely successful, indeed they often add to the chronicity by delaying appropriate measures and allowing further accumulation of fatigue or microtrauma.

The change in lifestyles and work practices from dynamic work to static work, from physical work to mental work and from manual work to computerized work, has been accompanied by a shift in the type of presenting musculoskeletal injuries. The overuse injury is becoming commonplace and now constitutes an important component in over 50% of musculoskeletal injuries. Overuse injuries are often poorly recognized as there is frequently no awareness of the link between the cause and the symptoms. The pain is often not clearly related to the ergonomic exposure and no ready association can be made. The symptoms are often attributed to a minor trauma or to a previous trauma, which may form part of the history but is probably not of sufficient magnitude to explain the symptom picture and its chronicity. This delay in appropriate diagnosis, and the subsequent delay in management, can contribute to chronicity.

There are two clear but overlapping stages of overuse injuries. The first involves muscle overload, subsequent muscle fatigue and microtrauma. In a one-off situation this will create a postexercise muscle soreness, which can last up to 3 days. If the muscle is further fatigued while still in its recovery state the fatigue and microtrauma starts to accumulate and the injury process begins. If the muscle is allowed to regain normal efficiency before further exposure, an adaptation process develops, which results in improved fitness levels. The greater the level of muscular fatigue, the longer the recovery period required.

When a muscle is given a daily exposure of work, the amount of muscle fatigue should be kept to a minimum, to allow rapid recovery of efficiency and avoid the accumulation of metabolites and microtrauma. This is the first principle in the management model: minimization of muscular workload. The factors responsible for muscular load are characterized in Figure 2.1.

MUSCLE FATIGUE MODEL

A person suffering from muscular pain will have developed and accumulated muscle tension

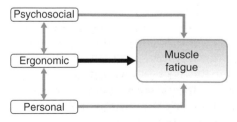

Figure 2.1 The muscle fatigue model – identifying and minimizing the factors relating to muscle tension will lower the risk of muscle fatigue and injury.

greater than their capacity for recovery. If as many sources of their muscle tension as possible are identified and minimized, their muscle tension levels will be reduced to below their symptom threshold and the recovery process can begin to take effect. The more factors that are identified and influenced, the better chance of recovery.

Ergonomic factors

The primary cause of muscular fatigue and injury is the generation of muscle tension without sufficient ability to recover. The greatest determinant of muscle tension is the workload performed by the muscle. This might involve static postures, including maintenance of posture or stabilization of the joints, or dynamic postures involved in mobility or manipulating tools. The physical work performed can be described as the ergonomic factors. These can be further summarized as:

- posture – deviation from joint neutral, or away from the centre of gravity, produces progressively increasing levels of muscle tension
- force – the degree of force required to effect the task is an important determinant of muscular workload
- repetition and duration of tasks are important factors.

Also in this category are environmental and work organizational factors, which can have a distinct bearing on muscular workload. The research literature has identified many of the types and durations of ergonomic exposures that are related to increased risk of injury. These will be discussed in some detail in later chapters. In summary: the longer the period spent in poorer postures, the greater the risk of injury. The greater the forces or repetitions used, the greater the risk of injury.

Psychosocial factors

While ergonomic factors are largely responsible for the muscular work-generated strain, they tend to be modified by psychosocial factors.

People who describe their job as high stress, tend to spend longer periods in poorer postures with fewer breaks. Workers who describe low job satisfaction tend to report more injuries; are more likely to take time off work and are less likely to return to work.

Psychosocial factors seem to be particularly responsible for 'switching on' a workload that was previously within the recovery threshold, and for the conversion from short-term fatigue to chronic injury. In practice, it is very difficult to separate ergonomic from psychosocial exposure. Jobs with high ergonomic exposure invariably have a high psychosocial index of risk factors, and vice versa. An example of this might be a machine-paced light industrial task as in a sewing factory or a production line. There might be constant repetition of the same biomechanical load; boredom from the repetitive nature of the task and the lack of autonomy; stress from the difficulty in keeping up with the pace of the production process; and low job satisfaction for all of these reasons.

Stress tends to lead to increased levels of muscle tension, and often when there is opportunity for a muscular break the muscles remain tense when under stress. This lack of 'electromyographic (EMG) gaps' has been linked to increased risk of injury. The development of an overuse injury is a stressful event for an employee and for their immediate co-workers. It can produce a cascade effect with symptom magnification and co-workers also developing symptoms. The quality of workplace and medical management of a symptomatic individual can have a marked effect on the levels of psychosocial stress following an injury. These can have a significant bearing on the reporting of an injury, the amount of time off work and the risk of chronicity and disability. A supportive and sympathetic environment, where people are listened to and conflict is avoided, is important for successful outcomes.

Psychosocial causes will be dealt with in greater detail in Chapter 5.

Personal factors

In a shared work environment one worker may develop headaches, one may suffer from episodic low backache and one may develop shoulder and arm symptoms; six others may be symptom free. It is the personal factors that determine who is predisposed towards developing certain injuries. Some of these factors cannot be influenced to any great extent, such as gender, age and anthropometric characteristics. Other factors can be as a result of lifestyle choices, such as fitness and smoking, or ergonomic exposure through hobbies – computer games, musical instruments, etc. Other factors can be historical, such as accident and medical history.

Stress is a normal part of everyday life but the reaction to it, and the coping mechanisms for it, can be affected by personality factors. Stress and relaxation need to be in reasonable balance to create a good environment for recovery. While the employer has a responsibility to provide a safe working environment, employees have a responsibility to manage their private lives so that they are capable of doing an effective day's work and are reasonably able to recover from this. It is important to educate patients about how they can manage their injury risk and to encourage them to take some responsibility for their health outcomes. This personal involvement helps them gain some control over their symptoms and helps avoid the feeling of helplessness and victimhood that can intensify the symptom picture.

LOAD MODEL

A complex interaction of ergonomic, psychosocial and personal factors determines the degree of muscle tension and fatigue. If the muscle tension becomes prolonged or cumulative, a number of changes take place in body symptoms:

- The prolonged mechanical exposure creates somatic dysfunction. Shortening of muscle groups, muscle imbalances and joint dysfunction become apparent. The joint dysfunction may be a change in mobility often seen in the wrist with extensor muscle overuse, or an alteration of joint position often seen in cervical facet joints.
- Biochemical changes due to reduced blood flow, oxygen supply and build-up of metabolites.

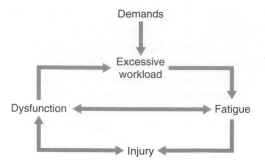

Figure 2.2 The fatigue–dysfunction cycle – a vicious cycle that leads to progression of symptoms.

● Neurological changes take place as a result of continuous afferent barrage, mechanical pressure and disturbance of the neural microcirculation.

The combination of these features further reduces work efficiency. Muscles have to work harder to produce the same work output, and a vicious cycle begins involving tension–fatigue–dysfunction–injury (Fig. 2.2). This process will be explored in more depth in Chapter 3.

In terms of chronicity, the major development is the progressive sensitization of the afferent nervous system and the reduction in stimulation threshold of the pain fibres. Pain and discomfort begin to be experienced at lower levels of mechanical exposure – things that used to be comfortable begin to create discomfort. This stage of injury is significant because the changes are very difficult to reverse. Careful management and understanding of the process becomes very important to prevent further progression and to manage the existing problem. Generally speak-

ing, the greater the level of neurological sensitivity, the more difficult the management and the more reduced the possibility of complete recovery. Management of the problem becomes the key issue, rather than seeking a cure. Figure 2.3 illustrates how this can be incorporated into the management model to show the progression from muscle fatigue to progressive neurological sensitivity and chronicity when the relevant issues are not addressed.

The LOAD (or chronic injury) model gives an overall picture of the nature of the injury and the symptom progression from muscle fatigue to neurological sensitivity to developing chronicity. It charts some of the common psychological and musculoskeletal effects that are associated with developing chronicity. It also demonstrates the traditional role of therapists and highlights the need to develop new management tools that offer more than just dealing with symptoms. Traditionally, therapists have worked at the musculoskeletal level, treating muscle, tendon and joint strains and neuromuscular dysfunction. Figure 2.3 demonstrates that while these treatments are likely to provide some temporary improvement in symptoms and coping mechanisms, unless the input cycle is addressed, and the exposure is reduced below threshold levels, chronicity is likely to develop.

The role of surgery is even more narrowly defined to reducing nerve compression while risking further insult to already oversensitized afferent nerves. Surgery is not likely to be successful unless the nerve compression can be clearly identified as being responsible for a large proportion of the symptoms, for example, in a

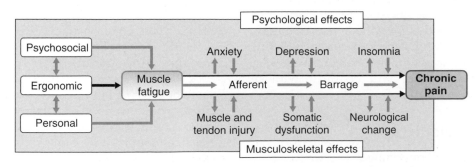

Figure 2.3 The LOAD model – the progression from muscle fatigue to chronic injury.

carpal tunnel syndrome. In a more chronic case of multiple site symptoms, the chances of surgery making a significant improvement diminish, while the risk of complications such as reflex sympathetic dystrophy increases.

The role of stress management and counselling is also limited. These can be very helpful for understanding and managing the role of stress, for dealing with the psychological manifestations of chronic pain and for developing appropriate coping strategies, but will not prevent chronicity unless the input cycle is also addressed. None of these therapies, used singly or in combination, is likely to improve the prognosis unless the exposure to musculoskeletal stressors is reduced to a level that allows a recovery process and the overload is removed from the neuromusculoskeletal tissues.

MANAGEMENT PRINCIPLES

Dealing with the input cycle of ergonomic, psychosocial and personal factors must be a treatment priority; reducing the biomechanical load is paramount. This can be achieved by reducing the workload or reducing work hours or, in extreme cases, by time away from work. This will give time to develop some management strategies but can sometimes create problems. Employers, who are sometimes not very sympathetic to overuse injuries, can be uncooperative and the patient's job may be at risk. Occasionally, patients will feel very threatened by being off work – that they are no longer important or that someone might take their job. People gain a lot of self-esteem from their work role and, if it is taken away from them, can suffer anxiety and stress. It is therefore sensible to help patients at work unless a crisis situation has developed, which requires some time out. More frequently, reduced work hours until the symptoms have been brought under control and the ergonomic exposure reduced to a manageable level is a better management option.

Workplace assessment is a priority to try and minimize the cumulative ergonomic workload while maintaining work output as much as possible. Identifying and minimizing the key sources of ergonomic exposure is a management priority. Mats Hagberg (1995), a noted ergonomist, stated: 'It is unethical to send a worker back to work after a work-related injury without a full workplace assessment'.

This remarkably sensible proposition has a laudable logic. Unfortunately, with a myriad of treatment processes based on symptom relief, workplace assessment is often overlooked. Musculoskeletal therapists need to take more responsibility for the input cycle of overuse injuries rather than examining patients in a controlled clinic environment and then sending them back into the environment that caused the problem in the first place. Education and advice are often very helpful, but the patient may have insufficient knowledge to make effective interventions. The identification of a close relationship between the ergonomics of work and the types of injury presenting at their clinic can give a great boost to practitioners' understanding of the injury process, and provide a great sense of satisfaction. There are a number of reasons why musculoskeletal therapists are very well placed to do workplace assessments:

- The understanding of muscle and joint function, and of the injury process, makes an easy transition to understanding the principles of good posture and ergonomics.
- Familiarity with a person's symptom picture and injury profile allows the practitioner to prioritize interventions and the equipment required.
- The patient-centred focus of musculoskeletal practitioners, and their understanding of how the person is affected by outside influences, enhances the recovery process. Most traditional ergonomists come from a systems or management or engineering focus.

Workplace assessment is very important, as people spend a large part of their life at work and it is likely to be the most significant single exposure involved in the production of the injury. However, there may well be other factors responsible for the progression of symptoms. The key to successful management is to identify as many factors as possible in the categories of ergonomic, psychosocial and personal inputs, and to mini-mize these. This maximizes the chance of a successful resolution. Clearly, this investigative work does take some time and the ability to provide time and develop good communication are essential prerequisites for managing chronic cases.

Patient education is an important part of the recovery process. The first step is to gain patient confidence by demonstrating that you understand the nature of their injury and the treatment and interventions required. The next step is to provide patients with some awareness of the nature of the problem and to let them know that the condition can be effectively managed. This will help alleviate fear and uncertainty, which can be potent enhancers of pain and dysfunction. The treatment and education processes should go hand in hand. Effective treatment for reversing symptoms and dysfunction should be accompanied by an education process that allows the patient to be aware of the nature of the dysfunction and develop patterns of managing it, such as exercise or relaxation. Hands-on therapy can be a valuable form of biofeedback and can help patients become aware of the condition of their bodies and provide them with an opportunity to to start to consciously control some processes they were previously unaware of.

Creating a positive environment for recovery is important. The most important principle is the avoidance of conflict. This is often easier said than done! Patients must feel listened to and believed, and they must be taken seriously. If their employer labels them as a trouble-maker, or thinks that it is not part of the employer's responsibility to assist recovery, it can be very difficult to make progress. Sometimes a health professional (usually doctor or specialist) will undermine patients with an authoritative manner, making them feel unimportant or as if they are not being listened to. Inappropriate medical care can be a major cause of chronicity in overuse injuries. Providing patients with pain relief and encouraging them to continue in an unsatisfactory ergonomic environment is poor medical management. Patients also need a supportive home environment where family and friends are understanding and supportive and prepared to accept modified roles. Often these interpersonal relationships with supervisors/ employer, medical professionals and family, require a degree of assertiveness and speaking up for oneself – not accepting a passive or victim-type role.

SUMMARY

The principles of the life overload adjustment disorder (LOAD) management model are:

- early recognition
- early ergonomic intervention
- appropriate management and therapy
- a supportive environment – avoidance of conflict.

If these principles are present then rehabilitation is straightforward and predictable. If one or more of these criteria are absent the prognosis becomes progressively more difficult. Chronicity and treatment failure can usually be explained by the absence of these criteria, which are frequently nothing to do with the treatment process.

3

Understanding the symptoms

The management of overuse injuries and the treatment strategies employed are partly dependent on the chronicity of the case. The prognosis and the coping strategies are also highly influenced by the extent of the symptoms. Chronicity is not just the length of time the injury has been present but is also related to the complexity of the symptom picture. There are a number of features that suggest increasing chronicity and complexity.

SYMPTOM ENLARGEMENT

Discomfort will usually first become apparent during certain activities that provide peak or prolonged exposure to the fatigued tissues. The feeling maybe an ache or pain, or it may be a fullness or awareness of a muscle that seems not to be able to relax. This may become apparent during the activity that provides the most exposure, such as playing a musical instrument or using a vibrating hand tool. In many cases, particularly with long periods of low isometric activity, the symptoms are not associated with the activity but become apparent during subsequent peak loading. For example, while prolonged use of a keyboard may cause strain and fatigue on the forearm extensors, this may not be sufficient to cause symptoms until the person attempts to pick up a full kettle or carry the shopping bags from the supermarket. This disassociation of the symptoms from the cause often leads to delayed recognition of the nature of the injury by the individual, and delayed diagnosis by the medical fraternity.

Sometimes the discomfort will first be felt at periods of rest, such as relaxing in the evening or when trying to sleep. The periods of reduced activity and reduced neurological distraction may increase symptom awareness at these times. Neck and back problems particularly seem to exhibit this feature. For example, waking up with a stiff neck and headache suggests an inability to completely recover at night from previous exposures (sleeping posture and pillow may also be secondary factors).

Initially, the symptoms may be episodic, with apparent recovery between episodes and prolonged periods free of symptoms. The symptomatic episodes may become more common and last longer. They may become provoked more easily as the tissues become more sensitive to an increasing numbers of exposures.

As the condition progresses, symptoms become apparent at an increasing number of activities and the person begins to think seriously about restricting their activities.

A significant step seems to be when sleep becomes disturbed by symptoms; either repeatedly waking up due to discomfort or being unable to go to sleep. Good quality sleep seems to be very important for efficient recovery of physical and psychological fatigue processes. When sleep is affected it seems to significantly hinder recovery and coping mechanisms.

Neurological involvement

Progressive neurological involvement is generally a sign of chronicity and can be increasingly difficult to reverse. A frank neuralgia may be related to a spinal problem caused by the intervertebral disc or facet joint, and may have a good prognosis rather than necessarily being a sign of chronicity. Any appendicular problems with neurological manifestations should always include some treatment to the spinal region that provides or influences neural outflow to the region. These spinal problems can often mimic appendicular problems. A diagnosed tennis elbow or carpal tunnel syndrome will often resolve with treatment directed to the cervical and thoracic spines.

In chronic overuse problems there is usually a subtle change in the quality of the pain as the afferent nervous system becomes progressively sensitized. The descriptors become burning, tingling or crawling sensations. Hyperaesthesia, paraesthesia and allodynia are signs of neural sensitivity and suggest chronicity. Changes in circulation – purple or blue limbs – suggest sympathetic nerve hypersensitivity and are suggestive of chronicity. Muscle strength can often be inhibited due to pain. This is often found in resisted abduction in rotator cuff strain, or resisted grip strength with extensor forearm strain. Strength usually returns following pain blockade or manual therapy. Continued muscle weakness in the absence of significant pain suggests neurological involvement and is suggestive of a more difficult prognosis. Where a muscle is permanently weak it will require higher EMG readings to perform everyday tasks, leading to accelerated fatigue processes.

Secondary spread

When a muscle group fatigues, the nervous system recruits other neigbouring muscle groups to try and spread the biomechanical load. However, these neigbouring muscle groups often work from a position of biomechanical inefficiency and can also become symptomatic.

An afferent barrage at spinal cord level will transmit a certain amount of stimulus to the neighbouring cord segment, leading to splinting reflexes and other changes at the neighbouring level. It is characteristic with overuse injuries for the symptoms gradually to spread to neighbouring muscles and joints. This can often lead to a confusing clinical picture, where the pain seems to apparently move around. Patients are often only aware of the most pronounced pain. When this pain is relatively diminished the next most prominent pain can suddenly be promoted to awareness. In overuse injuries there will usually be one or two prominent pain sites, but there may well be other sites that are almost as bad but of which the patient is not consciously aware.

Contralateral spread

About 10% of afferent nerve fibres cross over the spinal cord and begin to initiate reflex muscle spasm activity in the opposing limb. Symptom spread to the opposing limb is a common sign of chronicity in about 50% of cases. This can happen in the absence of significant biomechanical exposure to that limb. Once the pain becomes apparent in one muscle group it can also gradually spread.

The phenomenon of secondary spread in spinal problems has long been recognized by manual therapists dealing with spinal problems. Osteopaths used to call such spread secondary osteopathic lesions. The secondary and contralateral spread in soft tissue injury seems to be a more recent phenomenon and tends to be more common in patients whose work involves long periods of sustained or isometric contraction with a reduced variety of afferent input, than in patients with traditional manual work cycles. The work practices that encourage long periods of low-level isometric contraction are a feature of the modern workplace and with automation and computerization of systems. Just as it is physiologically advisable to vary muscle group activity, it seems to be equally important to provide afferent stimuli variation.

It is important to take a careful case history and perform a thorough clinical examination so the degree of chronicity can be carefully assessed. Many practitioners treat each newly presenting patient as if they suffer an acute problem. If there are clear signs of chronicity, such as a history of relapse, secondary spread of pain or neurological sensitivity-type symptoms, these patients should be managed according to the LOAD model of chronicity, in addition to being provided with symptomatic therapeutic relief.

STAGES OF LOAD

The presenting symptoms and the clinical picture give an idea of the complexity of the problem and clues to the management and the required levels of intervention. It is very helpful for both practitioner and patient to have some measure of this process. Accordingly, the following classification system can be used as a base for a management and education programme:

- Stage 1 – pain in a joint or muscle group when working in one position for a long period. The pain may occur at work, playing a musical instrument or when performing any activity that involves continual or repetitive use in a fixed posture. The pain eases promptly when the activity is stopped.
- Stage 2 – the pain starts to come on early in the activity and tends to continue after the activity is stopped. It becomes apparent in other non-related activities, domestic chores, etc. The pain is often more noticeable at rest.
- Stage 3 – pain comes on early in the activity and continues long after it has ceased. It starts to interfere with daily life and leads to activity avoidance – carrying bags, housework, etc. It can spread to other muscle groups and to the opposite limb; it can also disturb sleep patterns. A more complex symptom picture develops – tingling, numbness and muscle weakness. Other symptoms can include headaches, depression and circulatory changes. The patient begins seriously to consider reducing work and activity levels.
- Stage 4 – pain is constant and disabling. Work is very difficult and pain avoidance becomes a dominant feature of a person's life. Sleep can be severely disturbed, with accompanying depression and fatigue. Ordinary tasks become difficult. The pain is not consistent, with new sites occurring and old ones being revisited. Secondary effects of nerve symptoms and circulatory changes are more significant.

SUMMARY

- Stages 1–3 can be managed and treated successfully by work assessment, work management, therapy, exercise, etc.
- Stage 4 is very difficult and recovery can be prolonged, with little possibility of returning to the same workload. Good management and appropriate therapy can improve the quality of life and lead to a limited return to productive activity.

This completes the overview of the injury process. Subsequent chapters in Section 1 will explore in more detail the factors responsible for injury development and the pathophysiology of the injury process. To truly understand how injuries occur and to be confident in planning the treatment and management of them, practitioners must fully understand the nature of injury and how the pathophysiological mechanisms develop. Chapter 4 will provide some insight into the development of these processes.

CHAPTER CONTENTS

4

Understanding the physiology of the injury process

Something that is used up to, or beyond, its full potential will break at its weakest point. A high force can cause failure with a single application; a repetitive force can induce a fatigue failure as a result of forces that have previously been tolerated. In the human body these injury thresholds are modified by adaptive processes – the training effect and the recovery and healing processes. If runners gradually increase their mileage there will be an increase in strength of the trabecular structure and a resulting increase in bone strength. If runners increase their mileage at a rate greater than their adaptive processes can cope with, this will initiate a destructive process that culminates in a stress fracture. In the single force injury, the trauma and the injury are usually easily identified and the recovery process is not likely to become complicated. In the repetitive force injury, the process is more likely to be chronic, with all the inherent complications of chronicity, and recovery is frequently exacerbated by ongoing exposure to the stressor. Many injuries involve both peak forces and repetitive processes.

The traumatic injuries have generally been well understood and are usually well managed, but the repetitive-type injury, particularly when there is a very gradual development process, has generally been poorly understood and poorly managed.

A HISTORICAL PERSPECTIVE

Previous generations were more physically active and had a greater variety of physical activity than people today. As a consequence, repetitive or overuse injuries were less common.

However, Western society has moved away from a simple subsistence lifestyle towards production processes and trading economies. The demand for production has created a need for efficiency. Efficiency often requires repetitive applications of new technology. If a new technology creates greater efficiency there is a commercial demand for its application, often at the expense of health outcomes. The desire for continued efficiency has created an increasing number of work environments where there are repetitive processes and constrained postures. An increasing body of literature links these types of work with musculo-skeletal injury. In the past, different occupations were associated with overuse injuries related to that particular task, such as writer's cramp, telegraph operator's tendonitis or railway back. With the advent of the computer and its introduction into a broad spectrum of work environments on an unprecedented scale, there has been a substantial increase in overuse injuries to body parts associated with computer use. With the increasing adoption of the computer by different processes within the working environment, there is increasing evidence of a dose-related response between the time spent using a computer and the presence of fatigue and symptoms of overuse (Hochanadel 1995).

Overuse injuries were recognized long before the computer revolution. With the introduction of the steel pen as a replacement for the feather quill, Ramazzini (1713) gave a classic description of writer's cramp:

The remedies that afflict the clerks aforesaid arise from three causes: First, constant sitting, secondly the incessant movement of the hand and always in the same direction, thirdly the strain on the mind not to disfigure the books.

Pheasant (1991) points out that Ramazzini clearly identified the three principal causes of overuse injuries:

● fixed posture
● repetitive movement
● stress.

An article in the *Lancet* in 1875 lists a number of 'professional impotences' including: telegraphist's cramp, writer's cramp, hammer palsy, milker's cramp and bricklayer's cramp. The article attempts to explain the widespread phenomenon of writer's cramp and makes a clear distinction between intermittent and sustained muscle contraction fatigue:

The muscles are subjected to a prolonged strain, and are kept constantly in a state of contraction, often for many hours, are usually the first to fail and to drift into a state of chronic fatigue. In the other actions enumerated – milking etc – the muscles employed are not tired out by prolonged strain, but by constant repetitions of the same act; and constant repetition does not seem to induce the same state of chronic fatigue as quickly as sustained contraction, because in constantly repeated muscular contraction the muscle enjoys an interval of relaxation, and it is in this interval that the nutrition is maintained.

The article goes on to observe and attempt to explain the progressive nature of the fatigue process:

A muscle having become completely fatigued another is called upon to do its work … the progressive nature of the malady will be observed … once a muscle has failed those which are called upon to supply its place are sure to fail more quickly than the first.

These astute observations provide a succinct explanation of the muscle fatigue process, outlining the difference between cyclic and static contractions and the tendency for secondary spread of this type of injury. Modern research methods and sophisticated electromyographic (EMG) analysis have increased our understanding of the nature of muscle fatigue. Meanwhile, the modern work environment and the ever-increasing demands for work efficiency promote 'prolonged sustained contractions' and 'the progressive nature of the malady'.

A LITTLE MUSCLE PHYSIOLOGY

The ability to sustain exercise and muscular function requires muscle cells to be efficient utilizers of energy. If the energy demand cannot be matched by the energy supply, muscle fatigue rapidly follows. Sustained physical activity is supplied primarily by aerobic metabolism – the consumption of oxygen to drive the oxidation of carbohydrates and fatty acids. The mitochondria within the muscle fibres use the energy derived from oxygen consumption to resynthesize ATP from ADP and phosphate (the products of ATP breakdown). This process of energy production requires an adequate delivery of oxygen to the cell and an adequate fuel supply within the cell to support the oxygen consumption. The oxygen must be sourced from the blood supply to the muscle and must diffuse from the capillaries to the mitochondria in the muscle fibres. This oxygen supply must be matched by an adequate supply of chemical fuel – carbohydrates (glucose and glycogen) and fatty acids. Disruption of either fuel or oxygen will lead to rapid onset of muscular fatigue.

Muscle fibres

Skeletal muscles are made up of approximately equal portions of slow-twitch, or type 1, fibres and fast-twitch, or type 2, fibres.

Type 1 fibres have a relatively high blood flow capacity, a high capillary density and a high mitochondrial content, reflecting their aerobic function. They have a small motor unit size with a low-frequency firing pattern. Type 1 fibres are slow to contract and slow to relax and function very well where sustained low force output is required, as in maintenance of posture, provided there is sufficient blood supply. Type 1 fibres are usually positioned deep in a muscle, close to the bone where the blood supply is usually greatest.

Type 2 fibres are usually further divided into two subgroups. Type 2A fibres have a relatively high blood flow capacity, high capillary density and high mitochondrial content. They have a faster contraction and relaxation time than type 1 fibres, with larger motor units and a high-frequency firing pattern. They provide intermediate levels of power while being relatively resistant to fatigue. Type 2B fibres have a relatively low blood flow capacity, low capillary density and low mitochondrial content. They are largely anaerobic, produce high power and fatigue rapidly, requiring long recovery periods.

These muscle categories are generalizations and there are gradations of the fibre types and their properties. The relative proportions of types of fibres vary according to muscle type and role, and to individual characteristics – age, race, etc. While exercise training can enhance the role of different fibre types there appears to be little shift between the types of fibre and their distribution.

Motor units

The motor neuron and the muscle fibres it excites are known as the motor unit. The size of the motor unit varies considerably, from those responsible for precision tasks, which contain about ten muscle fibres, to large limb muscle motor units with over 1000 fibres. Rapid firing of nervous impulses to the motor units can cause mechanical summation, building the muscle tension to a higher level. Contraction strength can also be increased by recruiting more motor units. Low-level firing produces low-level contraction of the small motor neurons and, as more force is required, the larger motor units become progressively involved. The motor units recruited are those most efficient for the task. Muscle fibres consume energy to reaccumulate the calcium ions released with each nerve impulse. Energy is conserved if the required force can be maintained with as few impulses as possible.

Muscle fatigue

When muscular work is performed for prolonged periods, a fatigue process develops. Fatigue reduces the precision and strength of muscle contraction and increases the risk of accidental injury. In the absence of an accident, prolonged fatigue without sufficient recovery time can lead to musculoskeletal problems. Fatigue can be defined as the failure to maintain the required force, or as a reduction in the generation capacity, of the neuromuscular system. Studies of people with chronic myofascial pain have demonstrated lower strength and higher levels of fatigue than in normal subjects.

Muscle contraction occurs as a result of a series of related processes, a number of which can be subject to fatigue. The most significant disorders can be categorized as mechanical, metabolic or electrophysiological. The fatigue process depends on the type, duration and frequency of muscle contractions, and on the duration of the recovery.

Mechanical changes in fatigued muscle

Active muscle contraction develops a tension in the individual motor unit, the muscle and the associated connective tissues. The degree of tension can be influenced by the architecture of the muscle, the strength of contraction and the state of fatigue. Eccentric muscle contraction (exerting a braking effect) seems to generate higher contraction forces and increases susceptibility to muscle damage. High force development can cause muscle injuries such as rupture and tearing. Relatively high or prolonged force, insufficient to cause gross injury, can cause microruptures. If the microruptures are inflicted repeatedly, the regenerative processes are inadequate and degenerative and inflammatory processes can result. Microruptures of the myofibrils, known as Z-band streaming, are accompanied by increased levels of blood enzymes, creatine kinase and myoglobin. Extracellular changes can also occur with ruptures in elastin and collagen and alteration of the extracellular proteoglycans. Effusion from damaged blood vessels can liberate bradykinin and other metabolic factors, which can sensitize the free nerve endings.

Mechanical damage to muscle tissue will be accompanied by biochemical and inflammatory changes, which can affect the ability of the muscle to recover and its response to ongoing activation.

Metabolic changes in fatigued muscle

The energy required for muscle contraction is provided by the breakdown of ATP to ADP in the mitochondria. The ADP is restored to ATP by the provision of nutrients and oxygen in arterial blood. The blood removes the metabolic by products, particularly lactic acid and potassium, as well as heat, carbon dioxide and water.

The precise mechanisms of neuromuscular fatigue are not known, although there is much information about the fatigue process and the biochemical changes associated with it. A number of factors are known to be important and these may vary depending on the type of muscle contraction, the environment and the individual. Kumar (1994) describes several plausible causes of muscle fatigue:

- reduction or occlusion of blood supply, leading to hypoxia and lactic acidosis
- acetyl choline depletion
- potassium ion depletion
- phosphogen depletion
- glycogen depletion
- reduced heart rate
- disturbance in membrane permeability
- neuromuscular fatigue, as seen by median frequency shift on EMG.

Armstrong et al (1993) drew attention to disturbed calcium metabolism:

Increased calcium ion concentration in the intracellular space has been observed following repeated contraction. Increased calcium levels can increase phospholipase activity leading to membrane lipid breakdown and increases cell membrane permeability. This increases the accumulation of toxic metabolites and increases the sensitivity of the cell membrane to free radicals. Calcium overload can affect mitochondrial function.

Muscular effort is accompanied by a loss of potassium from muscle fibre cells. This can sensitize free nerve endings and alter the delicate potassium/calcium ratio necessary for efficient muscle contraction. The potassium can accumulate between the muscle fibres, decreasing membrane resistance, slowing action potential and conduction velocity and initiating a neurophysiological fatigue process (Caffier et al 1993).

Increased levels of metabolites, such as lactic acid, following intensive work produces a fall in tissue pH. This has been postulated as inhibiting the contractile elements and stimulating afferent nerve endings.

Edwards (1988) describes a 'unifying hypothesis' of: 'excessive contraction force per fibre leading to hypoxia, acidosis and metabolic depletion followed by calcium-mediated cellular damage'.

Several studies have focused on how myalgic muscle differs from normal muscle. Dennett & Fry (1988) examined specimens from the first dorsal interosseous muscle from 29 women with chronic overuse syndrome and from eight volunteer controls. They concluded:

Structural differences in samples from the women with overuse syndrome included increased type 1 fibres with type grouping, decreased type 2 fibres, type 2 hypertrophy, increased internal nuclear count, mitochondrial change and various ultrastructural abnormalities. These changes were related to clinical severity and point to an organic cause for the syndrome.

Larsson et al (1988) examined the descending portion of trapezius muscle in cases of chronic myalgia related to static work and compared them to controls:

Isolated pathologic 'ragged red' fibers were found only in the cases with myalgia (8 of 10) strongly suggesting mitochondrial damage. The phenomenon was confined to type 1 fibers. The frequency of type 1 fibers was increased. Levels of adenosine triphosphate and diphosphate were reduced in myalgic patients.

Clinically the condition appears as a maintained local, mainly static hyperactivity of the muscle. This might be primary as a more or less pronounced habitual neuromuscular hyperactivation, or secondary due to the occurrence of muscle tissue changes that may elicit local pain that, in turn, might lead to maintained hyperactivity of the muscle.

Bengtsson & Henriksson (1989), in a review paper of several Swedish studies of muscle changes in fibromyalgia, concluded:

1. There is rarely degeneration of muscle fibers or signs of inflammation.
2. There is morphological, chemical and neurophysiological support for the statement that the energy producing system in the muscle fibers is compromised.
3. Hypoxia is present in painful muscles.
4. Activity in the sympathetic nervous system is important for the maintenance of pain.
5. The muscular pain in fibromyalgia is nociceptive.

The authors state that the findings in fibromyalgia are similar to those found in work-related localized myalgia. They finally hypothesize:

Any conditions that could lead to the establishment of abnormal motor patterns or to constant muscle hypoxia could be regarded as possible causes of chronic muscle pain. Such factors could be improper use of the muscle in certain work situations, wrong postures, muscle tension of psychogenic origin and disorders of regulation of muscle micro-circulation.

Helme et al (1992) measured the capsaicin-induced flare responses in the affected and non-affected arms of 72 chronic RSI sufferers and compared them with 69 controls. They found a reduction in response on the affected limb and statistical analysis showed the severity of clinical pain was strongly associated with reduction in magnitude of flare size. They conjectured that this altered response may be due to a depletion of the neuropeptides that mediate vasodilation or a consequence of desensitization of the nociceptor following a period of chronic activation. They conclude: 'These findings provide objective evidence of altered nociceptor mechanisms in RSI subjects. And are consistent with the view that this chronic pain syndrome involves somatic pathophysiology'.

Dynamic and static contractions

In dynamic exercise, muscles are shortened and lengthened rhythmically. This pumping action, the contraction–relaxation cycle, acts as a vascular pump, increasing the blood supply to up to 20 times that of the resting state. This delivers oxygen and glycogen to the muscle and assists in removal of the waste products, principally lactic acid.

In static or isometric exercise, the constant muscle tension compresses the blood vessels, restricting the available energy supply, and allows a build-up of metabolic byproducts. Consequently, a static muscle contraction will fatigue very quickly, while a dynamic or intermittent activity can be performed for much longer periods. When the supply of oxygen is restricted the muscle starts to utilize anaerobic metabolism, which is less efficient, and produces less energy and increased levels of lactic acid. The recovery period for anaerobic metabolism seems to be much longer than for aerobic metabolism.

During static activity the amount of effort required, and the muscle tension generated, determine the available blood supply to the muscle. At approximately 20% of maximum voluntary contraction (MVC) the blood flow starts to diminish and at 60% MVC the blood supply is almost completely curtailed.

There has been a considerable body of research to determine the safe periods of muscle contraction before fatigue starts to set in. In a standard ergonomic text, Kroemer & Grandjean (1997) state that:

Field studies as well as general experience show that a static force of 15–20% of the maximum force will induce painful fatigue if such loads have to be kept up for very long periods of time. Many experts are therefore of the opinion that work can be maintained for several hours per day without symptoms of fatigue if the force exerted does not exceed about 10% of the maximum force of the muscle involved.

Recent research has suggested this view is inappropriate and that static contractions cannot be sustained even at low levels of loading. A series of studies by Sjogaard and co-workers (1988) on continuous and intermittent contractions at levels between 5 and 50% MVC found the pressure of blood flow during sustained contractions decreased at 10% MVC and became almost zero at 50% MVC. During intermittent contractions the blood flow decrease was of the same magnitude as during contractions, but during each relaxation phase blood flow increased to higher levels.

Sjogaard concludes that blood flow levels are sufficient to sustain contractions below 10% MVC but notes that, despite this, fatigue occurs during sustained contractions at below 10% MVC. Lactate accumulation was higher during continuous contractions but at 5% MVC for 1 h there was no evidence of lactate accumulation. Sjogaard warns that it is not possible to assess an exact level of MVC that blood flow restriction causes, 'as intramuscular pressure may vary considerably within a muscle group and between different parts of a muscle'. Sjogaard also notes that the position of the exercising muscle relative to the height of the heart is crucial, and that 10% MVC corresponds to maintaining the arms in a horizontal position without holding any weight.

Recent research has shown that there is a fatigue process at much lower levels of MVC than previously thought, and the recommended levels of static muscle activity have been lowered accordingly.

Caffier and co-workers (1993) tested EMG readings from the biceps brachii at levels of 4, 8 and 15% of MVC for periods of 1 h. They found that EMG readings progressively increased while conduction velocity and the mean power frequency of the EMG signal decreased. The changes increased linearly at all contraction levels and the researchers concluded:

Homeostasis in the working muscle was not preserved even at very low levels of load. … The skeletal muscle is not able to contract continuously without a growing disturbance of homeostasis, and a safe limit for sustained static contractions does not exist.

Hagberg & Sundelin (1986), in a study on word processing operators, found EMG readings of 3.2 and 3% MVC, respectively, in the right and left side of descending fibres of the trapezius. They found evidence of reduced fatigue and perceived discomfort after work periods with short pauses. Johnson et al (1996) investigated whether there was fatigue in the ring finger flexor digitorum superficialis of VDU mouse users playing solitaire. At an average loading of 0.6% MVC they found evidence of muscle fatigue after between 3 and 4.5 h; this persisted up to 40 min after mouse usage had ceased. Researchers have concluded: 'there is no load level low enough to allow an unlimited duration of contraction' (Caffier et al 1993). In a conference paper Westgaard (1997) reaches the same conclusion and points out that: 'another risk indicator has been the EMG activity levels in situations with an opportunity for rest, but without a conscious effort to relax'.

It seems that after long periods of static muscle contraction it becomes difficult to relax a muscle group, which develops a habitual tension in the presence of prolonged contractions. Practitioners will be familiar with the patient who no longer seems able to have conscious control over muscle relaxation. Even when lying in comfortable postures with no loading on a muscle these patients are unable to allow the muscle to relax. Other researchers have pointed out that in situations of high stress muscles remain tense, even when there are opportunities for muscle unloading and this lack of EMG gaps represents a risk factor for injury. 'A common finding is that workers with shoulder/neck disorders or who will contract disorders later have less gaps compared to workers without disorders or workers who stay healthy' (Hagg 1997).

The increasing drive for efficiency and automation have produced work practices where there are more static muscle contractions than in the past. Most activities take place in a single workplace with a relatively unvaried posture. The maintenance of posture is a major reason for static muscle contractions. Most tasks involve a mixture of both static and dynamic contractions. When standing, a number of muscles in the legs, pelvis, spine, neck and shoulders remain active in order to maintain balance. For this reason, humans often prefer to walk – a dynamic activity – or sit – fewer muscles are required to maintain balance in the sitting posture. However, working while sitting can produce high levels of static tension. Using a computer keyboard involves holding the arms in a position away from the centre of gravity and requires static contractions in the muscles of the scapular, shoulder, elbow, forearm and hand muscles. In addition, computer operators may have to assume unbalanced postures to view their work, particularly if they do not touch-type or use an effective copy holder, leading to high degrees of muscle tension in the head and neck extensor muscles. If the chair is poorly designed or poorly utilized it may be impossible to use the backrest, leading to a static contraction in the spinal extensors. Thus workstation design can make a remarkable difference to the amount of static muscle contraction and hence the degree of cumulative fatigue (Fig. 4.1).

In general, the further a body part is held from the centre of gravity, or a joint is positioned outside the middle one-third of its range of motion, the higher the degree of static tension required to maintain that posture. Particularly high levels of internal pressure have been observed in muscle

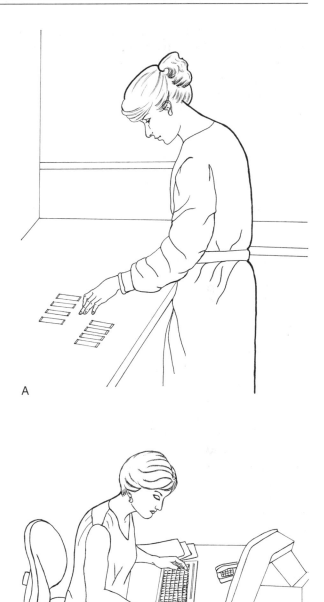

A

B

Figure 4.1 The design of the workstation can make a remarkable difference to the degree of static muscle contraction. A: A visually demanding task at a low workbench leading to high levels of static contraction of the neck and head extensor muscle groups, and high levels of shear force at the cervical facet joints. B: A poorly designed computer workstation leading to high levels of static contraction in the spine and neck extensors.

groups that are bordered by osseous compartments (supraspinatus and infraspinatus) or connective tissue (anterior and posterior tibialis). These can have a consequent effect on vascular perfusion and oxygen tension and as a result are particularly sensitive to prolonged workloads.

Electrophysiological changes – neuromuscular fatigue

The motor unit consists of a motor nerve and the muscle fibres innervated by that nerve; a single nerve can innervate anything from a few muscle fibres to over 1000. The contraction force of a muscle is determined by the number of activated units and the firing frequency of the motor units. The smaller motor units of a working muscle are activated first, with increasing size hierarchy as muscle activity increases. These low-threshold motor units have a high risk of damage at low load levels and have been identified as exhibiting red-ragged fibres. Relative ischaemia and accumulation of metabolites have been associated with increased low threshold afferent activity.

Increased levels of muscle tension due to increased psychosocial load can result in a magnified injury risk and inhibit the recovery process in situations that would normally provide an opportunity for muscle recovery.

At low loads, only a small number of muscle units are recruited and these generally work at relatively high individual loads, with more motor units being recruited for higher workloads. With monotonous or repetitive work the same motor units can be continually activated and can be subject to fatigue. These motor units, which perform a disproportionate amount of work, are known as Cinderella fibres.

The Cinderella hypothesis

The Cinderella hypothesis suggests there is a given order of recruitment of motor units during muscle activation, with small units generally being recruited before large ones. The hypothesis suggests that these low-threshold motor units are more likely to be activated at low levels of loading, and are likely to be at risk in sustained

activation of voluntary muscle to developing fatigue and associated degenerative change. Kaderfors et al (1998, 1999) found that low-threshold motor units in the trapezius muscle were active over a wide range of static and dynamic postures in situations simulating light work and computer use. The trapezius muscle is an important scapula stabilizer and, in situations where there is intense hand work, the trapezius muscle and the 'Cinderella fibres' are likely to be continuously active and prone to fatigue. Veierstad et al (1993) found that trapezius myalgia was more common in subjects who showed reduced micropauses on EMG study.

Motor unit substitution

Westgaard & Deluca (1997) found that there was a selective recruitment of motor unit fibres during prolonged isometric contractions. Using sophisticated EMG analysis of motor units of the trapezius muscle during typing tasks on a computer keyboard, they observed that lower threshold motor units ceased firing while higher threshold motor units were recruited:

We refer to this phenomenon as motor unit substitution. Our current belief is that the recruitment threshold of the motor unit, which has been active for some time and ceased firing, was increased by adaptation processes in the muscle membrane during its period of activity. Thus when the excitation to the motor neurone pool increased, the next motor unit in the hierarchy becomes or is maintained active.

The authors describe this as an adaptation process, but it could perhaps be more accurately described as a fatigue process. This theory suggests that, as motor units become fatigued by prolonged isometric contraction, they enter a rest phase, while other larger motor units become active in order to maintain task-related muscle strength. However, it is not clear whether these newly recruited motor units, which are larger motor units, are as physiologically efficient as the fatigued units initially chosen for the level of contraction. Clearly they are not first choice for the task at hand. The researchers point out:

This has profound implications for the field of ergonomics. It suggests that planned, but small and subtle changes in the activity level of a muscle may be advantageously used to modify the pool of motor units used in a work task, thereby reducing the risk of overuse injury to continuously contracting motor units, even in very low level contractions.

EMG readings during isometric contraction

Fallentin et al (1993) compared motor unit recruitment patterns from the brachial biceps muscle of male subjects performing muscle contractions at 10% and 40% of MVC. The 10% MVC readings demonstrated a quite different EMG profile to the 40% readings, with the mean number of motor unit spikes and the amplitude of the spikes increasing significantly:

> The progressive increase in spike activity was the result of a discontinuous process with periods of increasing and decreasing activity. The phenomenon in which newly recruited motor units replace previously active units is termed 'motor unit rotation' and appeared to be an important characteristic of motor control during a prolonged low level contraction.

Fallentin and co-workers noted that, as the period of contraction increased, there was a corresponding increase in spike amplitude, which was related to the increasing size of the muscle cell and the higher level of activation required. The authors note that this observation was not true of the 40% MVC readings. They also note that the fatigue of the motor units was at a level where blood flow and muscle biochemistry were relatively normal and concluded that: 'Fatigue or exhaustion probably related to an impaired excitation–contraction coupling due to the vast number of stimuli delivered to the muscle'. This contrasts quite clearly with high intensity contractions where muscle blood flow has demonstrable occlusion with dramatic metabolic change.

Johnson & Rempel (1995) found evidence of fatigue in the finger flexors at levels of 5% MVC for 5 min duration, with the fatigue indicators at the lowest levels 30–60 min after exercise.

In summary, there are quite different fatigue pathways for different types of muscle contraction. The high intensity, repetitive muscle contractions have a fatigue process based on vascular insufficiency and metabolic change.

Prolonged isometric contraction shows a gradual reduction in muscular efficiency, with increasingly greater motor unit recruitment required, and a fatigue process based on neuromuscular overload and failure of the excitation–contraction coupling. Hermans et al (1998b) conclude:

> From several literature studies it can be concluded that high load level tasks have relatively short force recovery times compared with submaximal low endurance tasks. In the latter case, the long lasting fatigue is due to the impairment of the excitation contraction coupling.

We can also note that the sustained low force fatigue has a much longer recovery time than the intermittent high force fatigue process.

In a laboratory analysis of ten subjects with unilateral rotator cuff tendinosus, Vollestad et al (1995) found that the injured shoulder showed a higher muscle activation, with a 50% higher EMG reading when subjected to a sustained exhaustive contraction at 25% MVC, than the non-injured shoulder. EMG recordings were taken from upper trapezius, middle deltoid and supraspinatus and infraspinatus. This study reinforces the findings that, as muscles become fatigued or injured, they become progressively less efficient, requiring progressively higher levels of activation to perform the same task. Thus we see the cumulative nature of overuse injuries and how a fatigued muscle group continues to deteriorate without additional exposure.

PERIPHERAL AND CENTRAL SENSITIZATION

The nociceptor system is normally very inactive, requiring intense or damaging stimulation before it becomes activated. However, once pain has been experienced, relatively minor stimulation may trigger the sensitized nociceptors. A large amount of research demonstrates that chemical mediators produced as a result of injury produce a peripheral nociceptor sensitization. A person will become more sensitive to exposures they used to be able to cope with. They can feel pain and discomfort, as well as other reflex changes, at gradually lower levels of exposure. In an acute injury this sensitization usually reduces with time, and the reduction in the concentration and effect of the chemical mediators and inflammatory processes progressively decreases. Some of the key mediators identified are: bradykinin, serotonin, histamine, potassium, adenosine, protons, prostaglandins, leukotrienes and cytokines. A number of different biochemical pathways for these effects have been described (Wright 1999). Where there is continued exposure to microtrauma or other stressors the peripheral sensitivity can persist. There are a number of plausible explanations for this, including:

- disturbed neurovascular circulation
- biochemical stress to neural structures from the neuromuscular fatigue, injury and inflammatory processes
- afferent overload
- neuromuscular fatigue as evidenced by EMG changes, the Cinderella hypothesis and motor unit substitution.

Prolonged increase in peripheral nociceptor activity can trigger a central sensitization at spinal cord level. There are a number of proposed neurophysiological and biochemical explanations for this (Wright 1999). The process is a complex one and seems to vary with the type of provocative stimulus. The increasing central sensitization leads to increased synaptic activity and neuronal excitability at cord level. This increased activity is thought to be responsible for the progressive involvement of segmentally related motor segments and increasing autonomic activity.

Woolf & Thompson (1991) have shown that repetitive stimulation of small-diameter primary afferent fibres creates a progressive increase in action potential discharge and a prolonged increase in excitability of neurons in the spinal cord, even after stimulus termination. There is an increase in peripheral sensitivity at the injury site and an increase in the excitability of neurons at the spinal cord.

In an excellent review article on pain and nociception, Charman (1994) elaborates on these processes. Dorsal root ganglion cells, at spinal cord level, continually synthesize a wide range of enzymes and peptides, including substance P and serotonin, which flow towards their peripheral nerve endings and spinal cord connections. Afferent C fibres monitor the changing state of tissues they innervate, both in health and injury, by 'tasting' the fluid medium and using neurotubular transport to convey tissue molecules to the dorsal root ganglion cells, which vary the type and concentration of substances they manufacture according to the chemical information arriving by retrograde flow. These substances cause further vasodilation, neurogenic oedema and sensitization of surrounding nerve endings, and also trigger the release of other proinflammatory agents, including histamine and serotonin. Prolonged C fibre activation by tissue damage leads to a leakage of these neuroinflammatory agents, which exacerbates the inflammation and leads to a reduction in dorsal horn thresholds to afferent stimuli. This applies particularly to joint injury, where normal mechanoreceptors' response to movement can trigger the increasingly sensitive dorsal horn cells. Thus normal mechanoreceptor activity can create a pain response.

This prolonged C fibre activation causes long-lasting widespread sensitization of spinal cord circuits, resulting in peripheral hyperalgesia and prolonged tenderness. Any regeneration of axons is highly sensitive and prone to spontaneous firing.

In an important review of the Australian RSI experience (which they call refractory cervicobrachial pain syndrome (RCBP)) Cohen et al (1992) point out that many of the terms used to describe chronic musculoskeletal pain include descriptors such as shooting, pulling, burning, tingling and numbness. After reviewing the possible pathophysiological processes they conclude:

There is a central disturbance of nociception in this syndrome, induced by continual afferent barrage from nociceptors and mechanoreceptors in anatomically relevant sites. These sites may be in the spinal zygapophyseal joints or related structures, or muscles, tendons and joint capsules in the upper limb and/or the dorsal root, the dorsal root ganglion and the peripheral nerves.

This afferent barrage can be readily related to the constrained work postures and movements executed by our subjects and may be sufficient to sensitize

WDR neurones so that mechanoreceptive afferent information is processed as nociceptive.

The authors state that manipulation of facet joints or proximal neural tissues in chronic pain cases may exacerbate the pain by triggering the sensitized nociceptors, and that treatment directed toward central (spinal cord) nociceptive mechanisms may be more successful. It is important for practitioners to recognize the chronically pained, neurologically sensitive, patient and adjust their treatment approach accordingly. There is increasing interest in pain blockade to interrupt the flow of nociception in chronic injury to prevent or reduce the secondary sensitization of nociception and allow chronic pain sufferers to become more active.

Edwards (1988) describes a second unifying hypothesis:

A disturbance of central control of postural motor units such that there is a failure of proper relaxation of low threshold units between periods of activity during the day and in sleep.

The increasing nociceptive sensitization is a consequence of the physiological fatigue of the neuromuscular system involving both biochemical and neurophysiological pathways. Once the nociceptive sensitivity has been established it can create a series of vicious circles (Johannson & Solka 1991, Johannson 1996).

Vicious circles

It is a characteristic trait of chronic musculoskeletal disorders that pain and tenderness often spreads to neighbouring muscle groups. Metabolites and inflammatory substances (lactic acid, bradykinin, serotonin, potassium ions and arachidonic acid) are produced during static or repetitive muscular activity. These substances stimulate the chemosensitive muscle afferents, which have been shown to be potent stimulators of the static and dynamic fusimotor neurons to the affected segment. This increase of reflex muscle spindle activity further stimulates the production of metabolites and inflammatory substances, creating a positive feedback loop or vicious circle. The muscle spindle afferents seem

to have an effect on secondary muscle spindle afferents, triggering a reflexly mediated increase in muscle tone in neighbouring muscle groups. These muscles become fatigued and further increase the afferent/efferent gain, creating a second vicious circle. The pathophysiological model of Johansson & Solka (1991) provides an explanation for the propogation of muscle pain and stiffness from their primary site to neighbouring and contralateral muscle groups. It also suggests that long-lasting exposures with the increased afferent load are more likely to trigger these effects and they speculate that arachidonic acid may be the key substance that triggers these changes. Djupsjobacka (1997) hypothesizes that the quality of the proprioception from the overactive muscle spindle system may be a key factor in causing the deterioration of precise motor coordination in fatigued or injured muscles, causing a further load on the overactive motor units (Fig. 4.2). This theory complements the motor unit substitution theory, where fatigued muscle spindles cease firing and are replaced by larger motor units in the hierarchy, which require an increased level of electrophysiological stimulation with a consequent loss of efficiency.

In a perceptive paper, Korr (1975) explores the role of the muscle spindle at an injured spinal segment. Through the CNS control of gamma activity, the muscle spindle length can be set at appropriate level for a given activity and turned up or down in adjustment to the motions and activities that are anticipated and subsequently performed. The effect of gamma gain can be subject to cerebral influences, which may occasionally be maladaptive. In muscle injury, muscle tension and anxiety states the gamma activity may be set too high for smooth and efficient coordination, resulting in a tense and jerky muscle action. Korr goes on to postulate that the basis of the spinal somatic dysfunction is a turn-up of the gamma gain in the motor neurons of the related spinal segment with the sustained high frequency discharge keeping the intrafusal fibres of the muscle spindle in a chronically shortened state. The higher degree of gamma activity will increase the friction between the joint surfaces.

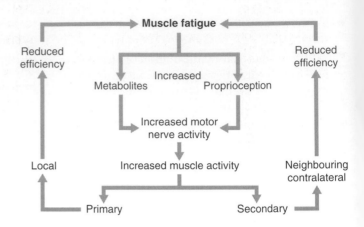

Figure 4.2 The muscle tension cycle: a schematic view of the proposed pathophysiological model and vicious circles proposed by Johannson & Solka (1991), Johannson (1996) and Djupsjobacka (1997).

Korr goes on to develop his hypothesis with the following rationale:

1. The high gain hypothesis is consistent with, and offers an explanation for, the steeply rising resistance to motion found in injured joints.
2. It explains the palpable ropiness and trigger points found in the muscles around the segment.
3. The compressed joints with diminished range of motion would be more likely to 'pop' when forcefully gapped than neighbouring joints with normal mobility.
4. The high gain spindle may contribute to the catch, twinge or grating sensations experienced at the affected segment.

Korr points out that a local sympathetic nervous system hyperactivity increases the level of afferent discharge from the spindles and envisages the creation of a vicious circle, with the increased spindle activity triggering further sympathetic preganglionic activity in the spinal cord.

The local effects of nociceptive sensitization and the vicious circles associated with them feed back into the organizational processes of the CNS and have important consequences for the reparative processes of the injury, the risk of reinjury and the development of chronicity.

The facilitated segment

In a fascinating series of experiments that began in the 1940s (and is outlined in Korr 1979),

Denslow and his co-workers found that, when subjected to pressure, certain areas of the spine showed exaggerated muscular responses as demonstrated by EMG. It took less pressure to elicit the first reflex muscular response in vertebral and paravertebral regions at these spinal levels. Denslow and colleagues found that these low-threshold segments could be identified by experienced palpators and were consistent over time with individuals. They also found that certain areas were more vulnerable than others – these were areas of high biomechanical strain, notably the junction of the neck and cranium, and the cervicothoracic and lumbosacral junctions. These chronic facilitated segments were preferentially excited at lower thresholds with greater responses, not only by local stimuli but also by distal or diffuse stimuli (noise, cold, etc.).

Responses occurred in these segments to impulses from many sources while at the same time nonlesioned sources remained quiescent. Under conditions where there was generalized muscular contraction the lesioned segments were relatively exaggerated. ... The easier opening of the motor pathways in lesioned segments suggested that this was a sustained form of facilitation ... had its origin in the sustained afferent bombardment by impulses from segmentally located source.   (Korr 1955a)

Continued investigation of these facilitated segments showed that there was a lowered threshold of associated neurological pathways of that particular spinal segment:

- sensory – lowered pain threshold and increased tenderness

- motor pathways – lowered reflex muscle response
- sympathetic pathways – low electrical skin resistance, lowered skin temperature.

Korr (1955b) concludes:

Because of the sustained facilitation of sensory, motor and autonomic pathways, the lesioned segment acts as a neurological lens, focussing and exaggerating the effects of impulses from many sources upon the tissues innervated from that segment; through that segment the individual is subjected to the exaggerated impact of life situations and environmental factors. To the facilitated segment and the structures which it supplies and therefore to the organism as a whole even ordinary innocuous life situations become relatively stressful and taxing and may continually demand and evoke the costly, reserve-reducing protective response.

This fascinating series of research papers, which began by identifying the characteristics of the palpably identifiable osteopathic lesion and went on to identify the neurological processes associated with it, provides an insight to the nature of the injury process. It shows the cumulative nature of biomechanical loading on the afferent nervous system and its effects on the motor and sympathetic nervous system, sensitizing the area to ongoing loading and further insult. While the research focuses on spinal segments it is clear that the afferent input and consequent effects could equally affect the segmental areas associated with the spinal segment. Peripheral injuries could also create an afferent bombardment, which could elicit a facilitated spinal segment that could in turn magnify the effects of the peripheral injury. This adds support to the vicious circle theory proposed by Johannson & Solka (1991). This research also suggests that injuries can create neurophysiological change within the related spinal segment and that this can create a spread of injury to tissues within the segment, or to predispose them to additional insult. This is relevant for the management of chronic injuries, where the therapist must address the related spinal segments and the segmentally related structures in addition to the injured tissues, dealing with any sources of aberrant afferent input and their associated effects.

The increasing role of the neuroendocrine immune network

Bengtsson & Henriksson (1989) pointed out that activity in the sympathetic nervous system (SNS) is important for the maintenance of pain. Charman (1994) explains the rationale behind this: raised sympathetic tone increases the availability of noradrenaline, which increases vascular permeability and inflammatory response and triggers local tissue production of prostaglandins, which are powerful inflammatory agents.

Korr believes the SNS can play a powerful role in the maintenance of an injury state. In a review paper (Korr 1973), he states:

In almost any kind of trauma the sympathetic nervous system is almost invariably bought into play. And very often it participates in a most inappropriate manner, which not only does not contribute to recovery from the injury but actually produces trouble that prolongs it. When the sympathetics are hyperirritable in a given area, in a given segment, in a given peripheral distribution, there is in that area a tendency for either exaggerated vasoconstriction or exaggerated vasodilation, or a mixture of the two, which contributes to chaos and the perpetuation of pathology. When you control the blood supply to a given area you control its life; you control its capacity for recovery, its capacity to resist infection, its capacity to survive and maintain its integrity as a tissue.

Stimulating the SNS will increase the sensitivity of cutaneous reception and muscle spindles and even cause them to fire spontaneously, falsely reporting stretch or contact, and causing exaggerated responses. … It exaggerates and exacerbates the disturbance, and tends toward positive feedback, toward the perpetuation of vicious cycles. The syndrome – the injury – becomes more and more disabling the more overactive the sympathetic nervous system becomes … .

The sympathetic stimulation produces chaotic feedback, yielding garbled information which is fed into the nervous system from the tissues and which, of course, can do nothing but create more and more chaos and cause the disturbance to persist longer and longer.

This colourful description by Korr of the potential deleterious effects of SNS involvement and the consequences of ongoing SNS stimulation in the injury process, highlights the need to identify

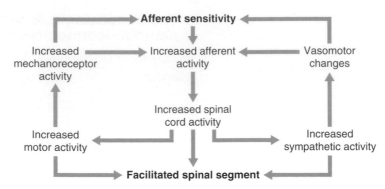

Figure 4.3 The afferent sensitivity cycle – a significant pathway to developing chronicity.

as early as possible the sources of aberrant afferent stimuli and the need to maintain healthy proprioceptive functioning (Fig. 4.3).

Once the CNS becomes involved in the injury process there is the potential for higher centres and other body systems to be influenced. A thoroughly readable explanation of the effect of nociceptive stress on the neuroendocrine–immune network is given by Willard (personal communication):

The axons of the β-afferent system can become sensitized, lowering their thresholds of activation and responding to low energy or non-noxious stimuli. In such cases the patient experiences allodynia, a painful reaction to non-noxious stimuli.

In addition to mechanical stimulation of nerve endings, specific chemicals involved with the inflammatory reaction and immune reaction can interact with receptors on the nerve endings. These chemicals such as histamine, bradykinin and prostaglandins stimulate the nerve endings to release substance P and other neuropeptides. Substance P is an irritant to the axons that secrete it and stimulates the release of histamine and further release of substance P. This chemical cascade results in oedema, inflammation and hyperalgesia.

Nociceptive information enters the dorsal horn through the small calibre axons of the β-afferent system. These signals influence the activity of the segmental interneuronal pool, thereby affecting neural activity in both the lateral horn (sympathetic nervous system) and the ventral horn (somatic nervous system). The persistent relay of nociceptive information from compromised tissues changes the tonic activity of the motorneurones and hence the tone in the associated skeletal muscles. This response is known as the splinting or guarding reflex of the musculature surrounding the injured tissue. The

increased sympathetic activity can influence vasomotor tone leading to vasoconstriction, and can affect changes in associated hormonal activity.

The dorsal horn of the spinal cord gives rise to two major ascending pathways known as the anterolateral system. Nociceptive information from the spinal cord is processed in the brainstem, thalamus, hypothalamus and several areas in the cerebral cortex. Thus via these links a general adaptation response can be initiated including the hypothalamic–pituitary–adrenal axis and the adrenal steroid hormones. With a breakdown in the hypothalamic–pituitary–adrenal axis the shift in body chemistry initiated by a noxious physical or emotional stimulus becomes difficult to reverse creating a chronic condition of general adaptation termed maladaptation.

Alteration of the axis affects psychological as well as physiological processes – elevated blood cortisol levels are a common feature of people diagnosed with melancholic depression, characterized by anxiety, vigilance, obsession, hyperarousal and feelings of worthlessness.

In summary, stressful, emotional or physical stimuli initiate a general adaptive response that the adult individual is incapable of controlling resulting in feelings of depression and anxiety as well as physiological changes.

Somatic events leading to nociceptive signals could either predispose or be a significant secondary factor to an emotional dysfunction such as some forms of depression or anxiety.

Repeated or prolonged insults are potentially the most dangerous and optimum physical stature and emotional balance will best assist in recovering a state of well being.

With the ascending pathways in the spinal cord and the involvement of the parasympathetic nervous system, the symptomatic possibilities that arise from the afferent barrage are increased. The CNS and the descending pathways also have a capacity to moderate the effects of afferent barrage and the symptomatic experience. According to Kendall (personal communication):

No stimulus or afferent barrage arrives in a blank central nervous system. At any given time afferents arrive in a CNS which is already in a particular state of excitability and that will be a function of many past and present factors. Stimuli arriving from the periphery interact with each other with greater or lesser importance attached to various signals.

Charman (1994) also provides a concise explanation of the ascending nociceptor pathways from the dorsal horn and the transition from nociception into pain experience.

Box 4.1 summarizes the mechanisms involved in chronic neuromuscular pain.

Box 4.1 Possible mechanisms involved in chronic neuromuscular pain, in approximate order of short-term to long-term effects

- Mechanical force – myofibrillar rupture, release of chemicals inducing inflammatory response.
- Prolonged increase of intramuscular pressure – reduced blood supply and oxygenation, build-up of metabolites.
- Metabolic crises – drop in pH and increase in lactic acid, extracellular potassium and intracellular calcium may increase pain perception.
- Neuromuscular fatigue – high loading on Cinderella fibres, inefficient motor unit substitution.
- Afferent sensitization – lowered afferent thresholds, increasing noxious stimuli, release of inflammatory agents.
- Segmental facilitation – reflex muscle spasm and vascular change to injury region and related segments.
- Progressive sympathetic nervous system and neuroendocrine immune network involvement.
- Increasing influence of higher brain centres and psychosocial aspects.

There is morphological and experimental evidence for the muscle fatigue pathways and the changes associated with myalgia. There is experimental evidence for a neuromuscular fatigue pathway resulting in afferent sensitivity. This latter pathway seems to be particularly relevant to the development of chronicity. There is no safe level for prolonged periods of static contraction.

OTHER TISSUES SUSCEPTIBLE TO INJURY

Tendon disorders

The stress experienced by a tendon depends on the muscle contraction force, the relative size of the tendon and its insertion, and the forces from adjacent anatomical surfaces. Tendon tensile strength is generally greater than that of muscle and ruptures of healthy tendon are less common. Tendon responses to excessive load can be mechanical – deformation and tears – or physiological – inflammatory and degenerative. The most common sites of tendon disorders in the working population are in the wrist, forearm, elbow and shoulder, and in the lower limb in sports participants.

The terminology of tendon dysfunction can be confusing:

- tendinitis or tendinosus is the term used for injury to the tendon
- tenosynovitis is used for any tendon sheath disorder, particularly common in the hand and wrist
- stenosing tenosynovitis is the term used when the movement of the tendon inside the sheath is affected, as in de Quervain's disorder affecting abductor pollicis longus and extensor pollicis brevis
- calcified tendinitis is used when hydroxyapatite is deposited in the tendon or sheath; it is well-documented in rotator cuff tendons
- peritendinitis refers to pain at the myotendinous junction.

Mechanical overload seems to be a major cause of tendinitis, with risk factors including repetition, high force and joint deviation from midline. Once a certain threshold of loading occurs, viscous creep occurs, which has been explained as cumulative microfailure between the molecular links between the tissue matrix and the filler material. Microdamage can accumulate faster than the recovery process with reduced collagen integrity, accumulation of debris and calcification. Impairment of circulation and nutrition caused by compression of the tendon against adjacent surfaces, thickening of tendon sheaths and reduced diffusion of nutrients can be regarded as an important contributory factor usually due to prolonged loading or anatomical impairment. Age is an important component with the older tendons having a lower injury threshold with frequent evidence of degenerative change and reduced vascularity.

The pathogenesis of shoulder tendinitis is generally well understood (Armstrong et al 1993). The tendons of the supraspinatus, biceps brachii and infraspinatus have zones of avascularity. These areas are the common sites of degenerative change. Impairment of circulation, and subsequent degeneration, is exacerbated by long periods of static tension or anatomical compression under the subacromial arch. Studies have shown a critical angle of 30 degrees of abduction or flexion at the shoulder joint (measured away from the body) with arm positions higher than this affecting circulation. For further discussion see Section 3.

Lateral epicondylitis is a common injury in the dominant arm of people aged 30–55 and is associated with repetitive or sustained use of the forearm extensor muscles. The pathology is not well understood but the predominant theory involves microruptures at the junction of the tendon and the periosteum of extensor carpi radialis brevis, with the formation of granulation tissue. Wrist tendinitis is commonly associated with repetitive work that involves high grip force and deviated wrist positions. The tendinitis or tenosynovitis is associated with friction stresses as the tendons pass through ligamentous compartments.

Management of tendonitis

The management of tendonitis is largely dependent on the site and the exposures identified. In general:

- ice to help limit inflammation
- deep frictions/massage to tendon to improve blood flow and remove debris and inflammatory products
- muscle release and stretching to reduce tensile stress

- joint mobilization to reduce any joint compressions or biomechanical inefficiencies. Controlled passive mobilization is helpful
- try and identify key exposures. Avoid poor joint positions with sustained or repetitive actions
- inner range cyclic exercises
- immobilization tends to weaken tendons and delay recovery. It should be avoided.

Nerve disorders

Nerve disorders are a common complication of injury and can occasionally be a primary injury.

Nerves can be affected by pressure from, or swelling of, adjacent muscles, tendons and tendon sheaths. These mechanical pressures can influence neurovascular circulation and create a physiological response that impairs nerve function.

A common site for nerves to suffer mechanical pressure or stress is as they exit the spinal cord through the intervertebral foramen. A common cause of pressure is intervertebral disc bulge or leakage of disc material (which then rapidly absorbs water and swells). The intervertebral foramen can be compromised by disc space narrowing or facet joint osteophytosis, which can increase the risk of mechanical pressure or irritation of the nerve root. Impaired conduction of nerves can be measured by nerve conduction velocity changes or changes in sensory threshold. Impaired circulation to the nerve results in tingling, numbness, pain and a reduction in motor control of the affected muscles.

Prolonged intracarpal tunnel pressure can lead to impaired nerve conduction, the effect being dependent on the degree of pressure and the length of the exposure. The changes to the nerve are caused by mechanical pressure and alteration in neurovascular supply to the median nerve. These changes are maximized during isometric contractions in positions of wrist deviation. Compression of the median nerve during wrist deviation is the basis of Phalen's or Tinel's test for median nerve sensitivity (see Section 3). Prolonged stretching of the nerve can cause impaired pressure or circulatory changes. This is commonly seen in positional paraesthesia, where subjects wake up with numbness in the upper limbs following awkward joint postures such as extreme elbow or wrist flexion. If prolonged, this can set up an inflammatory process with micro-ruptures and tissue scarring. This can occur where nerves cross mobile joint surfaces such as the:

- anterior shoulder and chest wall – thoracic outlet or pectoralis minor syndrome
- elbow – the ulna nerve in the cubital tunnel
- wrist – carpal tunnel syndrome
- hip – the sciatic nerve between the piriformis and pelvis.

Direct pressure on the nerves has been demonstrated to block inward and outward axoplasmic flow in the median nerve and can be a problem, particularly with subcutaneous peripheral nerves in which the pressure is higher than systolic pressure; for example, the sharp edge of a desk over the carpal tunnel when writing or using a keyboard or 'Saturday night palsy' – falling asleep in an awkward position in a chair causing pressure in the ulna nerve.

Microscopic studies of tissue in the carpal tunnel have shown thickening of fibrocytes and connective tissue in the median nerve. The pattern of these changes corresponds with the pattern of stresses produced between the tendons, nerves, flexor retinaculum and carpal bones.

The effect of exposure on the neurological tissues is moderated by the individual response. Individuals with low blood pressure will be more affected by mechanical pressure causing impairment of neurovascular circulation. Hormonal status has been demonstrated to increase the pressure in the carpal tunnel. High levels of oestrogen increase fluid retention during pregnancy. Metabolic disorders such as diabetes mellitus may make the nerve more sensitive to pressure increases.

Nerves can also be affected by exposure to vibration and cold. Vibration has been shown to cause protein leakage in the neurovascular blood supply, which can result in localized oedema and increased pressure. Vibrating tools that produce higher force muscle contractions in the affected limbs in an effort to stabilize the involved muscle groups can also lead to increased exposure levels.

The use of gloves, particularly those that reduce proprioception, lead to higher grip forces and can also contribute to increased exposure levels.

Thus, the types of exposure that affect muscle and tendons also affect neural function. These include awkward joint postures, prolonged or repetitive muscle contractions, prolonged localized pressure and vibration. The neurovascular changes are very much dose dependent – the degree of pressure and the length of exposure – highlighting the need to avoid static postures with isometric muscle contractions and prolonged doses of repetitive neuromuscular function. A healthy neuromuscular mechanism needs a healthy neurovascular blood supply, frequent postural alterations, varied cycles of muscular contraction and mixed proprioceptive activity. Neurovascular variety avoids prolonged episodes of fatigue and accelerates recovery.

Articular cartilage

Articular cartilage is a thin lining (1–7 mm) of hyaline cartilage that lines both surfaces of the synovial joints. It is moulded to the underlying bone, often altering the congruity of the bony surfaces. When combined with synovial fluid it provides a smooth, wear-resistant, low-friction lubricated surface that is slightly compressible and elastic, and is ideally suited to resist large compressive forces, generated by compression and shear and created by gravity and muscular forces. Joint cartilage consists of four distinct zones, which consist of collagen fibres, chondrocytes and proteoglycans. The bonding of the proteoglycans to the collagen is thought to provide the dynamic properties of articular cartilage.

The largely inextensible collagen fibrils are thought to be maintained in a taut form by the water swollen ground substance, thereby providing an instantaneous elastic response to compressive loading. Superimposed on this is a more time-dependent response to compression resulting from the movement of interstitial water out of the region of local deformation.   Broom (1985)

The articular cartilage has no nerve supply and no active blood supply. It is thought to derive its nutrition from the synovial fluid and the synovial membrane.

Synovial fluid transport around the joint, and nutrition to the articular cartilage, is assisted by movement and alteration in the compressive pressure of the joint. Immobilization tends to reduce cartilage nutrition and delay recovery processes.

Constant pressure on the articular cartilage can produce deformation of the cartilagenous structure and a decreased ability to dissipate load. In an important experiment that compared compressive stress on articular cartilage during short-loading of 20 s and creep-loading of 2 h, Adams et al (1999) found that:

Localised concentrations of compressive stress do exist within articular cartilage and are intensified by sustained loading.
The localised peaks of compressive stress which are intensified by peak loading may have important consequences.
... they may deform chondrocytes
... the steep stress gradients associated with the peaks imply high shear stresses within the matrix and these may possibly damage the collagen-proteoglycans interface upon which cartilage integrity depends.
... the high stress peaks may possibly elicit joint pain by pressing unevenly on the subchondral bone.

In theory, sustained compressive loading or areas of peak compressive stress could accelerate the deterioration of articular cartilage. Evidence for this includes:

- Increased levels of degeneration in load-bearing joints in asymmetry, such as the hip and knee on a long leg side or the spinal facet joints in scoliosis or asymmetry.
- The most common sites of spinal facet degenerative change are in the lower cervical spine and the lower lumbar spine. Both parts of the spine have considerable compressive force of the facets during flexion moments with the added leverage of the head and trunk, respectively.
- Facet degeneration seems to accelerate in cases of disc degenerative change or narrow-

ing, which seems to increase the proportion of weight borne by the articular surfaces of the facets.

The absence of nerve endings in the articular cartilage means there are no warning signs of cartilagenous fatigue or damage. The fatigue-injury cycle of articular cartilage is not a short one, as in muscular fatigue, or even a medium-term one, as in neuromuscular fatigue, but seems rather to be long term, and a process that contributes to the degenerative process of articular joints.

SUMMARY

There is a significant understanding of many of the pathways to injury:

- Acute injury often involves mechanical compromise of muscles, tendons and ligaments.
- Subacute injury shows increasing involvement of different muscle fatigue pathways and neuromuscular fatigue processes.
- Chronic injuries show increasing peripheral sensitization at the injured site, with progressive involvement of efferent reflex arcs to the injured and neighbouring regions.
- Very chronic injuries show increasing sympathetic nervous activity and can be profoundly influenced by psychosocial and environmental factors.
- Prolonged postures, prolonged loading of joints and prolonged isometric contractions tend to inhibit physiological recovery and may be associated with accelerated fatigue, delayed recovery and increasing risk of chronic injury, including neurological and degenerative change.
- Postural variety with a variety of isotonic muscle activity, variation of proprioceptive pathways and efficient metabolic transport optimize healthy physiological and recovery processes.

5

Ergonomic factors

We have evidence that the more risk factors combined in the same job, affecting the same tissues, the greater the risk of WMSD. We have evidence the longer the duration to the exposure the greater the risk of a WMSD. We have evidence that reducing the physical and psychosocial risk factors decreases the severity, and may also decrease the incidence of WMSD.   Silverstein (1995)[1]

Injuries are usually caused by physical loading of some sort – actions initiated by muscles, using bones and tendons as levers, articulated at joints. The loading can be very short and intense, cyclic, prolonged, or a combination of these. The different factors that determine the demands of the tasks involved – the posture adopted, the amount of force required, the duration of the load and the environmental factors such as temperature and humidity – are ergonomic factors. This is a limited definition of the term ergonomics, which can also cover many other aspects of the work environment such as psychosocial factors and systems management.

POSTURE

Overall body posture and individual joint posture are important determinants of injury risk. A number of work postures have been identified with an increased incidence of injury. These will be covered in greater detail in Section 3. Posture is an interface between the job we are required to do and the tools we have to complete the task. Good posture requires education as

---

[1] WMSD corresponds to work-related musculoskeletal disorder (WRMSD), as described in Chapter 2.

to how to complete these tasks using the tools appropriately.

Individuals often do not have a natural sense of what constitutes good posture. When asked to demonstrate a comfortable posture, a person will usually identify a familiar posture as being comfortable, even though this may have a high biomechanical loading. Some body tissues, such as articular cartilage and intervertebral discs, have minimal afferent nerve endings and provide no feedback on levels of loading or fatigue. The unfamiliar, which may have a much lower biomechanical loading, will often be rejected as good posture because it feels different and there is a low neurophysiological adaptation to this new posture. If you ask someone to assume a good posture, the posture he or she adopts will be based on cultural and learned habits rather than on an assessment of internal neuromuscular information, such as joint loading or muscle activity. People may be provided with excellent equipment but may set it up in ways that increase their joint loading based on a mistaken view of what constitutes good posture. The key point is that a person has to be appealed to on an intellectual level to understand the need for good posture, and educated in a practical environment as to what is good posture. Once these are established, the person must be prepared to trial the posture through the familiarization and adaptation period. Frequently, when setting up individuals with a slightly forward-sloping seat for sitting at desk-based or VDU tasks, the unfamiliar nature of the posture encourages them to question the validity of it. When the physiological benefits are explained, and they are encouraged to try it, they soon adapt and there is usually a very high uptake of this posture, with the consequent benefits.

What is good posture?

Good posture should involve:

- minimum joint strain or biomechanical loading
- economy of energy – minimal muscular loading

- avoidance of prolonged, repetitive or awkward movements.

The soft tissues around a joint – articular cartilage, muscles, tendons, ligaments and joint capsule – are usually in their greatest balance in the middle third of their range of motion. As this range is extended, there is increasing soft tissue stress. People in a relaxed state, such as sleeping, usually adopt joint postures in this mid-range (Fig. 5.1). If the demands of gravity are removed, the joint positions move into their own natural balance and the same phenomenon is found. However, as soon as people start assuming postures to do work these joint postures start to become compromised by the demands of the task. Even standing requires quite a high workload to maintain balance and defy gravity. In the standing posture the lower body – pelvis, hips and knees – move into extension to keep the body position close to the centre of gravity and minimize muscle tension. However, this is not a comfortable position to maintain for long and people transfer weight from one leg to another to try and introduce some flattening of their lumbar curve and some pelvis, hip and knee flexion (Fig. 5.2).

Relaxed sitting generally uses less energy than standing because there are more points of support and balance and less muscular energy is required to maintain the posture. However, performing a task while sitting can compromise this relaxation. Head and neck posture will be compromised by visual demands; upper limb postures will be compromised if the hands are used.

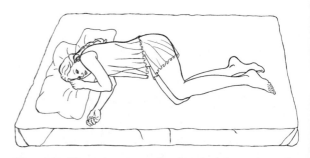

Figure 5.1 When choosing a sleeping posture most people usually place their joints in the middle third of the range of movement – the joint comfort zone.

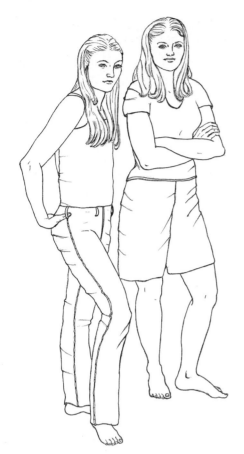

Figure 5.2 Relaxed standing posture usually involves placing one pelvis, hip and knee into flexion, and regularly alternating legs. This reduces biomechanical loading.

The further a body part is moved from the centre of gravity, the more muscle tension is required to move it to or hold it in that position, unless that part of the body is supported against gravity. To minimize muscle tension, a person must:

- keep their joints in the middle one-third of the range of movement as much as possible
- keep their limbs close to the centre of gravity as much as possible
- try and support body parts that move away from the mid-range or centre of gravity.

People tend to hunt for comfort around these parameters, usually naturally alternating the biomechanical demands on different body parts. For example, when people are standing, arms

hanging by their sides have the least gravity but there is a muscular load on the upper arm and shoulder girdle. They may attempt to unload this by folding their forearms. This tends to relieve the shoulders but creates some tension in the forearms. Next they may attempt to support the limbs by putting their hands in their pockets.

It is normal and healthy to move the joints through their full range of motion. There are positive vascular, lymphatic, neurological and other homeostatic processes that benefit from movement. The difficulties start to become apparent when people do stereotyped, repetitive movements or they sustain postures that are physiologically demanding.

Sitting posture

People are increasingly spending more and more time sitting – for work, for travel and for relaxation. The more labour-saving devices perform manual tasks, the more people sit. Sitting has become the predominant daily posture for a large proportion of Western society. Sitting fundamentally changes the posture and the demands and constraints placed on the musculoskeletal system. It changes the natural spinal curve from a three-curve structure to a single curve, which profoundly alters the biomechanical forces and physiological homeostasis of the spine. A number of effects on other body systems are also caused by the sitting posture:

- circulation – reduced muscle pump effect of circulation, particularly venous return from the lower limbs
- digestion – increased abdominal pressure, can increase incidence of reflux, constipation and carcinoma
- respiration – increased thoracic cavity pressure can affect quality of breathing and oxygenation
- physical inactivity – can be regarded as a risk factor for obesity, osteoporosis and arteriosclerosis.

A person who works in a sitting position tends to move certain parts of the body to perform certain tasks, chiefly the head and neck to maintain visual contact and the upper limbs to manipulate tools. The ramifications of this will be covered in Section 3. It is possible to sit and fulfil good biomechanical requirements for task work and to maintain the joints in their natural comfort zones.

Joint comfort zones when sitting for work

The aim is to provide good spine and pelvis posture while still being able to easily access work tools and maintain good visual angles and distances:

- spine and pelvis – 110–130 degrees
- lumbar spine – retain some natural lordosis
- thoracic spine – a slight kyphosis
- head and neck – erect and close to the centre of gravity
- visual angle – 10–30 degrees below horizontal
- shoulders – relaxed in line with the trunk
- elbows – 90–100 degrees
- wrists – straight with wrists extended up to 20 degrees
    - forearms supported where possible
- knees – 60–120 degrees
- feet – flat on the floor or on footrest.

Sitting for relaxation, when the arms are not required to manipulate tools, is generally improved by more reclined postures where spinal weight is more supported. If people want to watch TV in the reclined position they may require neck/head support to maintain a comfortable posture. Aaras et al (1997) found greater neck flexion angles when viewing a VDU task while standing and greater spinal flexion when sitting. They recommended alternating between sitting and standing postures to minimize joint stress. This will be explored in further depth in Section 2.

FORCE

The forces applied to the joint structures can be an important determinant of the risk of injury. If the force exerted exceeds the tolerance of the tissues, injury results. The force is determined by a number of possible components including the load, the distance, the joint position required and

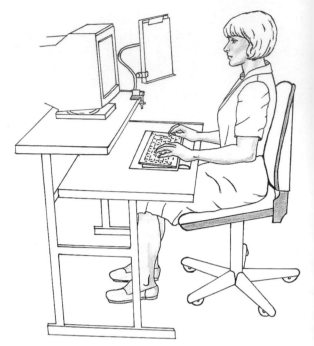

Figure 5.3 Joint comfort zones for task-related sitting posture while working at a computer.

the activity involved. Repetitive forces tend to reduce the tolerance of most tissues such as muscles, tendons, intervertebral discs, vertebral end plates, etc.

The load

The load refers to the object being manipulated. The weight of the load is a significant determining factor for the risk of injury. Most occupational safety legislation sets maximum limits for recommended lifting, based on this recognized risk factor. The size, shape and position of the load will also determine how easy it is to lift or how much the posture needs to be compromised to affect the activity.

When attempting a musculoskeletal (MS) load, a person generally has an expectation of the force required and their MS system prepares for the expected loading in a reasonably efficient manner. If the load differs from expectations, for instance, if the weight of a lift has been underestimated or a step has not been noticed, this dramatically increases the MS forces generated and the risk of injury. An unstable load, and a variable load, thus represent risk factors that can dramatically modify the risk of injury. Experienced load handlers will usually carefully assess the requirements of the load and the task and try and avoid sudden peak forces, as far as possible.

Distance

The distance required to reach to the load away from the body, or against gravity, and then the manipulation of the load at that distance are dramatic modifiers of the force required to manipulate the object. Lifting a heavy object close to the body can be relatively straightforward, but place the same load at a distance from the body and it can become a very high-risk activity (Fig. 5.4). It has been estimated that a load is 12 times greater when lifted at a distance from the body than when the load is kept close to the body and the trunk remains upright.

Lifting a child close to the body may be straightforward; lifting the same child from their seat in the centre of the back seat of the car is a much more significant load. Using a well-sited computer mouse with forearm support can produce a relatively low MS load; placing the mouse at an awkward height or distance, without forearm support, dramatically modifies the degree of load on the forearm, shoulder and neck. The load on the MS tissues then includes the weight of the part of the body extended to the object plus the magnifier of the distance involved.

Joint position

We have established that there is a lower physiological load when the joint is in its comfort zone in the middle third of the range of movement. Among the reasons for this are:

- the biomechanical load can be distributed between the range of supporting musculature around the joint
- the musculotendinous units generally provide efficient force vectors, with less friction or pressure, when there are no significant changes of direction

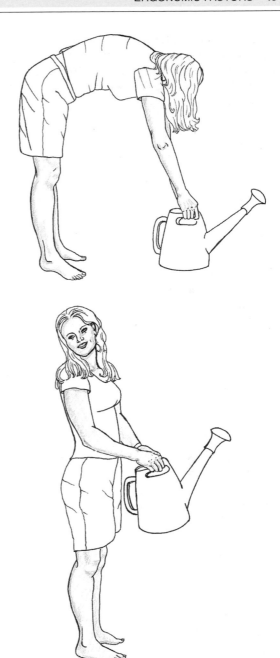

Figure 5.4 Lifting a load at a distance from the body can magnify the forces at the low back by up to 12 times. In addition to the load of the object, the weight of the trunk has to be lifted as well.

- the joint architecture provides efficient distribution of loads throughout the articular surfaces

- nociceptive and mechanoreceptor afferent stimuli are minimized
- in the mid-range of joint movement there is usually more efficient homeostasis of vascular and neurological processes, which become progressively compromised as we move to joint extremes.

Moving a joint in one plane away from its comfort zone tends to localize the forces to the particular prime movers of that action, and their antagonists, which may also be involved in maintaining the joint position. These become selectively loaded. As the movement away continues, these prime movers have to work even harder to overcome the passive resistance of the other tissues. It often introduces joint angles that reduce the efficiency of the musculotendinous unit and create additional muscle tension, friction and leverage, while affecting neurological and vascular homeostasis. This can have a marked effect on the level of musculotendinous loading and the rate of fatigue. If we introduce movement in another plane, this further localizes the stress to a smaller portion of the MS structure and creates even stronger leverages.

The wrist provides a good example of this process. In the mid-range there is an efficient and strong wrist grip. However, when it is moved into flexion or extension the wrist grip reduces noticeably, despite considerable muscular effort. Thus more effort is required to perform the same task in a poorer posture. In addition, the increasing angle of the flexor and extensor wrist tendons produces considerable stress on these structures. Furthermore, the dramatic increase in pressure in the carpal tunnel inhibits the efficient physiological processes of the median nerve, and this can be an important factor in carpal tunnel syndrome (Rempel 1996).

Another important example is the movement into flexion of the lumbar spine, which dramatically increases the loading. This loading is further increased if an element of rotation is introduced that changes the symmetrical nature of the stress introducing localized peak loads, and leads to an increased odds ratio of low back pain (LBP) (Punnett et al 1991).

Joint postures near the limit of their mobility often place a load on the ligamentous structures. This ligamentous tension can often substitute for the muscle activity that would otherwise be required to hold this extreme joint posture. This is often seen in slumped spinal or neck postures. While this can be valuable in providing an opportunity for muscular recovery it can also create additional problems. The taut ligament is at risk from any sudden increase in the magnitude of load. The ligaments are also subject to a fatigue loading and exhibit a creep effect. This can produce a wedging effect of the intervertebral discs at this level, and this alteration in dynamics has been postulated to be a significant risk for disc injury (Adams & Dolan 1995, McGill 1995).

Cumulative effect

The classic study by Armstrong et al (1987) shows that risk factors are not just cumulative but that they can also magnify or multiply to a remarkable magnitude. Using videotape analysis, Armstrong and colleagues studied 652 workers at seven manufacturing plants and compared the incidence of wrist tendonitis with the characteristics of the job. They categorized the jobs as low or high force and low or high repetitiveness. They found the following risk ratios:

- low force/low repetition – risk ratio 1 – % affected 0.6
- high force/low repetition – risk ratio 6.1 – % affected 3.1
- low force/high repetition – risk ratio 3.3 – % affected 3.3
- high force/high repetition – risk ratio 29.4 – % affected 10.8.

The combination of high force and high repetition had a remarkable increase in the risk of injury.

The corollary of this is that identification and reduction of risk factors may have a remarkable benefit by reversing or reducing this multiplication factor.

The magnifier effect of different risk factors combined in the same job has been clearly demonstrated in the literature. The executive summary of the comprehensive NIOSH review (NIOSH 1997b)

Table 5.1 Evidence for causal relationship between physical work factors and MSDs

Body part *Risk factor*	Strong evidence	Evidence	Insufficient evidence	Evidence of no effect
Neck and neck/shoulder				
Repetition		✓		
Force		✓		
Posture	✓			
Vibration			✓	
Shoulder				
Posture		✓		
Force			✓	
Repetition		✓		
Vibration			✓	
Elbow				
Repetition			✓	
Force		✓		
Posture			✓	
Combination	✓			
Hand/wrist				
Carpal tunnel syndrome				
Repetition		✓		
Force		✓		
Posture			✓	
Vibration		✓		
Combination	✓			
Tendinitis				
Repetition		✓		
Force		✓		
Posture		✓		
Combination	✓			
Hand–arm vibration syndrome				
Vibration	✓			
Back				
Lifting/forceful movement	✓			
Awkward posture		✓		
Heavy physical work		✓		
Whole body vibration	✓			
Static work posture			✓	

This information is in the public domain and may be freely copied or reprinted.

shows a table of the causal relationship between physical work factors and musculoskeletal disorders (MSDs) (Table 5.1). It shows clearly the increasing evidence of risk when multiple ergonomic risk factors are present. Where the evidence exists for combinations of risk factors (elbow, hand/wrist tendonitis, carpal tunnel syndrome) combinations of exposures provide the strongest evidence of the association between risk factors and injury.

DURATION

The duration of work, or the duration of an exposure, is one of the key determinants of the overall injury risk. The duration determines the cumulative biomechanical force and the degree of fatigue experienced. The duration can be short and intense, leading to acute disorders, or prolonged with low or moderate intensities, leading to chronic or degenerative disorders. All functions of the human body are a cyclic relationship between work and rest and recovery. Sufficient recovery periods are indispensable if effective performance and efficiency are to be maintained, and injury avoided. Fatigue can be localized to a particular muscle group, generalized, or primarily psychological. New, unfamiliar tasks tend to be more fatiguing than accustomed tasks.

Rest breaks

There are different types of breaks that allow recovery or at least add variety to the workload.

- Variety of workload gives an opportunity for some exposed tissues to get relative rest.
- Structured breaks.
- Unstructured breaks, such as taking the opportunity to talk to a colleague or to have a drink of water.
- Pauses in workload provide an opportunity for a break in well-designed workstations. Computer work has frequent pauses provided there are comfortable and easily accessible surfaces to unload the weight of the arms and a good back support to unload the weight of the trunk. Telephone headsets maximize the opportunity to rest some body regions when taking phone calls.

If pauses are optional, or breaks are deducted from the pay schedule, there is often a reluctance to take them. It is often much easier to continue work than to stop and abandon the work process, particularly with machinery or electronic based tasks. People often become so involved with a task that they are reluctant to stop. It is important to assess what is a reasonable workload at any particular task, or a reasonable concentration span, and ensure there are sufficient breaks to accommodate these tasks. It is difficult to make generalizations for recommended periods of exposures for many tasks. There are so many variables that can be involved, such as individual factors and environmental factors, as well as the demands of the task. It is important to be flexible and allow people to work at a comfortable pace rather than a predetermined pace. For a good review of recommended work/rest and break schedules for different industries and shifts see Konz (1998a).

The first marker of fatigue is usually deterioration in work efficiency – a slowing of process time and an increase in error rates. An important marker of overexposure is the development of work-related symptoms. Where there are work-related symptoms in a workplace then, clearly, some people are being overexposed to some tasks. Hence it is also important to establish an environment that encourages the reporting of early symptoms, and early modification of the exposure.

It is vital to establish a break culture where people learn the importance of breaks to the process of productivity, and are made aware of the responsibility to ensure that they maintain a healthy balance between work and rest.

Type of exposure

Static loads and postures have been linked to increased risk of developing MS symptoms, even at low levels of loading. The pathophysiological mechanisms for this are discussed in Chapter 4. Even low static loads in optimal joint postures cannot be held for long periods of time. A number of writers have represented the injury risk from different types of physical workload as a U-shaped curve. Those with long periods of static postures have a high risk of injury; those who are moderately active with frequent postural variation have a low risk of injury; those who have high physical workloads or high frequency repetition have a high risk of injury (Fig. 5.5).

One of the major factors for the increasing incidence of injury may be that, as the industrial and electronic revolutions continue to change society, people's postures are also changing, as they adopt

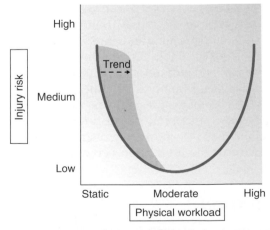

Figure 5.5 The relationship between types of workload and injury risk.

increasing static postures in all areas of life – work, transport and recreation. This has the effect of increasing the volume on the left side of the graph in Figure 5.5 and squeezing the U. As static joint postures move away from the joint comfort zone and become suboptimal, or as the MS load increases, the period available before the onset of fatigue becomes relatively less. Static loads have relatively poor physiological efficiency and the need for postural and task variation are paramount. Where these are not possible, micropauses, pauses and breaks are necessary to allow physiological recovery and to delay or diminish the onset of fatigue. Where jobs involve static activity without significant variation, the need for well-designed workstations and good management practices are essential. Breaks should be taken before the effects of fatigue become apparent. If the break is delayed until there is fatigue or performance deterioration, the recovery period is longer and often the break is not sufficient to recharge the batteries, resulting in an accelerated fatigue process, with a performance decrement and a prolonged recovery period. The fatigue process increases exponentially with time – the greater the level of fatigue the relatively longer the recovery period becomes. However, recovery from fatigue is also exponential – there is maximum benefit in the earlier phases of the recovery period. Thus, three breaks of 5 min have more benefit than one break of 15 min as: (i) recovery is better; and (ii) fatigue is not as advanced (Konz 1998b).

For static work that requires intense concentration, 30 min seems to be the ideal time to work, followed by a 5 min break. For tasks that require less concentration and a little more variety, but which are still mainly static postures, up to 1 h work followed by a 10 min break is reasonable. For tasks that have good variation without requiring prolonged, intense psychological demands, the standard morning and afternoon breaks are acceptable, although research has shown improved efficiency with more frequent breaks. For dedicated word processing tasks, longer breaks or more task variation are recommended. For general VDU tasks the consensus of the literature seems to recommend taking breaks every 30–60 min, depending on the intensity and the psychological demand of the work. Johnson et al (1997) found that there were effects of fatigue in the finger muscles (flexor digitorum superficialis) in subjects working in well-designed workplaces after 3 h typing, even when they took a break for 7.5 min per 30 minutes:

Significant levels of muscle fatigue were measured after 3 hours of typing and persisted up to 40 minutes after typing had ceased. Similar levels of fatigue were found in both hands despite the right hand performing twice the number of repetitions as the left. Therefore it appears that muscle fatigue is dependent on typing duration and force rather than on the repetition itself.   Johnson et al (1997)

Johnson et al found that heavier force keyboards produced significantly greater levels and duration of fatigue.

People with a previous history of injury, or who are not well adapted to a particular work task, will require reduced periods of exposure with increased opportunity for recovery.

For clerical tasks there is a significant exposure for prolonged static muscle tension in the cervical musculature from head and neck posture for viewing purposes; and finger and wrist flexors from gripping the writing implement. These demands can be minimized by providing an appropriate height, and angled, work surface, which significantly reduces neck flexion, joint torque and cervical musculature EMG readings (see Section 3). The hand and wrist can be aided by a good quality, low friction pen with a comfortable grip that has a good gripping surface area.

VDU tasks have a considerable capacity for prolonged static muscle tension, with the continuous nature of the tasks creating high visual demands and prolonged static tension in the upper limbs. A number of studies have identified an exposure–response relationship between keyboard work and the development of symptoms. Some authors recommend a threshold of computer work of 4 h a day, above which the risk of injury increases dramatically. The configuration of the computerized workplace is of major importance for minimizing these loads. However, even with well-designed workstations, the ability to effect pauses, micropauses and regular breaks is essential.

Active breaks

For people who have static loading or are involved in monotonous tasks, active breaks are more beneficial than passive breaks. An active break will encourage circulation, oxygenation, concentration, muscle stretching and a better balance of proprioceptive activity. A 5 min walk, or climbing a flight of stairs, will be more beneficial than sitting down and having a cup of tea. It will encourage recovery and delay fatigue. A sedentary worker should also try and have some moderately vigorous activity at the end of the working day to encourage neuromuscular relaxation and recovery, as well as improving fitness.

Cyclic loading

Cyclic loading, with its more physiologically efficient contraction/relaxation cycles, allows better fluid dynamics and more varied proprioception and tends to delay onset of the fatigue process. It also allows some time for recovery between loads. If the cyclic loading is varied over a number of different body regions there is a general process of fatigue rather than a local process. Inevitably there is an element of both local and general fatigue. Repetitive loading cycles at relatively high rates of maximum voluntary contraction (MVC) or high joint torques can lead to rapid onset of fatigue. Monotonous or repetitive work has to be planned carefully, with attention given to workstation design in order to minimize the exposure to muscle fatigue and joint stress. The ratio of work to recovery has to be carefully assessed and allowances made for individuals and changing circumstances. Generally, the longer the period of exposure, the slower the available output and the greater the risk of fatigue.

Generalized fatigue

With mixed tasks where there is no significant local exposure, prolonged workloads may lead to generalized fatigue. Symptoms of generalized fatigue may include:

- weariness, lack of enthusiasm, distaste for work
- reduced alertness, sluggish thought processes

- slow perception and decision-making
- reduced output
- depression or mood instability.

Generalized fatigue can be delayed by application of stress, or states of high arousal or motivation. However, this will delay the need for recovery rather than replace it. Continued work at these states of stress or arousal can create a state of chronic fatigue or exhaustion.

Efforts to increase output by increasing work hours or increasing work intensity can often be disappointing due to reductions in efficiency due to fatigue, and increased risk of illness or injury.

ENVIRONMENT

The environment in which work is performed can be an important determinant of the total exposure to musculoskeletal strain. Any suboptimal environmental factors can contribute to the overall exposure and accelerate accumulation of fatigue and strain. This section will briefly cover the key environmental exposures and provide guidelines for their management.

Lighting

Research has shown that in many workplaces productivity can rise, and the error rate fall, by improving the quality of lighting. Poor lighting can increase the rate of visual fatigue, general tension and can create poor posture in a bid to improve vision. Lighting levels are dependent on the visual acuity required for the task. General guidelines are:

- moderately precise – packing, carpentry, engineering – 200–300 lux
- fine work – reading, writing, book-keeping – 500–700 lux
- precision work – technical drawing, sewing, delicate electronics – 1000–2000 lux.

For VDU work 300–500 lux is recommended; for general office work a range of 500–700 lux is considered appropriate. Over-bright lighting (over 1000 lux) can lead to visual strain caused by reflections, high glare, contrast between light and shadow, etc.

General guidelines for lighting

- Lighting sources (windows and lights) should be placed parallel or overhead rather than directly in front or behind.
- Walls should be light coloured to allow an even distribution of light.
- Sharp contrasts between dark flooring or furniture and reflective table tops should be avoided.
- No light sources should be in the visual field when working.
- Light sources should never flicker. Some people seem to be sensitive to fluorescent light flicker.
- It is better to use more lamps of low power than a few of high power.

Glare and reflections are very visually fatiguing. Good placement of workstations and light sources is important. A light source from behind can cause reflected glare on a VDU screen. Light sources in front can create glare. Glare from windows can be reduced by using blinds or tinted film. Ceiling or wall lights can be shielded to reduce glare or reflection.

Noise

Noise levels are best kept to a minimum, particularly where a high degree of concentration is required. Telephone and dictaphone work demand auditory acuity and these tasks can be very stressful if there is background noise.

Temperature

Low temperatures can be a significant problem for sedentary work, where very little body heat is generated. It can lead to significantly increased levels of muscle tension. A warmer working environment is preferred for sedentary work. The recommended air temperature is 20–21°C for summer and 20–24°C for winter. Drafts can be a very irritating factor for sedentary workers, producing significantly increased tension levels especially at neck and shoulder level – they should be eliminated.

Comfort levels of temperature are subject to considerable personal variation and can be influenced by clothing, posture, fat levels, metabolic rate and personal preference.

High heat and high levels of humidity can create difficulty in controlling body heat. It can lead to increased levels of stress and lower work efficiency.

Electromagnetic radiation

Radiation remains a controversial subject. It is a specialist area and, even among specialists, it is difficult to get a consensus view as to safe levels and what, if any, health risks are associated with exposure. Most Health and Safety Regulations state that it should be 'reduced to negligible levels' (Health and Safety Executive 1992). Some general guidelines to minimize exposure levels are:

- Position monitors carefully. Most radiation comes from the rear and sides of a screen. Workers should sit at least one arm's length from the front of a screen and two from the rear or sides of a screen.
- Arrange desks carefully to avoid radiation from a co-worker's screen. Walls do not provide effective screening.
- More modern monitors generally have lower radiation levels. Liquid crystal screens (as in flat screens and lap tops) do not give off radiation.
- Turn off computers and other electrical equipment when not in use.
- Photocopiers and plain paper fax machines also give off radiation and these should be at safe distances.
- If in doubt, seek specialist advice.

SUMMARY – AVOIDING FATIGUE AND INJURY

- Good workplace design.
- Interesting and varied tasks.
- Comfortable postures with optimum neuromuscular efficiency.
- Work at comfortable pace.
- Opportunity for structured and unstructured breaks.

- Avoid prolonged hours.
- A comfortable environment.

This chapter began with a quote from Barbara Silverstein, a noted ergonomist who specializes in public health policy, regarding the presence of risk factors and the risk of WMSD. It finishes by summarizing her plan for dealing with these risk factors:

1. Employers must provide information to all employees and their supervisors regarding early symptoms and risk factors so they can participate fully in the identification, control and prevention of poorly designed jobs.
2. Employers must look at their workplaces for high-risk jobs, determine the underlying causes, and involve employees in identifying and minimising solutions.
3. Employers and end users must provide critical feedback to designers and suppliers whose end products contribute to WMSD so future designs can be improved.
4. Health care providers and their societies must work together with employees to familiarise themselves with the disorders, the risk factors and appropriate treatment, and how the workplace can participate in the treatment by keeping the employee at work and reducing exposure.
5. Business, engineering, industrial design, health sciences and educational institutions (from primary school onward) should incorporate ergonomics and the evaluation of healthy work into curriculum and practice.

Silverstein (1995)

6

Psychosocial aspects

Despite a society in which increasingly little physical work is done, people's awareness of discomfort, treatment costs for injury, and disability caused by musculoskeletal (MS) problems, continue to escalate at an alarming rate. The traditional medical model of identifying the injury – often very difficult with MS problems – and providing treatment aimed at promoting or restoring MS integrity, may work well for acute injury but seems unable to prevent a rapidly increasing rate of disability.

New paradigms are needed for assessing injury, and new models for treating and managing injury. Researchers need to stop looking for simple solutions to complex, multifactorial problems.

It is recognized that psychosocial factors are important in the development of injury, the costs associated with the injury and the risk of developing chronicity.

INTRODUCTION

The term 'psychosocial factors' is a basket one referring to non-physical aspects of the patient's environment, including stress, work organizational factors and personal traits. Psychosocial factors are difficult to measure objectively and the information regarding them is usually gained through interview and self-report methods. This introduces a significant degree of subjectivity to the reports and raises the question as to the divide between the workplace and the individual. Psychosocial factors are difficult to quantify and therefore it becomes difficult to determine a safe level. One person's stress may be another person's ideal level of stimulation.

The role of psychosocial factors in the development of MS pain is an area fraught with misconceptions. These have largely arisen out of the difficulty in clearly delineating the pathophysiology of injury, and a difficulty in developing diagnostic criteria for overuse or chronic injuries. This has led some investigators to believe that some conditions have no physical basis and there has been an obvious temptation to ascribe the injury process to psychological and behavioural processes. This changes the focus from the job to the individual and frequently there has been a type of victimization of those workers involved, as if they were somehow responsible for their own injury. This is quite common where a diagnosis of fibromyalgia is made, which then becomes a reason for deciding that the condition is not work related and for denying employer responsibility and worker compensation. This is frequently nonsense, based on a poor understanding of pathophysiology, a poor understanding of the role of psychosocial factors and the 'creation' of vague definitions (i.e. 'fibromyalgia', which is simply a descriptor for chronic pain with no insight into the aetiological or pathophysiological processes). Chapter 5 has shown that the pathophysiology of injury, although complex, is logical, understandable, and backed by a reasonable body of research, which for the most part fits with clinical observation. This chapter will show the role of psychosocial factors in the injury process and will demonstrate that they play an important role in the pathophysiology of injury and that we have come a long way to understanding that role.

Linda Rosenstock, Director of NIOSH – the largest Health and Safety organization in the world – has stated that, after the most comprehensive review of the occupational epidemiological literature to date (NIOSH 1997):

In workplaces with high rates of work-related musculoskeletal disorders there is little scientific evidence that the principal reason for the excess number of injuries or illnesses is the workers' psychological reaction to their workplace. However, there is evidence, particularly in office settings, suggesting that both physical and psychosocial [work organization] factors may be important contributors to musculoskeletal disorders.   Rosenstock (1997)

Troup (1989) has expressed similar conclusions:

Although psychosocial factors are seldom causal to back disorders, it should be emphasised they may nonetheless modify the development and natural history of musculoskeletal diseases.

That psychosocial factors are important in the production of injury, that secondary psychosocial factors can be a result of and complicate an injury and that psychosocial factors are a key component of the conversion of acute to chronic injury, are not doubted in informed circles. However, there is very little evidence that psychosocial factors alone are causal to an injury.

THE ROLE OF STRESS IN THE WORKPLACE

Stress arises when people have difficulty coping with the demands placed upon them. The effects of stress and the ability to cope with stress are highly individual. They can be affected by such things as age, gender, experience, ambition, motivation, personality and other lifestyle factors.

There has been a significant amount of research outlining the role of psychosocial stress in the injury process and the relationship between different psychosocial exposures and the incidence of musculoskeletal disorders. There is a distinct relationship between poor ergonomics and high psychosocial stress (Carayon 1995). Job demands place high physical and mental workloads on the individual. Continued work pressure tends to reduce the opportunity for breaks or rests. The modern automated work environment is associated with many types of work pressure:

- high workload
- fast work pace with few pauses
- reduction of work variety
- time pressure
- being always in touch
- equipment failure
- restructuring.

People who describe their jobs as high stress spend longer periods in poorer postures, have less variety of work and take fewer breaks than those in lower stress jobs. When under stress, individuals exhibit behavioural changes that increase the neuromuscular workload. They may hit the keys harder or grip the tools tighter; they have faster, less efficient body movements, with higher levels of EMG readings and greater joint forces. A poor work environment invariably has a poor ergonomic and a poor psychosocial environment (Fig. 6.1).

Lim (1995) studied 129 office workers using a computer for an average of 7.1 h per day. He analysed information regarding the psychosocial and physical work environment, psychological stress and upper extremity musculoskeletal discomfort (UEMD). The results showed: 'An increase in work pressure is related to an increase in the experience of anxiety and fatigue. Anxiety is a significant predictor of UEMD and UECTD [upper extremity cumulative trauma disorder]'. Anxiety was found to be highly related to awkward work postures:

The presence of a relationship between ergonomic risk factors and psychological stress suggests that both ergonomic risk factors and psychological stress can influence each other. Poor ergonomic conditions may lead to stress experienced while stress can alter ergonomic working conditions.
Results of the study support the hypothesis that psychological work factors are related to psychological distress which in turn is related to UEMD.   Lim (1995)

There is now a large body of literature that links high stress index to increased incidence of mus-

culoskeletal disorders. This chapter illustrates the difficulty in separating and untangling the effects of high stress from increased ergonomic exposure to determine precise risk ratios. For practical purposes (i.e. workplace assessment and management), there is no need to separate them as long as the relationship is well understood and both factors are given the appropriate consideration. The neglect of one aspect is at the expense of the other.

Factors that modify stress in the workplace

The demand–control–support model suggests that psychological demands have more adverse consequences if they coexist with a lack of ability to influence decisions regarding the job (low decision latitude) and low social support (Karasek & Theorell 1990, Theorell 1996). There is some support for this idea in the research literature: that the workplace organizational environment influences the type of stress and the ability to cope with stress.

Where workers feel little opportunity to influence their work environment they feel trapped, with little opportunity for advancement. The feelings of stress can be magnified. The ability to cope with stress can be modified by the degree of social support available. Social isolation tends to magnify feelings of stress and the physiological changes associated with them. Social isolation can be due to external factors such as excessive competition, attitude of co-workers, poor language skills, or it can be a personal characteristic – feeling left out. Social isolation is becoming increasingly common in modern, high technology workplaces where personal interaction has been replaced by interaction with computers and other machinery. In these situations the relationship with the supervisor or employer can assume paramount importance (Fig. 6.2).

Many chronic pain sufferers appear socially isolated. This may be because socially isolated people are predisposed to developing chronic pain or because chronic pain is a socially isolating experience. Whatever, chronic pain sufferers do enhance their coping mechanisms by making

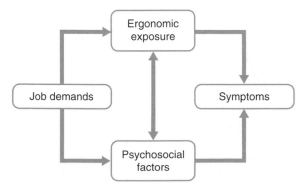

Figure 6.1 The relationship between job demands, psychosocial stress, ergonomic demands and symptoms.

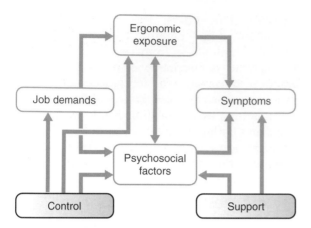

Figure 6.2 The role of job control and social support.

a deliberate effort to socialize. Immigrants into a country, particularly where there are language difficulties, are often in a very difficult psychosocial environment. They frequently are unable to make use of their skill levels and become stuck in boring jobs with little opportunity for advancement. They are often socially and culturally isolated. This leads to high levels of stress and high levels of internalization of stress. If there is an injury, the effects of it can become magnified.

Psychosocial factors and MS disorders

In an exhaustive and award-winning review paper, Bongers and her co-workers (1993) reviewed the epidemiological literature with the objective of establishing whether there was evidence of psychosocial work factors and MS disorders. They concluded that:

Monotonous work, high perceived workload, and time pressure are related to musculoskeletal symptoms. The data suggests that low control on the job and lack of social support by colleagues are positively associated with musculoskeletal disease. Perceived stress may be intermediary in this process. Stress symptoms are often associated with musculoskeletal disease, and some studies indicate that stress symptoms contribute to the development of this disease.

However, in this paper Bongers is quite clear that this: '... does not present conclusive evidence due to high correlations between psychosocial factors

and physical load and to difficulties measuring dependent and independent variables'.

Since the Bongers study there has been an effort to design better quality research, and to separate the relative risks of physical and psychosocial exposures.

In a more recent review of the literature, which was described as: 'the most comprehensive review of the occupational epidemiological literature to date' (NIOSH 1997b), the authors summarize the findings as follows:

While the etiologic mechanisms are poorly understood there is increasing evidence that psychosocial factors are related to the job and work environment of WRMSD of the upper extremity and back. Though the findings of the studies reviewed are not entirely consistent, they suggest that the perceptions of intensified workload, monotonous work, limited job control, low job clarity, and low social support are associated with various work-related musculoskeletal disorders. ... A number of studies have found associations even after adjusting for physical demands, the effects of these factors may be in part or entirely, independent of physical factors. It is also evident that these associations are not limited to particular types of jobs (e.g. VDU work) or environments (e.g. offices) but rather seem to be found in a variety of work situations. This seems to suggest that psychosocial factors may represent generalized risk factors for WRMSDs. These factors while statistically significant in some studies have only modest strength. The evidence for the relationship between psychosocial factors and upper extremity disorders appear to be stronger for neck/shoulder disorders or musculoskeletal symptoms in general than for hand/wrist disorders.

NIOSH (1997b)

A number of features of the work environment have been linked to increased risk of MS disorders. These factors have generally been found to be associated with both office-based and manual tasks:

● monotonous work, low use of skills
● lack of variety
● monitored or machine-paced work
● fear of job loss
● high workload
● time pressure and deadlines
● lack of job control
● insufficient work breaks
● low social support

- poor employer or supervisor attitude
- equipment failure
- environmental stress – noise, humidity, temperature, etc.

In an excellent review paper of the psychosocial aspects of using VDUs, Smith (1997) finds some additional risk factors that specifically apply to computer users:

- Computer users in lower paid, less skilled jobs have greater amounts of psychological distress than those in higher paid, more skilled ones.
- When jobs are transitional in from one technology to a new one, those employees in lower paid, less skilled, jobs report more stress due to the new technology than employees in more skilled, higher paid jobs.
- Older employees perceive greater job changes than younger employees, and also report more stress when technology changes.

Physiological effects of psychosocial stress

There are a number of plausible links between psychosocial stress and the increased risk of injury:

- higher biomechanical loading – longer periods spent in poorer postures
- increased levels of muscle activity during tasks
- Few electromyographic (EMG) gaps – opportunities for breaks and pauses show continued muscle activity – inability to relax
- lack of relaxation when away from work
- stimulation of sympathetic nervous system and increased output of hormonal activity associated with stress
- disturbance of sleep patterns and the restorative processes associated with sleep.

For further details of these pathophysiological responses to stress see Chapter 4. The most significant effect of these physiological effects is to increase the neuromuscular load and to reduce the ability of the homeostatic processes to recover and adapt to the increased load. According to Smith & Carayon (1996):

Chronic exposure to cumulative trauma stressors while the organism is undergoing psychological stress may create micro damage that cannot be fully repaired due to the impaired immune response, and over time this may lead to permanent tissue damage.

So, overuse, cumulative and chronic injuries are largely a neuromuscular phenomenon and psychosocial factors are an important determinant of the total neuromuscular load, and the recovery processes from neuromuscular fatigue and injury. However, it is not quite as simple as this. Stress and the psychosocial environment can also cause many behavioural effects that can modify the course of an injury once it is established. The coexistence of high psychosocial stress levels and symptoms can significantly increase the risk of early symptoms developing into a more serious, and potentially disabling injury.

Psychosocial factors that modify the injury

A number of psychosocial effects can complicate the risk of chronicity. If people do not feel safe to discuss MS symptoms with their employer for fear of being victimized or regarded as a nuisance, there is an increasing risk of chronicity as the factors that cause or exacerbate the problem are less likely to be identified, reported and modified. A safe reporting environment, with encouragement to report early symptoms and with early job modification, is the optimum scenario for minimizing the pain and disability of overuse injuries. Even if this optimum is achieved, some personality types are reluctant to speak up for fear of being regarded as a nuisance. They soldier on, blithely ignoring the consequences. This is irresponsible and can have adverse consequences for the person and the employer. A good education programme and a peer support network will usually highlight the need for collective responsibility of managing work-related risk factors.

Symptom perception

The experience of some sort of MS sensation is a very common experience during the working or non-working day. It may be a muscle tightness or fullness, a feeling of fatigue or a fasciculation. It does appear that the appearance of symptoms is more common in computer users and that there is a dose-related response to the amount of computer use per day and the presence of symptoms. Hochanadel (1995) surveyed 3326 computer users; 49% of the respondents described symptoms associated with computer work, of which 46% stated it affected their work performance. Closer examination revealed a clear dose–response effect of computer work and symptoms:

- 0–2 h per day 21% reported symptoms
- 2–4 h per day 50% reported symptoms
- 4–8 h per day 68% reported symptoms.

The perception of the symptoms, and the significance accorded these symptoms, is related to the degree of arousal of the individual and the amount of competing stimuli in the immediate environment. There is some evidence that a monotonous job may increase awareness of symptoms, whereas a highly stimulating job may delay the perception, or the attribution of significance to symptoms. Once the symptoms reach consciousness, most people will attempt an explanation for the symptoms experienced. If they are felt to be unimportant or of no great consequence, little action will be taken unless symptoms persist or worsen, when their significance will be re-evaluated. If the symptoms are perceived as alarming, or the first sign of a more serious condition, it is more likely that some further action will be taken. At this stage people's response to symptoms can vary widely. There are a number of features that may influence their response to symptoms once the symptoms are established:

- the degree of severity of symptoms – duration and intensity
- whether symptoms affect work performance
- the ability to control symptoms by modifying work – degree of autonomy
- association of symptoms with a disabling or serious condition
- whether co-workers have suffered similar problems and the outcome
- do they want to be at work – job satisfaction, monotony, etc.
- do they feel safe to report the symptoms – consequences for employment, income, job security

- individual factors such as personality type, personal circumstances, etc.
- the overall levels of work-related stress. These can either delay the reporting of symptoms due to fear of consequences or magnify the stress and cause an exaggerated response.

Smith & Carayon (1996) succinctly describe the process of heightened symptom perception caused by stress:

Pain that is really non-clinical and a normal part of the general adaptation process to work activity may be perceived by the employee as much more significant due to heightened psychological stress. If the person were not under psychological stress the pain may not be perceived as significant and go unreported and untreated.

Symptom epidemics

There are many cases of repetitive strain injury (RSI) epidemics, which can involve a particular workplace or even an entire nation, when there is a dramatic increase in the reporting of overuse injuries. Hochanadel (1995) noted that there is a very high, self-reported incidence of symptoms related to high intensity of computer use – he reported 68% in subjects using a computer over 4 h per day. In the author's own surveys, an overall figure of 50% of people in a workplace are taken to have some kind of work-related symptoms that can be influenced by work – the occasional headache, visual fatigue or aching shoulder. For the most part, people manage these quietly, without registering an injury. If there is a dramatic change in the psychosocial environment – restructuring, fear of job loss or the effect of new technology – there can be a dramatic rise in symptom perception and symptom reporting. This has a cascading effect – as one person goes down the people around have increased levels of anxiety and concern and will report symptoms that were previously unreported, and this can reach epidemic proportions. It has been rather unkindly attributed to mass hysteria, but one researcher (Hocking 1997) neatly compared it to an iceberg, where there is a small number of reported cases above the water and a large number below the surface that are not reported and mostly not per-

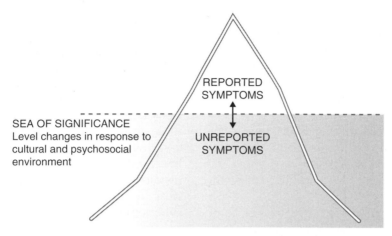

Figure 6.3 Epidemics of RSI are usually caused by a re-evaluation of the perception of previously unreported symptoms – 'the tide going out on the iceberg'. The re-evaluation is usually triggered by a change in the psychosocial environment.

ceived as significant (Fig. 6.3). Circumstances may change and the cases below the surface can have a deterioration of their condition, perhaps due to changes in work practices, or the perception of their symptoms may increase, or individuals may re-evaluate the seriousness of their symptoms in light of changing circumstances. More cases start to appear above the surface (the tide goes out).

The real problem is not usually a sudden increase in serious RSI cases, it is a change in the psychosocial environment, plus a sprinkling of fear of the consequences and a dash of ignorance. Once the real issues are dealt with the tide starts to return and the number of cases returns to the norm.

Symptom disassociation

An insidious injury may have a multitude of contributory or cumulative causes. If the person does not easily relate their symptoms to any obvious cause it then becomes difficult for them to link the problem with the most likely cause of their symptoms. The nature of overuse and chronic injuries is that they can be influenced by many exposures and sometimes the symptoms can appear remote from the exposures. This disassociation tends to delay recognition of the cause of the problems and delay making the effec-

tive modifications to exposures. For example, the forearm paraesthesia that often occurs in the early morning, even though it is related to work exposures; the headaches that come on in the evenings and seem unrelated to anything in particular. In this type of case the problem is more likely to become medicalized and the prognosis can be influenced by the knowledge and skills of the health professional in dealing with gradual onset, cumulative or chronic injuries. The role of the practitioner is to assess the injury and attempt to unravel and modify the exposures, in addition to addressing the symptoms.

Medicalization of the injury

The health professional is an important component of the management in a severe or chronic injury and their ministrations can be the key to effective management or, alternatively, they can have a major adverse effect on the outcome. There are a number of psychosocial effects that can arise from medical involvement:

● Once patients have seen a health professional they may no longer feel responsible for the outcome of the injury. They are in the hands of the professionals and may be demotivated to help themselves.

- The practitioner may apply an inappropriate medical model. The relief of symptoms without effective management of risk factors or modification of exposures will increase the risk of chronicity by disassociating the pain from the exposure and providing a false sense of wellbeing.
- Referral of patient to a specialist will often continue the inappropriate medical model, with a continued search for pathology and medical intervention that may not address the real issues.
- The search for pathology may reveal some positive findings such as degenerative change (arthritis) or anomalous differences that are involved only peripherally but will be given exaggerated significance – 'The doctor said I've got arthritis'.
- The practitioner may advise time away from work, which may help reduce the symptoms. However, without an effective management plan the return to work will probably aggravate the symptoms. It becomes increasingly difficult to return to work as time goes by.
- Patients are often well rewarded by being away from work by provisions for sickness benefits or accident insurance. This reduces the incentive to return and they may begin to develop a disability mentality. It becomes easier to stay at home and manage disability rather than return to work.

There are key intervention points in this process and, with poor management, these are missed and the patient becomes increasingly fatigued, depressed and worn out by the injury and the process of dealing with it. The frustrations of developing a chronic condition, the ongoing pain and the lack of a clear understanding of the injury all create a disastrous psychosocial situation, which gradually mitigates toward disability.

Injured people need clear guidelines to successfully negotiate the medical maze. They need knowledgeable and genuinely helpful, multi-skilled practitioners, able to recognize barriers to recovery and modify these and refer for help as necessary. There is also urgency – every delay can create an increased level of chronicity of

both physical and psychosocial effects, which becomes progressively more difficult to reverse.

Applying an acute model of pain relief and rest to a chronic or cumulative injury is not just wrong, it is bad medicine. Applying symptom-relieving manual therapy without addressing potential injurious factors, and the patient's ability to manage these, can also mitigate toward chronicity by assisting patients to cope with a level of exposure beyond their recovery threshold. Patients with insidious, cumulative and chronic pain need a clear management structure, something more than symptom relief and hope for the best.

The claims process

It seems simple enough. If you develop a pain that prevents normal work, you seek compensation from an agency that has been paid from your taxes or from employer contributions to compensate for loss of earnings or loss of productivity. In reality, the claims process can create a very adversarial climate, where clinical and psychosocial information can be interpreted in a number of different ways. There are many parties involved in the claims process, each having a different agenda.

Employers may seek to limit their insurance costs and discourage claiming at all. The presence of a claim, however small, often creates friction and distrust between employee and employer, which makes for a deteriorating psychosocial atmosphere at work.

The insurance company will often refer to its own medical assessors. These medical assessors often have a particular viewpoint, which is to help reduce the company liability. Much of the advice given by these so-called experts is not based on objective evidence, such as functional evaluation tests, but on preconceived beliefs by the examiner. Often the patient is subjected to new labels and a new emphasis on some aspects of the condition. In fact, the specialist is not usually an advocate for the patient, seeking a successful outcome for the patient, but more interested in writing a report for the insurance agency and seeking a successful outcome for them. The two roles do not easily coincide. The patient can become very confused by the new labels and the subtle shifts of emphasis involved, which often emphasize the personal role in injury causation. It can be extremely stressful:

- trying to learn and understand the new terms
- trying to come to terms with an injury model that conflicts with your own
- feeling disbelieved – that your pain is not a real injury.

A number of possible negative psychosocial scenarios can arise. Certainly there is increased stress. There is often symptom magnification due to stress and the need to prove 'I am really injured'. It can also be alienating – that this person has made a judgement about your injury after a fairly cursory interview and examination and you have no opportunity to discuss the report or the findings, which inevitably includes some errors, omissions and misinterpretation. The patient can feel abandoned by the system and the sense of self-esteem and self-worth start to deteriorate. The issues undergo a subtle change of focus: from rehabilitation and a return to work, to a battle of wills and attempting to win the battle with the perceived adversary. This often involves more independent specialists and legal involvement. The further removed the process comes from the workplace and the initial injury, the more complicated the injury becomes, with increasing disassociation of symptoms and cause and increasing psychosocial complications. The descent into depression and disability becomes more and more inevitable.

CREATING A POSITIVE PSYCHOSOCIAL ENVIRONMENT

Stress is not all bad! Stress can be stimulating, rewarding and motivating. It can contribute to personality development and job satisfaction. It can enrich both work and private life. The important point is that stress must be kept in balance. Short periods of defined stress must be balanced with recovery periods. An exam scenario, which creates significant psychological demands that reach a peak and then rapidly diminish, allows recovery. Frequent deadlines, such as the daily deadlines of newspaper production, are more difficult to manage and require careful attention to stress management and the work–relaxation cycle.

Omnipresent stress, which remains constantly in the background without prospect of diminishment, is probably the most difficult to manage – it is difficult to get away from. It is insidious, the more you think about it the more significant it becomes. These types of stresses, such as job dissatisfaction or difficult relationships, can have a cumulative effect that gradually wear coping mechanisms down. They often manifest by exaggerated reactions to minor events. Ongoing stress requires particular attention to management of the stress and the long-term coping mechanisms in place to deal with unremitting stress, such as exercise and relaxation techniques. These kinds of stresses also require good social support to keep them in perspective and to review the management methods of dealing with them.

There is a very individual tolerance to stress levels based on many personality, environmental and lifestyle factors. What seems like a manageable stress level can suddenly become intolerable with a relatively small complication, such as a family sickness or bereavement. Most people can cope with excessive stress for short periods (with some neurophysiological cost) but not for prolonged periods. People cope better when they see an end in sight and less well when they resign themselves to a long-term stressor.

CREATING A POSITIVE WORK ENVIRONMENT

In an inspired approach to the problem of stress and the psychosocial environment, Smith (1997) outlines the need for holistic management of organizational factors, as opposed to focusing on one or two parameters. The following summary is based on his strategy:

- **Supportive environment for employees**. This enhances employee's motivation to work, feelings of security and reduces feelings of stress. It is particularly important in times of change or incorporation of new technology.

- **Employee participation in decision making processes**. This can provide feedback on production processes and change implementation. It assists early warning of problems and highlights solutions. It helps employees feel valued.
- **Good job content.** A healthy job should include physical and intellectual variety. There should be opportunity to develop skills with career opportunities that reflect technical and performance merit.
- **Autonomy.** Job control over tasks and decision making has powerful psychosocial benefits.
- **Realistic workload.** Automation often creates a demand for increased production and high volumes of information processing. Workload should be achievable at a comfortable work pace in a normal work schedule without sacrificing breaks, variety or social interaction.
- **Opportunities for socialization.** Automation has increased interaction with machines and reduced human interaction. This can lead to social isolation. Jobs should have periods when there are structured opportunities for social interaction between colleagues and with supervisors.
- **Good ergonomics.** Poor ergonomics can create and magnify psychosocial difficulties. Good ergonomics can have powerful psychosocial benefits in addition to prevention.

Even the best workplace environment will sooner or later have to face the issue of symptomatic workers. It is best to have a policy for this where workers can be rehabilitated, with full employer support, in the work environment. Big employers can have inhouse facilities where the goals of the employer, the employee and the rehabilitation staff neatly coincide. Smaller employers can contract out these facilities, ensuring that the involved services fit a holistic model as outlined in these pages. At all times the employee must feel valued, supported and part of the 'family'. Regular expressions of interest from the employer are important. Employers with active injury management programmes have shown fewer claims and reduced periods of disability.

CREATING A POSITIVE MEDICAL ENVIRONMENT

In an excellent review on psychosocial risk factors for the avoidance of low back pain chronicity (Kendall et al 1997) the authors state:

The research literature on risk factors for long term work disability is inconsistent or lacking for many chronic painful conditions, except low back pain, which has received a great deal of attention and empirical research over the last five years. Most of the known risk factors are psychosocial, which implies the possibility of intervention especially when specific individuals are recognised as being at risk.

The authors, in their full text *Guide to assessing psychosocial yellow flags in acute low back pain – risk factors for long term disability and work loss* have produced an excellent set of guidelines for better early behavioural management of low back pain. While these are designed specifically for low back pain, they apply equally for management of musculoskeletal problems generally. They are reproduced here in full:

Suggested steps to better early behavioural management of low back pain problems.

1. Provide a **positive expectation** that the individual will return to work and normal activity. Organise for a regular expression of interest from the employer. If the problem persists beyond 2–4 weeks, provide a 'reality based' warning of what the likely outcome (eg loss of job, having to start from square one, the need to begin reactivation from a point of reduced fitness, etc)
2. Be directive in scheduling **regular reviews of progress**. When conducting these interviews shift the focus from the symptom (pain) to the function (level of activity). Instead of asking 'how much do you hurt?', ask 'what have you been doing'. Maintain an interest in improvements, no matter how small. If another health professional is involved in treatment or management, specify a date for progress report at the time of referral. Delays will be disabling.
3. **Keep the individual active and at work** if at all possible, even for a small part of the day. This will help to maintain work habits and work relationships. Consider reasonable requests for selected duties and modifications to the workplace. After 4–6 weeks, if there has been little improvement review vocational options, job satisfaction any barriers to return to work, including psychosocial distress. Once barriers to

return to work have been identified, these need to be targeted and managed appropriately. Job dissatisfaction and distress cannot be treated with a physical modality.

4. **Acknowledge difficulties** with activities of daily living, but avoid making the assumption that these all indicate all activity or any work must be avoided.

5. Help to **maintain positive co-operation** between the individual, an employer, the compensation system, and health professionals. Encourage collaboration wherever possible. Inadvertent support for a collusion between 'them and us' can be damaging to progress.

6. **Make a concerted effort to communicate having more time off work will reduce the likelihood of a successful return to work**. In fact, longer periods off work result in reduced probability of ever returning to work. At the 6 week point **consider suggesting changing vocational direction, job changes**, the use of 'knights move' approaches to return to work (same employer, different job).

7. Be alert for the presence of individual beliefs that he/she should stay off work until treatment has provided a 'total cure'; watch out for expectations of **simple 'technofixes'**.

8. Promote **self-management and self-responsibility**. Encourage the development of self-efficacy to return to work. Be aware that self-efficacy will depend on **incentives and feedback** from treatment providers and others. If recovery requires development of a skill such as adopting a new posture, then it is not likely to be affected by incentives and feedback. However if recovery requires the need to overcome an aversive stimulus such as fear of movement (kinesiophobia) then it will be readily affected by incentives and feedback.

9. Be prepared to ask for a second opinion, provided it does not result in a long and disabling delay. Use this option especially if it may help clarify that further diagnostic work up is unnecessary. **Be prepared to say 'I don't know'** rather than provide elaborate explanations based on speculation.

10. Avoid confusing the **report of symptoms** with the presence of emotional distress. Distressed people seek more help and have been shown to be more likely to receive ongoing medical intervention. Exclusive focus on symptom control is not likely to be successful if emotional distress is not dealt with.

11. **Avoid suggesting** (even inadvertently) that the person from a regular job may be able to **work at home**, or in their own business because it will be under their control. This message, in effect, is to allow pain to become the reinforcer for activity – producing a deactivation syndrome with all the negative consequences. Self-employment nearly always involves more hard work.

12. Encourage people to recognise from the earliest point **that pain can be controlled and managed** so that a normal, active or working life can be maintained. Provide **encouragement for all 'well' behaviours** – including alternative ways of performing tasks and focusing on transferable skills.

13. If barriers to return to work are identified and the problem is too complex to manage refer to a multidisciplinary team.

The psychosocial environment is more positive when there is cooperation from the employer and between the various healthcare personnel and agencies. It is easier to be more confident in a positive psychosocial environment when it is clear that patients are taking responsibility for their personal issues, the workplace ergonomics have been addressed and there is an effective therapist involved in the treatment and management of the problem.

There will always be good and bad days; these are not the same as relapses, though patients often get very despondent on a bad day. It is up to the treatment provider to stay positive, monitor progress and be constantly vigilant for barriers to recovery.

Good psychosocial management is important for all patients, acute or chronic. It is particularly important to apply good psychosocial management to chronic or recurrent injuries which will always be subject to some psychosocial influences or belief structures.

Kendall et al (1997) emphasize this point:

Treating chronic back pain as if it were a new episode of acute back pain can result in perpetuation of disability.
This is especially true if treatment providers:

- rely on a narrow medical model of pain and emphasise short term palliative care, with no long-term management plan
- discourage self-care and fail to instruct the patient in self-management
- sanction disability and don't provide interventions that will improve function
- over-investigate and perpetuate belief in the 'broken part' hypothesis.

DOMESTIC PSYCHOSOCIAL STRESS

There is surprisingly little research on the role of domestic stress in the causation of musculoskeletal injury.

Bongers et al (1993), in their award-winning review paper, concluded:

… that studies investigating the relationships between musculoskeletal symptoms and psychosocial relationships outside the work environment, such as life events or social support in the family, did not report a strong relationship between these events and musculoskeletal symptoms.

However, if we accept the cumulative nature of overuse and chronic injuries, we can see a role for domestic stress in contributing to injury production. If, outside work, life is regarded as an opportunity for recovery of work-related exposures then the presence of domestic stress may at least inhibit that recovery and may lead to additional stress exposure. This double loading effect will have a contributory effect in the accumulation of ergonomic and psychosocial exposures and their interplay. Feuerstein et al (1985) found that, when comparing chronic, recurrent lower back pain patients to controls, increased family conflict was predictive of increased psychological distress and increased pain, while increased family organization and independence were associated with lower levels of anxiety and depression. They conclude that: 'the present findings support the role of family conflict in the modulation of pain'. It may well be that our compensation systems and our research funding systems do not really encourage full expression of the role of domestic psychosocial stress in the accumulation of injury. A common scenario is the working mother with preschool children who, after a busy day's work, goes home and continues to be busy managing the domestic environment. She will frequently be under time pressure with tired children, meals and the demands of a busy domestic environment. Her sleep may well be disturbed. Children can have frequent illnesses such as asthma or recurrent ear infections, which can create peak stresses. Similar situations can occur with needy family members such as the elderly or disabled. Although it is not reflected in the statistics, domestic stress can be an issue in some cases. It beholds the practitioner to try and recognize these scenarios. All chronic or ongoing cases should be reviewed regularly for the presence of barriers to recovery and a psychosocial review should be part of this. Psychosocial reviews can be completed by questionnaire, although these can be a bit alienating and there is sometimes a reluctance to complete them, or they can be done by discussion. Once the practitioner has the patient's confidence it can be quite straightforward to ask 'how are things at home?' and lead a discussion. In these situations it is not necessarily the role of the practitioner to decide the intervention but to identify the risk factor and explain its possible role in the injury process. This creates the opportunity for discussion that will often help facilitate change.

SUMMARY

The psychosocial environment can influence the:

- risk of injury
- reporting of an injury
- decision to take time off work and the ability to return to work
- risk of chronicity and disability.

Effective psychosocial management in the workplace can reduce the incidence of symptoms and the reporting of injury. Effective psychosocial management of reported injuries can minimize pain and disability and enhance recovery. Improvement in psychosocial management of symptoms and psychosocial risk factors in at-risk patients are probably the most significant changes that can be made in MS healthcare. This makes for good business and good medicine.

7

Personal factors

A person's injury risk depends on a number of individual factors. These can be hereditary, developmental or lifestyle.

- Hereditary factors might include a predisposition to arthritis or a tendency to hypermobility.
- Developmental or acquired factors might include poor posture such as kyphosis or scoliosis or a history of previous injury.
- Lifestyle factors might include the amount of exercise, the diet and smoking.

These different categories may intersect. For example, people may have an inherited tendency to obesity, which can be exacerbated by poor diet and lack of exercise. They may have a history of illness such as hypertension or chronic bronchitis, which can also be influenced by lifestyle decisions.

Explaining the personal factors related to in an injury is important because it helps develop a sense of individual responsibility. It helps people to understand that they have some control over events, that they can influence their outcomes for better or worse. They are not merely victims of circumstance but they have the opportunity to improve their situation. This is particularly the case with chronic injuries that require a more active management approach.

An employer has an ethical responsibility (and in most Western economies a legal responsibility) to provide a safe work environment. Employees have an equal responsibility to manage their private lives in such a way that they are capable of performing a day's work with a minimum risk of injury. This means managing their own health, fitness and private life in such a way that they arrive at work reasonably rested and capable of working. Many factors affect people's capacity to work, their risk of injury and their risk of chronicity. This chapter will explore some of these influences.

AGE

There are a number of risk factors for injury that increase with age:

- Most tissues show a reduced ability to tolerate loading – they can become injured at lower thresholds.
- The recovery, reparative and wound healing properties reduce with age.
- Degenerative changes in soft tissues and joints are more liable to injury and reactive inflammatory change.
- Loss of elasticity in tendons and ligaments reduces joint mobility.
- There is a gradual reduction in muscle strength after the age of 30. Peak muscular strength deteriorates 12–25% between 45 and 60 years, more marked in the lower than upper limbs (Millanvoye 1998).
- Eyesight deteriorates; balance and coordination become slower.
- The ability to learn new tasks becomes more difficult.

There are quite individual variations to the risk of injury associated with ageing based on such things as fitness, medical history and smoking. It is quite possible for a 50-year-old to be less of an injury risk than a 25-year-old. The effects of ageing can be off-set by experience, wisdom, caution and other compensatory factors. For practical purposes there is little deterioration in function until the 50–60 age bracket, unless the subject is expected to perform at or near maximum workloads.

There are some benefits associated with ageing. Experience can be a great teacher:

- Experienced workers have usually learnt to perform tasks with greater efficiency – economy of energy, with reduced peak forces.

- They are more likely to know their physiological capacity and to stay within this.
- While peak muscular strength deteriorates, muscle endurance remains relatively stable.
- Back injury disability seems to peak in the 35–45 age group. Thereafter the injury rate and the disability rate seem to reduce. There may be some protective factors in the degenerative changes in the spine – the reduction in mobility may reduce localized peak forces, disc dehydration and changes in the nucleus pulposus seem to substantially reduce the incidence of prolapsed discs.

SEX

There are a number of features related to sex that affect the risk of injury. Women on average have around 60% of the peak strength of the average man – relatively less in the upper body and relatively more in the lower body. Women have better mobility and dexterity. With their smaller digits women seem to be better at tasks that require fine motor coordination. Men tend to be taller with proportionately longer limbs. There are large individual variations from these averages.

While these sex differences may affect the predisposition to injury, there are also differences in the type of jobs that each sex is selected for that are reflected in injury statistics. Males tend to be selected for jobs that require high strength and as a result are over-represented in the low back pain (LBP) statistics. However, in jobs that are traditionally female and which have high peak spinal loads, such as nursing and childcare, there are very significant injury and disability rates due to LBP. Women seem to be over-represented in injuries to the neck, shoulder and upper limb. They seem to be more at risk of developing chronicity in these regions. However, women tend to be chosen for the tasks that require precision fine motor coordination, such as sewing machining and word processing. It may be these demanding, prolonged static postures that create the injury risk. Male tradesmen have a high incidence of arm overuse injuries and the more dynamic nature of these tasks may reduce the tendency toward secondary spread that we commonly find in static loading.

Women are more prone to developing injuries due to pregnancy, childbirth and nursing young children. These are often not represented in the statistics as they are not 'economically productive' tasks.

There is some evidence that women are more likely to seek treatment than men. This may be due to cultural factors (male stoicism) and to the fact that women have a significant amount of injury, related to domestic activities, which are often not compensatable and therefore under-represented statistically. Discussion of sex differences inevitably involves generalizations and the characteristics of the occupation, the tasks involved and the individual are probably more valid in determining injury risk and injury management.

MEDICAL HISTORY

We all have a medical history. Some features of our medical history may predispose to some types of injury:

- Anaemia will reduce muscle oxygenation and accelerate fatigue processes. It will also slow down recovery. Iron deficiency anaemia is remarkably common in women.
- Thyroid disorders can affect muscular metabolism and recovery processes.
- Diabetes can increase the risk for carpal tunnel syndrome and other peripheral neuropathies.
- Inflammatory problems can be an important predisposition or complication of musculoskeletal injury. Rheumatoid arthritis and ankylosing spondylitis often manifest with task-related joint pain and delayed recovery from relatively minor trauma. The presence of tissue type HLA B27 should alert for the possibility of inflammatory complications, as should Crohn's disease or psoriasis.
- Viral and bacterial infections are often associated with fatigue and myalgia, not just during the illness period but for months after the infectious symptoms have cleared.

MUSCULOSKELETAL HISTORY

Most people have had musculoskeletal insults as part of their life experience. A history of previous injury increases the likelihood of reinjury. The nociceptive threshold at the site of injury and its related spinal cord segment often remains more sensitive to future exposures. Generally, the more severe or chronic the injury, the greater the sensitivity, particularly with spinal injuries. The injured spinal segment acts as a 'neurological lens', reacting to any stressors with localized muscular reflex tension (see Chapter 4). If there has been direct neural involvement this is more likely to create neurophysiological sensitivity. Severe injuries may involve a change in normal architecture or biomechanics such as hypermobility, hypomobility or instability, which may predispose to further strain or degenerative change.

A person may be well adapted to a particular musculoskeletal exposure then, following a trauma that apparently recovers, they become more sensitive to the previous exposure (see Chapter 1). This is quite a common feature of whiplash – there is an apparent recovery from the whiplash but the individual becomes much more sensitive to neck, shoulder and upper body muscle tension.

The injury history is only part of the case history and the practitioner should avoid the temptation to always attribute symptoms to past injuries, they should look for other contributing factors as well. Everyone has an injury history of some sort and this needs to be taken into account in devising treatment plans and creating a healthy work environment.

FITNESS/EXERCISE

The amount and type of exercise that a person gets can be an important factor in determining their state of health and risk of injury. All musculoskeletal tissues are capable of adaptation. The more work they are required to do, the better adapted they become at doing it. The structural integrity increases: so bone becomes stronger and muscles, tendons and tendon insertions develop greater structural strength.

Connective tissues have been found to change in response to increased biomechanical load. The collagen type, diameter, orientation, packing and cross-linkages change, and the amount of glycosaminoglycans increases. Their ability to withstand force increases and they become less susceptible to fatigue failure.

Muscles have very powerful properties of adaptation – they become more efficient at transferring chemical energy into mechanical energy and are able to develop and sustain much higher levels of force. A number of different components contribute to this improved efficiency:

- improved aerobic capacity
- improved blood flow
- increased muscle capillarity
- increased mitochondrial content of muscle cells with improved control of energy metabolism
- muscle hypertrophy – an increase in myofibrils, with more actin–myosin bridges, generates greater levels of force.

Some of these features provide general health benefits and some are specific to the muscles or the fibre types being exercised.

Many other body systems show efficiency adaptation to exercise programmes including the cardiovascular system, pulmonary system, nervous system, immune system and endocrine system. For discussion of these effects see Shankar & Nayak (1999).

People who exercise regularly will cope better with increases in workload or peak forces. They will have greater reserves of available work capacity before becoming fatigued, and will probably have a higher failure point of some musculoskeletal tissues.

Injured or degenerative joints are characterized by reduced joint mobility and reduced muscular strength and endurance. There is consistent evidence that adherence to a regular exercise programme will increase joint mobility, strength and endurance, and reduce pain and disability. For a good review see Nicholas (1999).

Exercise has been shown to produce a post-exercise analgesic response. Bartholomew et al (1996) documented the pain thresholds of 17 healthy males completing an unstructured exercise programme lasting 20 min using a pressure device over the medial surface of the tibia. They documented a significant reduction in postexer-

cise pain thresholds. The results were consistent for both aerobic exercise and resistance exercise. Other researchers have found a postexercise analgesic response 20 min and 40 min after exercise and that this response occurs independently of the endorphin response. The ability to carry on participating in a sporting event despite significant injury has been observed, and this suggests a combination of physical and psychological response. It can also be observed that the pain threshold dramatically reduces when a football player ventures into the opponent's penalty area, seemingly suffering great pain with minimal provocation! The sporting field shows a graphic example of how a reward situation can either increase or reduce pain thresholds and pain behaviour.

There are well-documented psychological benefits from exercise, including improved confidence and self-esteem and reduced depression and anxiety. These are excellent characteristics for managing stress, dealing with difficult work situations and provide a good psychological environment for injury recovery. For a good review see Thirlaway & Benton (1996) who conclude: 'there is good support for the hypothesis that physical activity improves mental health'.

There has been an increasing trend toward worksite fitness programmes. In an excellent review of the subject, Shephard (1996) lists the following benefits:

- reduced employee turnover
- enhanced productivity
- reduced absenteeism
- enhanced corporate image and employee recruitment
- fewer accidents and injuries
- reduced medical costs and premiums.

Choi & Mutrie (1996) describe additional benefits from exercise for women. Menstruation, pregnancy and menopause all benefit from regular exercise. Most of the benefits of exercise are documented for moderate levels of exercise and many of the benefits are reversed for people who overexercise (Griffiths 1996).

The physiological benefits of exercise have to be balanced against the injury risk of the exercise itself. Some types of high impact exercise, and sports, are associated with an increased risk of injury and degenerative change, particularly if there is high impact and high frequency. The exercise-related injury may not be of a type that interferes with work productivity. A runner may develop muscle strains in the Achilles tendon but this would not affect their ability to do office work.

Other types of sport, or leisure pursuits such as contact sports, may create a high risk of traumatic injury, such as fracture or concussion, which may impact on the work environment.

A large Japanese study involving 21 924 male workers in manufacturing companies demonstrated a reduction in absenteeism due to illness and injury amongst workers who exercised regularly (Muto & Sakurai 1993). The workers were categorized into four groups: 1, no exercise; 2, less than once per week; 3, once or twice per week; 4, more than three times per week. The number of days' absence among the exercise groups was 48%, 43% and 26% less respectively than among non-exercisers. The number of days' absence due to musculoskeletal problems was 68%, 54% and 58% less.

Regular exercise therefore appears to have a protective effect against work absence due to musculoskeletal injury and ill health. An exercise programme benefits musculoskeletal injuries with improvements in function and reduction in pain levels. Regular exercise appears to benefit all groups. With injured subjects the question is not whether to exercise but what type and at what intensity is most beneficial. Injured workers often require supervision and motivation to begin and maintain exercise.

PHYSICAL CHARACTERISTICS

Personal physical characteristics can influence the risk of injury. Particularly tall people will have longer leverages and will create higher joint forces, which can increase the risk of injury. Tall slim people do not always have the muscle development to compensate for these higher moments, hence they can generate greater muscle contractions and fatigue more quickly.

The tall person often has to 'make do' with lower desks, work benches, seating, etc., which can result in poor postures in addition to high biomechanical loading. These poor postures are a major cause of chronic joint problems for tall people. Tall people gain huge benefits from good ergonomics, but they are often unable to purchase off-the-shelf products that are suitable for them. It is important to specify their requirements clearly, for example, high backed chair with extra height gas lift, a workstation height of 80 or 85 cm rather than the standard 72 cm. Short people can also be at a disadvantage. They may have difficulties with extra reaching, or elevating the arms and shoulders to work surfaces. Reducing the height of the work surface can make a substantial difference to a person with chronic neck and shoulder problems.

High body mass index can be a risk factor for injury and degenerative change. It contributes to increased joint loading and joint compression. It is a known risk factor for chronic LBP and accelerated degenerative change in weight-bearing joints.

ANATOMICAL VARIATIONS

There are a number of anatomical variants that can contribute to the risk of musculoskeletal disorders.

- Anomalies at the lumbosacral articulation such as complete or partial sacralization or lumbarization have been associated with increased chronicity of LBP (see Section 2).
- Cervical ribs and fibrous bands at the thoracic outlet have been linked with thoracic outlet syndrome.
- Leg length inequalities and scoliosis have also been linked to increased incidence of LBP and attendant chronicity.
- Congenital spinal stenosis can be a factor in lower limb radiculopathy.
- Hypermobility, and resultant instability, can increase the predisposition to musculoskeletal injury.

This area is very controversial. The cause and effect relationship between congenital anomalies and the risk of injury, or the presence of symptoms, is very difficult to establish. Good data are difficult to find.

In practice, the anomaly may present during an investigation to determine why a patient fails to fully respond to a relatively normal injury. To what extent the anomalies are responsible for the ongoing symptoms, or the risk of relapse, can be difficult to assess.

SMOKING

Smoking has been linked to the presence of many musculoskeletal conditions including LBP, neck and shoulder pain, hand pain and paraesthesia. It has been linked to increase incidence and increased risk of chronicity. The postulated mechanisms are reduced oxygenation, delayed recovery processes, and the mechanical strain of coughing.

Andersson et al (1998) collected data on smoking and pain symptoms from a random sample of the Swedish population (1806 subjects) with a 90% response rate. When comparing smokers to non-smokers they found an increased incidence of chronic LBP (odds ratio of 1.6) and chronic widespread musculoskeletal pain (odds ratio of 1.6). The findings were true for both sexes and there was a dose–response relationship between daily cigarette consumption and chronic LBP.

PERSONALITY

There are certain personality types that are more prone to injury than others.

High achievers

Feuerstein (1996) noticed that a certain pattern began to emerge when he studied patients who presented with chronic or recurrent upper extremity disorders.

Many of the patients reported that they continued to work with pain for months because of their interest in keeping their job, the need to achieve at work, their perception of their important contribution of their work to the organisation, or a strong work ethic. These individuals also tended to report difficulty pacing their work and a need to perform perfectly/optimally day in and day out. They also displayed a certain heightened reactivity, increased level of intensity of effort and increased need to improve their health **now** so that they could return to work immediately.

Feuerstein called this pattern of behaviour 'workstyle'. He hypothesized that this workstyle may predispose an individual to an increased risk of developing an injury, particularly when coupled to other ergonomic risk factors. He also suggested that workstyle can increase exposure to biomechanical stressors by its association with increase in force, repetition, awkward postures and inadequate breaks. This pattern of behaviour may be triggered by excessive work demands (perceived or real), continual deadlines, heightened competitiveness and a burning desire to succeed.

There are a number of features of this high-achieving personality type that can predispose to injury and more importantly are particularly prone to chronic injury. It is important to recognize this type of person and treat them appropriately:

- They are hard workers and, often, high achievers.
- They are reliable and conscientious – they rarely take time off work.
- If a job needs doing urgently they are the people you turn to – they will skip breaks and lunch times, do overtime if necessary and take work home.
- Their sense of identity and self-esteem are very closely related to their working life.
- They are competitive and take great pride in their ability to perform consistently under pressure.
- They frequently diminish or ignore early symptoms of injury.
- When they do succumb to injury or fatigue it is very significant – they have literally seized up or ground to a halt.
- The prospect of not working is difficult to imagine.

The important feature of these cases is often the delayed diagnosis. By the time the injury surfaces it is already chronic. Their high work rate and strong coping mechanisms have diminished the early warning signs. If these people are not managed appropriately early on they continue to deteriorate at an alarming rate. The management strategy involves:

- Identifying them as high risk for chronicity and explaining why.
- Highlighting the need for best practice ergonomics and workplace design.
- Highlighting the need for regular breaks, work variety and sensible work schedules.
- Educating the employer, who may have become reliant on the employee's ability to cope in a crisis or under deadline. This expectation may no longer be appropriate.
- Limiting contact time to particular at-risk exposures if necessary.
- Encouraging them to stay at work. If there is a need to reduce work exposure, reduce their work hours and modify their tasks.
- Keeping a watch for obsessive behaviour, which may be manifest in their home environment as well as at work. Over-zealous cleaning, obsessive sport or fitness regimens may be risk factors.
- Not trying to change their personality. Recognize their personality type and explain the risks. If a person has an at-risk personality there is even more need to follow safe work practices and a balanced lifestyle. Once these personality types are educated about ergonomics and safe work practices they will often convert the entire office.

Canaries

Canaries are the first people to sing out in an office when they feel they are working beyond their optimum capacity. They have relatively low coping skills and are at increased risk of reporting an injury. People with a low coping threshold like to work at a steady controlled pace and respond poorly to increased stress levels or work surges. They often exhibit an exaggerated response to stress; they often have heightened pain sensitivity and can be quite reactive. They tend to speak up quickly if they have a problem and will frequently seek help or take time off if necessary. This personality type can be over-represented in injury statistics and costs due to their willingness to report an injury and seek help. This effectively provides an early warning system and provides an appropriate opportunity for managing the problem at an early stage, avoiding a more difficult problem.

This personality type responds very well to attention, ergonomic intervention and care generally. They feel much better as soon as they feel the problem is being dealt with but tend to have heightened responses if they feel the problem is not being addressed.

In a poor work environment they are often unfairly treated because they are the first to speak up and 'make a fuss'. This victimization can have a disastrous effect on the person and the psychosocial environment generally. On the other hand, these personalities can be seen to provide a valuable role in dealing with workplace health and providing a safe environment.

Clinically, these types are good responders to therapy but are prone to developing treatment dependency.

Self-esteem

People with high self-esteem have less tendency to focus on pain and can often keep a better perspective on their symptoms and any problems that may arise. They are more confident at dealing with conflicts and keep healthy boundaries without feeling compromised.

People with low self-esteem may find it difficult to speak out if they develop symptoms. This inward focus of discomfort may magnify the symptoms and increase perception of injury. They may find it more difficult to deal with the issues that arise as a result of their injury and are more likely to play the role of the victim of circumstances, or 'poor me'.

Providing and encouraging an early warning system for fatigue or discomfort, and encouraging reporting of work practices that can be improved, will assist these at-risk personalities to seek assistance when it is needed.

Activities

The activities that people do in their personal time can either add to their musculoskeletal exposure, contributing to the fatigue processes and the injury risk; or they can assist recovery, improve fitness and reduce the injury risk. Someone who uses a computer for 4 h per day at work and then spends a large amount of time on the internet at night will be much more likely to develop symptoms than somebody who has mixed tasks at home involving some active aerobic exercise and some relaxation. Another example might be the person with a precise, visually demanding job such as laboratory analysis, who then spends evenings doing knitting or crocheting or other visually demanding handiwork. This would increase the risk of developing neck and shoulder symptoms. A person with a very physically active job such as forestry pruning or landscaping would be better advised to spend the evenings recovering, rehydrating and refuelling rather than engaging in further strenuous physical activity. The monotonous or repetitive job, or the job that has long periods of constrained postures, that is, the jobs that have relatively high exposures of any particular at-risk activities will be most at-risk from private exposures.

Static work is a known risk factor for developing neuromuscular tension and fatigue. Vigorous active exercise is a method of reducing this risk factor. Employers who have jobs that are very static can encourage their workers to exercise by providing on-site facilities for exercise or structured exercise sessions. Smaller employers can subsidize gym or sports club membership. These have been shown to be cost-effective preventions to assist workplace health.

SUMMARY

It is very important that individuals accept that the way they lead their personal life can influence the risk of injury, the incidence of recurrences, and the level of discomfort. There are always some improvements people can make that can affect their injury patterns. When people accept this it empowers them and gives them powerful practical and psychosocial tools to improve their destiny.

8

Principles of treatment and management

This chapter will give an outline of the key management and treatment principles of the injured patient. It will not be a definitive technique guide – there are many good technique texts and practitioners are expected to have some familiarity with their favoured techniques. Instead, it will be my personal interpretations of the available literature filtered by my bias as an osteopath and an ergonomist, my instinct as a manual therapist and my 20 years' clinical experience. It will be a summary of what works for me, in my environment, with the type of patients I attract. I will outline two approaches for treatment. The first – the manual therapy model – is a series of manual techniques based on identification and removal of musculoskeletal dysfunction and the provision of manual techniques for the relief of pain. It has been used throughout history and has been an integral part of the healing arts for at least 4000 years. Manual therapy techniques are particularly useful in the acute or subacute injury where they address the painful tissues – the most common cause of patient presentation.

The second – the clinical ergonomics model – is based on looking at the cause of dysfunction and removing the inputs responsible for the injury process. This involves a systematic search for 'exposures', that is ergonomic, psychosocial and personal factors that intersect to create musculoskeletal symptoms; and the subsequent modification of these exposures. This is based on the LOAD injury model presented in Chapter 2. Manual therapy is the first choice of therapy for the acute or traumatic type injury while the clinical ergonomics model is important for the

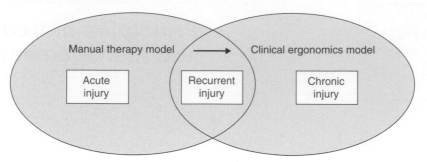

Figure 8.1 Different management approaches are necessary for different types of injury.

cumulative or chronic injury. Many injuries will benefit from both approaches: the manual therapy technique provides symptomatic relief while the clinical ergonomics approach assists rehabilitation and long-term management (Fig. 8.1).

THE MANUAL THERAPY MODEL

Manual therapy consistently rates the most effective of the treatment modalities tested for musculoskeletal pain. It is difficult to assess how much of this is due to the enhanced placebo response or to genuine therapeutic effect of the procedures. It also needs to be recognized that there is a very high individual component in each treatment situation, based on the skills and the personality of the operator, the environment in which the therapy is performed, the nature of the injury and the personality of the patient. Given the nature of these individual factors it is important to develop a flexible treatment model that is adaptable to the occasion.

Manual therapy has been shown to be particularly effective for the acute injury, where it seems to break the pain–spasm–dysfunction cycle and accelerate the natural healing process. It appears to be less effective in chronic injuries where there is a sensitization phenomenon at peripheral and spinal cord level that leads to exaggerated afferent perception and response. In the more chronic injury a more complex treatment model is required to address the afferent input, the central processing of this information and the psychosocial factors involved. That is not to say that the manual therapy does not have a role to play in the management of chronic injuries. It can

be very valuable in improving biomechanical function and reducing nociceptive or mechanoreceptor activity to the cord level. It can also help turn down the natural exacerbations that the chronic pain patient experiences. To use exclusively manual therapy techniques will inevitably have a limited effect, and it can be argued that the failure to see the limitations of manual therapy can contribute to chronicity.

I like to think of a patient as three dimensional. The first dimension is the history of the patient prior to their arrival, including medical, family, social and work history. The second dimension is the person that presents to you for examination and treatment – it is a snapshot in time. The third dimension is the environment that they venture out into after your involvement. Each dimension can provide a wealth of information, but must be kept in its proper context. In chronic cases a good understanding of all three dimensions is important to create effective change and to ensure that the effective change has some longevity.

Case history

A thorough case history is an important part of any injury management. Sometimes it appears relatively simple with a straightforward cause and effect. Other times a patient will arrive with a complex and detailed history involving multiple trauma, ongoing exposure and a long and complicated treatment history. In these cases it is important to realize that the salient points should be recorded, so a treatment process can begin, but the full picture can emerge over a period of time as the patient/practitioner relationship develops and different features of the case become apparent. As the symptom picture changes (and hopefully improves) new barriers to recovery emerge and different features of the case history assume new levels of prominence. For example, the most prominent pain site may improve and a previously less significant region emerge and assume a greater prominence. Another example might be the realization of a major psychosocial conflict in the work environment, which needs to be addressed before recovery can be effective.

History of any sort is never definitive but merely a perspective. Different perspectives are appropriate at different times. Good case history taking is an ongoing process that continues as long as treatment continues. It never finishes.

Good case history taking is enhanced by good communication and a trusting relationship. It takes time for a trusting patient–practitioner relationship to develop and some case history details, particularly of a psychosocial nature, are better left until this is well established.

The immediate needs to be established by taking the initial case history are:

- are there any contraindications for treatment?
- is further referral appropriate at this stage, e.g. X-rays or blood tests?
- to establish a working diagnosis – to commence treatment
- what are the main exposures, is any urgent intervention required?

Clinical examination

There are many excellent publications on clinical examination and it is not my intention to cover this in detail. In short:

- assess overall posture – lower limb posture, pelvic level, spinal curves, shoulder and upper limb posture, head position
- test appropriate active movements – range and symmetry
- test appropriate passive movements – range and symmetry
- resisted muscle strength. Test for overall strength, quality of contraction and presence of pain

- test reflexes, neurological functioning and neurological stretch and other appropriate orthopaedic tests
- perform a palpatory examination.

Palpation is an art. At best it can provide a diagnosis, or confirm a working diagnosis. It can elicit a great deal of information about the injury, the state of the soft tissues, the feel of the joint, the degree of degenerative change, the reactivity of patients and their ability to consciously relax.

As you perform a palpatory examination, ask yourself: 'Do the palpatory findings match the symptom picture?', 'Is the pain more likely to be referred?'. There are many cases of subacute or chronic pain that give little in the way of clinical signs, such as gross mobility change or resisted muscle weakness. Frequently there are no relevant objective findings on which to base a diagnosis. Palpation provides the ability to provide findings, albeit with some subjectivity, and link them to the case history and clinical examination. Like all arts, some people are more talented than others at palpation and the skill requires some development. It also requires a good knowledge of anatomy in order to identify the tissues involved. Developing a sense of tissue layers is important to differentiate deeper tissues from overlying tissues, such as the supraspinatus from the overlying trapezius or the piriformis from the gluteus maximus.

You then need to consider whether the physical findings confirm your working diagnosis. The case history and physical examination will give an idea of the chronicity and the severity of the problem. The physical finding will not necessarily be the same at subsequent examinations and it is important to retest the salient features to assess changes in the symptom picture and progress made. If there is a test that seems reasonably indicative of the injury, I will retest this before and after each treatment to assess results, e.g. grip strength for forearm and wrist tendonitis, resisted shoulder abduction for rotator cuff problems, straight leg raising test for sciatica.

With an overuse-type injury you have to be careful not to expose the injured tissue by over-zealous testing. Be sensitive with your testing.

Overuse injuries commonly do not test weak on initial resisted muscle test, although they fatigue very quickly. I prefer not to test a muscle to fatigue as it disturbs the injury, increases the symptoms and makes the examination and treatment process more difficult.

I work in an environment where patients pay for treatment, and are well motivated and honest. I do not find any problem with malingerers. In my 20-year career I have identified one malingerer and he admitted it very quickly. Any discrepancies between the case history and the clinical picture should be probed.

I think manual therapists who have more time to take a thorough case history and examination and generally see the patient more than once are very well placed to make decisions regarding work status and whether modification of work exposure is required. Once I feel I have an understanding of the case, I am quite happy to make recommendations for my patients for the benefit of their GP, specialist or employer.

It is very important to glean from the case history and the clinical examination the type of injury involved – traumatic or insidious, acute or chronic – and the previous successful and unsuccessful modalities tried. The management plan should be based on a clear understanding of the nature of the injury and the patient with the injury, rather than based on a preconceived treatment plan used with every patient.

Placebo effect

The term 'placebo effect' is generally used to describe a response that is a result of the treatment process rather than a specific pharmacological or physiological property of the treatment. In the past it has been used to describe sham treatment effects, and it has often been used to discredit treatments that are difficult to prove. However, the placebo effect can also be a powerful and legitimate healing tool that can provide real and long-lasting benefit to patients.

Turner (1996) describes three possible reasons for improvement in the patient's condition:

1. The natural history of the condition may lead to improvement. Pain usually subsides with time,

irrespective of treatment. In more chronic conditions there are fluctuations of pain and people tend to seek help when the condition is in a more severe phase. In this situation there is increasing likelihood that they will improve toward the long-term mean level of pain.
2. They will improve due to the specific effects of the treatment.
3. They will improve due to non-specific effects of treatment (other than the specific active components). These are commonly known as the placebo effect.

Turner et al (1994) list these possible effects as due to:

- physician attention, interest, and concern in a healing setting
- patient and physician expectations of treatment effects
- the reputation, expense and impressiveness of the treatment
- characteristics of the setting that influence patients to report improvement.

Some writers estimate that up to a 70% improvement in symptoms can be attributed to the placebo effect. It seems to be particularly high where there is a high personal input into the process such as manual therapy and surgery. The placebo effect can be cumulative with repeated exposures, long lasting and can continue after the placebo has ceased. It has also been associated with side-effects.

The placebo effect can be highly individual, some people respond readily to it and others are quite capable of effectively negating it. Efforts to identify groups who respond more readily to placebo have been unsuccessful.

Factors that encourage a good placebo effect are:

- a supportive and professional environment
- friendly and caring staff
- good communication, and the time to listen properly to patient concerns
- confidence that the practitioner is competent, sympathetic and knowledgeable about the condition
- removal of fear and anxiety – education about the nature of the problem and that the symptoms are normal
- touch seems to have special benefits in developing confidence and trust

- patient involvement in the treatment process using exercises and advice – so they feel they have some control over symptoms.

The placebo effect is not some sham effect that we should attempt to discount – it is born as a result of good practice. I am frequently surprised that good practitioners who have spent much time and money developing their skills do not pay enough attention to these basic principles. Clearly, different practitioners using similar techniques can have quite different placebo responses based on the environment in which they perform their skills, their personality, their communication skills and the confidence they place in the procedures they use.

Dr James Fisk, in an unpublished manuscript, exhorted his medical colleagues to learn from the successes of alternative medical practitioners:

We now know enough to say with reasonable conviction that this effectiveness is largely due to their ability to invoke the enhanced placebo response, allay the fears that make us feel and be sick. So why are we not utilising this effective form of therapy, even attempting to make it more effective? The profession particularly at the general practitioner level is in urgent need of more effective placebo stimulators, and communicators, people trained to understand the fears which assail us, and the ability to explain and allay such fears.

The placebo effect will never be a substitute for good clinical management and effective therapy, but it can provide a very good start.

Placebo effect and manual therapy research

Much of the popularity and success of manual therapy can be attributed to the enhanced placebo effect. We would expect a higher placebo response to manual therapy than we would expect from therapies that are more passive such as ultrasound or medication. This has generally been borne out by research (Koes et al 1992). There is some criticism by epidemiologists that until the placebo effect can be negated there is no evidence that manual therapies are effective. It will always be very difficult to control for the enhanced placebo effect. A random trial is considered more effective if the participants (subjects and examiners) are not able to pick the difference between the control and the therapy tested. It is inherently difficult to make someone think they have had a manual treatment when, in effect, they have had a control treatment (such as massage), without creating some kind of treatment effect.

If one accepts strict research methodology there is little, if any, treatment that is more effective than the enhanced placebo. It may be that treatments are relatively ineffective (although the enhanced placebo can have a powerful therapeutic effect) or it may be that our research tools are insufficiently sensitive to recognize the positive treatment effects and distinguish them from various placebos. However, people continue to be injured and continue to seek treatment that they perceive will benefit them – there is an ethical responsibility that we recommend the therapy that is most likely to have a positive influence. It is not acceptable to stand on the sidelines and say there is not sufficient evidence to recommend any treatment. There lies the inadequacy of evidence-based medicine: the lack of evidence may not be because the treatment is unhelpful but because the research methods are insufficiently sensitive or inappropriate for the paradigm being examined. It is only since the 1990s that there has been a reasonable consensus that manipulation has a beneficial effect for acute low back pain (LBP) and that it is starting to be recommended as the treatment of choice, but it has been producing effective results for thousands of years.

Some of the important questions when evaluating a therapy are:

- Does the therapy make logical sense given the pathology as we understand it?
- Is the therapy sympathetic to the healing processes that we are familiar with?
- Does the therapy enhance the natural placebo effect?
- Is the therapy safe?

These are important questions, which become increasingly relevant when there is an absence of academic consensus as to the effectiveness of treatment for a particular condition.

Manual therapy strives to create a natural symmetry of anatomical structure and a symmetry of mobility. It strives to create a harmonious working relationship between different body systems and between musculoskeletal tissues. This is not always achievable – many people are naturally asymmetrical and remain problem free with this natural asymmetry. Manual therapy also provides a philosophical approach that aims to improve joint function, reduce joint distress and provide a platform for recovery. If we accept the principles of biomechanics and try to minimize the peak forces on anatomical structures and if we accept the principles of ergonomics – trying to maintain cumulative load within the recovery processes of the human body – we can see that we have a powerful, logical framework to establish a system of therapy that conforms to established scientific principles and functioning of the body in so far as we understand it. It remains to the researchers to establish more appropriate and more sensitive models to follow these paradigms. Evidence-based medicine is all very well, but by definition it is likely to follow rather than to lead best practice. It is more important to move forward with the best of the tools that are available rather than wait for the evidence – waiting for the perfect can sometimes be the enemy of the good.

Many of the studies done on manual therapy techniques pick out one treatment modality, such as manipulation or a specific exercise, and try to test the efficacy against a control. Once again, this has inherent difficulties. Manual therapists have a range of tools at their disposal and will pick the appropriate ones based on the type of patient and the presenting condition. Singling out a particular modality to be used in all cases will deny not only the individuality of the approach (based on the individuality of the patient, the injury and the practitioner) but also the benefit of a more philosophical approach, with a range of tools at the disposal of the practitioner.

Manual therapy is popular with the public, despite having been discriminated against by medical agencies in the past. It is associated with high success rates, which are in good measure due to the enhanced placebo effect. Efforts to break it down to components for rigorous testing will always compromise it.

Qualitative aspects of clinician–patient interactions can significantly influence patient symptoms. For many chronic pain problems, patient and provider expectations and interactions may be even more important influences on patient outcomes than the specific treatments applied. Healers since ancient times have recognised and emphasised the importance of psychosocial influences in influencing patient outcomes. Unfortunately today's focus on the biomedical model, new technology, and laboratory and imaging tests has caused many to lose sight of the importance of clinical observation of the patient and of attention in treatment to the beliefs, expectations and psychosocial factors that affect the patient.   Turner (1996)

Placebo effects act synergistically with active treatment effects and natural history to influence patient outcomes. Physicians should use these nonspecific effects to their (and their patients') advantage.   Turner et al (1994)

Koes et al (1992) made a valiant effort to try and sort out some of the issues regarding the effectiveness of different treatment modalities for musculoskeletal problems. They undertook a randomized clinical trial on 256 patients that focused on the relative effectiveness of physiotherapy and manual therapy compared with continued treatment by the GP and detuned ultrasound for patients with non-specific back and neck complaints lasting at least 6 weeks. The patients were randomly assigned one of the following. The average number of treatments is shown in brackets:

- physiotherapy – exercises, massage, heat and electrotherapies (14.7)
- manual therapies – mobilization and manipulation (5.4)
- GP treatment – medication, postural advice, exercises, advice about activity, etc. (1)
- placebo – a physical examination followed by detuned short-wave diathermy and detuned ultrasound (11.1).

The patients were followed up at 3, 6 and 12 weeks. There was a higher drop-out in the placebo and GP groups as patients switched to groups that were thought to offer better results. When these were factored into the results, as the score at the point they dropped out of their respective group (assuming they were failing to

Table 8.1 Mean improvement in main complaint – 10-point scale

Type of therapy	Follow-up (week)		
	3/52	6/52	12/52
Manual therapy	2.1	3.0	3.8
Physiotherapy	1.7	3.0	3.4
Placebo	1.1	1.8	2.3
GP	1	1.5	2.4

improve), there were clear distinctions in the results. The physiotherapy and the manual therapy groups improved the most but they could not be separated at any of the outcome measures at the follow-up periods, although the number of treatments was considerably less for the manual therapy group. The placebo group performed better then the GP group. The researchers commented that the lack of referral and lack of follow-up in the GP groups may have provided a negative placebo effect. Table 8.1 is a representation of the results; for more details see the original paper (Koes et al 1992).

The researchers concluded that: 'It seems useful to refer patients with non-specific back and neck complaints lasting at least 6 weeks for treatment with manual therapy or physical therapy. Patients also respond remarkably well to placebo therapy'.

The Koes et al (1992) paper demonstrates the results of the enhanced placebo effect of spending time with patients. It shows additional benefits for physiotherapy and manual therapy, with a similar result with considerably less treatment for manual therapy.

Therapy

This part of the chapter briefly describes the general treatment methods used in manual therapy. A more detailed description of techniques relevant to the different body regions appears in Sections 2 and 3.

The aim of the initial visit is to get a good case history and clinical examination, to make a working diagnosis and to initiate appropriate management. Treatment on the first visit is usually abbreviated. I will ask the patient which

is the most painful region and confine my treatment to that area; for example, neck and shoulder or low back and pelvis. I will usually treat conservatively the first time. Adverse reactions to treatment are very common with manual therapy, occurring in around 50% of cases. They are most common on the first visit and produce a temporary increase of sensitivity around the injured region. This can vary in degree, based on individual susceptibility and treatment approach. Hence the need to err on the side of caution on the initial treatment. I often regard a treatment reaction as a positive occurrence as it shows evidence of an inflammatory phase followed by a healing process – it seems to stimulate the recovery process. A treatment reaction is usually followed by a marked improvement in symptoms 24–48 h later.

Muscle release techniques

Tense muscles with palpable taut bands (trigger points), muscular fatigue and reduction in circulation are an inherent part of most musculoskeletal injuries, particularly chronic ones. Reducing muscular tone and improving circulation is an important part of manual therapy. I use a neuromuscular technique (Chaitow 1996), which is a manual, deep massage technique, which I find most effective. It is used on tense and contracted muscles and associated trigger points. It involves using deep pressure with thumb, fingers, palm or occasionally elbow, using some sort of lubricant (I use sunflower seed oil) along the line of the taut muscle fibres. I usually pass along the taut muscle three times, increasing the pressure each time and feeling for the muscle release (Fig. 8.2). There are some regions where the muscles are very short, such as suboccipital muscles and the deep hip rotators, where it seems more appropriate to work the muscle transverse to its fibres. This technique can be quite hard on the practitioner's hands and forearms and must be used wisely.

I also use a modified form of this technique, which I describe as deep friction to other less contractile soft tissue regions, such as tendons, ligaments or insertion points onto bone. Some

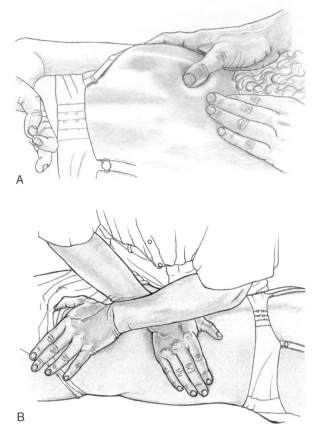

Figure 8.2 A: Neuromuscular treatment being applied to the middle fibres of trapezius; B: Neuromuscular treatment being applied to the erector spinae and quadratus lumborum.

examples of these are the rotator cuff tendon complex, the common extensor tendon at the elbow and the Achilles tendon insertion on the calcaneus. This involves using a gradually increasing pressure and small oscillatory movements over the region concerned. I would perform this intermittently for about 2–3 min.

Other soft tissue release techniques include trigger point acupuncture, acupressure, inhibition, ice spray and stretch, and a variety of deep massage techniques.

Mobilization

An injured joint will show signs of dysfunction. The features of this are:

- muscular and soft tissue shortening
- restriction in normal mobility
- change in bony position, e.g. pelvic torsion or upper cervical complex rotation.

These changes can cause abnormal biomechanics, increased proprioception, and altered fluid dynamics.

A restoration of normal mobility and normalization of soft tissue tone will allow a joint to revert to normal position, function and physiology. Mobilization techniques are an effective way of restoring normal mobility. They can be used with long lever, short lever, muscle energy, post-isometric relaxation or other techniques. As well as restoring normal mobility, it is important to pay attention to accessory joint mobility, such as joint distraction and joint glide. Mobilization involves working within the range of available joint motion and encouraging additional mobility at the restricted range of motion – extending the barrier toward full mobility. This is best done rhythmically to a joint that has the soft tissues warm and relaxed with preparatory soft tissue release. The barrier of joint motion, whether an anatomical or dysfunctional barrier, will be rich in proprioceptive activity. You have to be careful to not overstimulate this area and create a reactive spasm. The soft tissues should be prepared with soft tissue release, the hold either side of the joint should be firm and supportive with the region voluntarily relaxed. The movements should be smooth and rhythmical, without sudden movements or extended periods spent at the limit of mobility (Fig. 8.3).

Muscle energy technique

The muscle energy technique (MET) involves taking a joint to a functional barrier of mobility in one or more planes of movement and then asking the patient to perform a gentle (approximately 1 kg) isometric contraction against operator resistance back toward the midline of joint mobility (Fig. 8.4). This is held for approximately 3 s. A post-isometric relaxation then allows a small amount of extra mobility before moving to the functional barrier once again. This can be repeated three to four times, until there is no

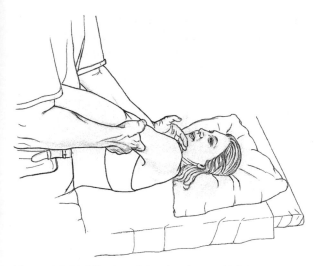

Figure 8.3 Mobilization of the glenohumeral joint.

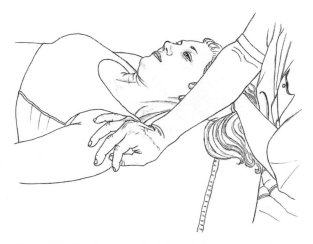

Figure 8.4 Muscle energy technique to increase cervical sidebending.

further gain to be made. This is a very effective way of improving mobility using minimal operator force while making the patient aware of the importance of the contraction–relaxation cycle of muscles. Care must be taken not to use large forces at the limit of joint mobility when the proprioceptors are engaged.

MET has the ability to relax the involved muscle, to 'turn down' the overactive proprioception in and around the muscle and to allow an increase in joint mobility.

Manipulation

Manipulation involves taking a joint to its physiological limit of motion and providing a quick movement or thrust. This is usually described as 'high velocity and low amplitude'. The thrust is designed to create a separation of the articular joint surfaces. The sudden change in pressure usually causes an audible pop, thought to be due to vaporization of the fluid on the joint surfaces. The efficacy of manipulation for different conditions, notably low back pain, will be discussed in Sections 2 and 3.

In skilled hands manipulation can be an excellent tool for providing an immediate improvement in joint function. An effective manipulation provides an immediate improvement in joint function, increase in joint mobility and reduction of pain. This is reasonably consistent and measurable. There are a number of theories how manipulation works. The most persuasive of these involve neurological inhibition of nociception and inhibition of reflex muscle contraction. For a good review of the subject see Katavich (1998).

Manipulation has in the past been quite controversial and has tended to be the domain of alternative medicine. The osteopathic and chiropractic professions have built large professions on the back of skilled teaching and application of these techniques. Not for nothing was the term 'million dollar roll' coined for the treatment of LBP. However, as evidence of the efficacy of manipulation grows, the alternative medical practitioners have become more acceptable to mainstream medicine, now tending to be called 'complementary medicine', and manipulation is being increasingly used in traditional medical and paramedical circles. Manipulation works effectively in a good proportion of spinal problems and it can work quite dramatically. It is very nice to have a treatment technique at your disposal that can make a patient arise from the treatment couch and exclaim with genuine surprise how much better they feel. It is a skilled technique requiring good teaching, good coordination, a sensitive touch and careful administration. The consensus of evidence is that it is particularly effective for acute back pain, reducing the period of morbidity and the incidence of recurrence. Its efficacy for chronic back pain is more controversial. It can create a temporary improvement but this needs to be augmented with a comprehensive rehabilitative approach.

Ice

Ice treatment is a very useful therapy for providing symptomatic relief and for assisting with the healing process. It can be used for pain relief, by using cold stimulation to 'close the pain gate' at spinal cord level. It also reduces sensory nerve conduction and velocity, and reduces muscle activity. It generally turns down the acute inflammatory response in the injury situation. Its use as an anti-inflammatory in acute injuries is well known. The lower tissue temperature creates a local vasoconstriction, reduces capillary permeability, increases viscosity and reduces tissue oedema.

Application of ice produces an initial vasoconstriction to preserve core body heat and secondary vasodilation to restore body heat to the chilled region once the cold stimulus is removed. This rapid increase in circulation provides a powerful stimulation to the healing process, but only occurs if the tissue temperature is low enough to produce this effect. This vasodilatory effect can be used in the chronic injury scenario to provide an increase in blood supply to improve tissue oxygenation and metabolite removal – to stimulate the recovery process. Some schools of thought emphasize alternate hot and cold applications to enhance this effect, always finishing with cold to prevent oedema.

Ice can be used at all stages of an injury from the very acute to the chronic. It can be used as a local anaesthetic agent to reduce local sensitivity prior to treatment – it pays to have it handy in the clinical situation. It can be used to the same effect to desensitize traumatized tissues and begin gentle rehabilitation exercises – with careful supervision.

Methods of application. Ice can be used in many forms, from the reusable ice pack to ice cubes in a plastic bag or a damp cloth. I often use a damp tea towel, frozen. After removal from the freezer it can be softened by running it for 10 s under trickling water, and then wrung out. The advantage of this is that it is very malleable and can be use on curved surfaces such as the neck or the knee and it maintains a high contact area. When using something very frozen it is best to wrap it in a damp towel to prevent ice burns and to move it frequently. Within 24 h of a very acute injury, ice can be used up to 30 min at a time; in a subacute injury, for 15 min per session; in a more advanced injury I will use it 5 min on then 5 min off for 2–3 sessions once or twice per day.

Occasionally people react badly to ice and find it increases their pain levels; these cases prefer heat treatment.

Heat

Heat is an effective muscle relaxant and can provide immediate comfort for a stiff sore joint. It causes a peripheral vasodilation and a reddening of the area. The heat sensations will also provide some inhibition of pain fibres by closing the pain gate. Heat gives immediate relief and comfort but tends to not be as long lasting nor have the secondary effects of increased circulation as ice. Some people tell me that the pain is often worse 30–60 min after application of heat, in which case it is preferable to finish with ice application. Heat is effective for join stiffness and the early morning or disuse stiffness. Heat should not be used in inflammatory situations, where it can increase oedema.

Ancillary treatment

At the initial presentation I will generally treat a patient twice per week for the first 1–2 weeks, and thereafter once per week unless the patient remains particularly acute or needy.

I give all patients some home therapy to do on a daily basis. This will vary on a case-by-case basis and depends on progress. There are great physiological and psychological benefits in having patients involved in their therapy. They will feel very well cared for. The home therapy usually consists of:

Exercises. I will always include some exercises. Exercise has a number of roles – it can:

- improve comfort
- reduce dysfunction, such as muscle shortening, muscle imbalance or joint stiffness
- improve strength, coordination and stamina
- assist in providing joint stability.

There is a natural tendency for the sensitized soft tissues to shorten after an injury, and exercises can help restore these contracted tissues. Exercises can help maintain the gain from manual therapy and reduce the tendency to relapse. Exercise will also benefit circulation and provide a valuable form of biofeedback.

General exercise. As a general rule, people do not get sufficient and varied exercise. Exercise has powerful benefits to improve and maintain good health (see Chapter 6) and some vigorous or aerobic exercise should be done on a daily basis. At any stage of an injury there is always some exercise that can be done to promote healing. I will try and give each patient advice about the appropriate exercise for him or her. Injured joints progressively lose function with gradual loss of strength, efficiency and early onset of fatigue. Exercises can help restore joint integrity, stability and function.

Self- or partner massage. I will often show patients the key trigger points to massage themselves. This is particularly helpful when they finish work. This will help relax the soft tissues, improve circulation and help stimulate natural recovery processes. For pelvic and spinal problems using their body weight and rolling on a small ball such as a tennis ball will help stimulate those hard-to-reach points.

Relaxation. If stress and associated muscle tension are major factors a relaxation technique can be helpful; there are a number of possible forms.

Ice or heat. A treatment routine is often very beneficial. For example, if there is a significant work-related exposure I will often give a treatment programme for patients to do when they return from work. This may include:

- 5 min ice

- 3 min massage
- 5 min ice
- 5 min stretching exercise.

This programme will give patients the opportunity to optimize their post work recovery periods before they are due to start work the following day.

If night pain is a major problem, a prebed routine may be advisable.

I will often give patients simple exercises to do throughout the day, particularly if they do not get much postural variation. This emphasizes body awareness and provides valuable movement, stretching and vascular pump as well as providing healthy proprioception.

Gaining some improvement in the initial treatment phase with a combination of placebo, good therapy and patient involvement is usually relatively easy. In an acute, short-duration-type injury this is usually sufficient to effect recovery. Many practitioners build busy clinics around good management of these acute-type problems. Effective management of acute injuries is important to prevent chronicity, although there will always be a sector of patients that need more than just short-term improvement. These cases may have significant ongoing exposures or previous histories that encourage ongoing symptoms and chronicity. These will be the real therapeutic challenge, where a greater range of skills and knowledge is required by the practitioner to convert a short-term gain to a long-term success story.

The path to recovery in a chronic case is never linear and many plateaux and relapses will need to be surmounted as part of the recovery process. These are part of the learning experience, where the patient and practitioner learn where the barriers to recovery are, what the appropriate levels of exposure are and develop and modify management plans accordingly.

The plateau effect

A good practitioner working in a good practice environment will find it relatively easy to gain an initial improvement. There is an enhanced placebo effect, a therapeutic gain, as well as the natural healing process. In acute injuries this may be sufficient to effect recovery. In chronic injuries that have been symptomatic for 3 months or longer, the patient must be carefully monitored to make sure the progress is maintained and the condition stabilized:

- priority 1 – recovery
- priority 2 – stabilization
- priority 3 – management to enhance recovery and reduce risk of relapse.

In reality, the typical recovery of a chronic case may be as shown in Figure 8.5.

The first significant plateau or symptom trough can be quite a telling moment. Patients can arrive with all their hopes dashed: 'I'm just as bad as at the beginning – back to square one'.

It is all too easy for the practitioner to join in the despondency and refer them back to the GP or for some other type of treatment. I have had many new practitioners work with me in my clinic and they rarely have the confidence to persevere with the tricky patients or have a suitable management framework in which to place them. I generally try and defuse the situation with a positive approach and a smile – I often suggest that after a few good weeks we had been due a bad week. I will reassess them and compare them to their initial presentation. You can usually show them that, despite a relapse, they have made significant progress. Patients are often very poor assessors of their own progress and require a practitioner who can take a

long-term view and remain a little detached from the inevitable fluctuations in symptoms. I will usually vary the treatment to deal with the change in symptomatology and amend the exercises or home treatment to help traverse the trough. The troughs often have a high psychosocial component. Patients will usually recover in 1–2 days and be back on their improvement pattern. However, you must ask what it was that caused this symptom exacerbation?

- Were they becoming overconfident and increasing the exposure, such as lifting, bending or a long motor vehicle journey?
- Was it a psychosocial stressor?
- Was it a change in the weather?

Most people try to be as active as they can following an injury. They are often not aware of the limits to their activity until they have been exceeded. Once a barrier to recovery has been identified, it can then be addressed and managed in such a way as to gain continued improvement. So each trough in the recovery period is also a learning experience that enables the injury to be better managed by both patient and practitioner. When patients gain an understanding of the injury and become aware of the appropriate limits and boundaries of their activities then they are able to improve their management of their condition and feel more confident and less disabled. The emphasis changes from seeking a cure to promoting effective management.

A person's exacerbation threshold will not remain constant. It will vary depending on the other influences present in their life and their environment. It is this variation that can be manipulated in a person's favour to allow a continued recovery.

There is usually a reason for each exacerbation that the patient is able to identify and accept. When the patient is well-managed the exacerbations will be short – 1 or 2 days – and will not be accompanied by distress. The practitioner's role becomes gradually less important and only occasional treatment may be required.

I have a checklist that I work through with chronic patients when they reach their plateau. This covers the things that I want to teach them

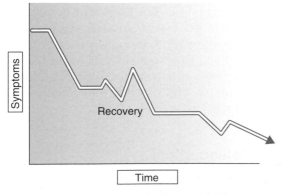

Figure 8.5 The plateau effect – the peaks and troughs of the recovery process.

and the tools that will help them manage their problem in the future.

Plateau breakers – checklist

- Exercises
- Relaxation techniques
- Stopping negative thoughts
- Breathing techniques – for relaxation and avoiding hyperventilation
- Exercise programme
- Bed, pillow, sleeping posture
- Nutrition – healthy diet
  - reduction in caffeine and other stimulants
  - nutritional supplements
- Work-related ergonomic exposures
- Sitting posture
- Motor vehicle posture
- Home-related ergonomic exposures.

Be careful not to overload patients with too much information in one go. Concentrate on the key intervention you wish to make. Try and support it with handouts and diagrams that they can refer to. This helps remind them and reinforces the key information. Remember – a picture is worth a thousand words, particularly with advice about posture and exercises.

The initial recovery is usually prompt, 50–75% improvement in about four visits, but continued improvement and stabilization can be prolonged. It is important to remember that the worst 10% of back pain patients occupy approximately 85% of expenses related to back pain. The principal cost is time off work. In New Zealand the off-work costs are approximately ten times the cost of therapy. The longer people are off work, the less likely they are to return to work. If the practitioner is able to effect the return to work of injured patients, or to assist in keeping them at work, then treatment, even if prolonged, is a highly cost-effective procedure.

Identifying the chronic patient

Two types of chronic patient present in clinic:

1. The first presents as an acute injury but subsequent events show that the injury is destined to become chronic. This may be because of the severity of the injury and the continued biomechanical exposure. It may be because a person has a low coping threshold and allows the symptoms to become magnified.

2. There will also be the person with the long history of disability doing the rounds of different therapeutic possibilities looking for a solution.

In both cases, early identification of the nature of the problem, identification of the barriers to recovery and institution of appropriate management can save an awful lot of meandering around the medical system with increasing medicalization of the problem. This may include a lot of expensive and often pointless imaging, and even unnecessary surgery.

Avoid overmedicalizing the problem. Most overuse or insidious-onset injuries are not related to an easily identified pathology, they are related to dysfunction. A lot of unnecessary imaging or referral to specialists encourages a disease orientation. This is not necessarily productive and tends to delay appropriate therapy and self-help management. Degenerative change in the joints is a normal part of the ageing process. This can be accelerated if there has been trauma or high biomechanical exposure. It is particularly common in the large weight-bearing joints, such as the hip and the knee and the areas of the spine that have high flexion moments, such as the lower cervical and lumbar spines, where large forces are required to hold the body against gravity. A degenerative joint has to be managed carefully. It is not as flexible or resilient as it used to be. It will not enjoy long periods of time at end-range of mobility or with joint compression. When managed sensibly, a degenerative joint does not have to be a source of pain.

Refer a patient for further investigation if there are clear clinical reasons. These can be:

- neurological symptoms
- inflammatory problems
- unexplained weight loss
- history of cancer
- severe unremitting night pain
- continued deterioration.

Time can also be a great enemy to efficient recovery. The longer people spend in chronic pain, without clear information as to the nature of the problem and without appropriate management, the more difficult it is to reverse the neurophysiological and psychosocial factors related to chronicity. Doing the rounds of different practitioners can be an important part of a patient's learning experience, as each practitioner may have different lessons to teach, and it helps the patient build a picture of the problem and how it fits into the medical maze. However, the patient doing the round often has unrealistic expectations and is looking for a quick-fix solution: 'If you can just move this bone, or loosen this muscle, or cut this bit out, everything will get better'. If this simplistic view is inappropriate, point out the need for a more holistic approach to the problem.

When patients have a clear-cut, chronic history, avoid recycling them as acute patients who have just received their injury. This tends to encourage the simple fix-it solution and they tend to continue the round of practitioners, becoming more chronic and not gaining the benefit of effective long-term management in addition to temporary symptomatic recovery.

THE CLINICAL ERGONOMICS MODEL

It may be clear from the outset, or it may become apparent during the course of therapy, that manual therapy alone will not provide an adequate recovery. The clinical ergonomics model then gives us a different perspective for management of the injury. It concentrates on the input cycle into injury and attempts to modify the risk factors responsible for symptoms. This involves a careful search of the three categories of exposure – ergonomic, psychosocial and personal factors – and attempts to modify them. The risk factors for these categories have been discussed in previous chapters. The more risk factors that can be identified and modified, the greater the possibility of optimizing long-term improvement and recovery. Many of these modifications will be extensions of topics mentioned in the ancillary

treatment and plateau breakers sections. In reality, the incorporation of the clinical ergonomics model into practice should not be regarded as one of a change of direction or a completely new approach but can be done quite seamlessly with an increasing emphasis on patient management in addition to, or instead of, manual therapy. A range of skills can help establish a much more holistic approach to clinical management. The practitioner becomes not just a purveyor of techniques but has the opportunity to become an ergonomist, a counsellor, a teacher and a motivator. Each person must develop the skills they feel comfortable with and refer or import the skills that they feel are beyond their modus operandum. For example, some psychosocial problems may be better dealt with by a counsellor or mediator rather than a therapist. An exercise programme may have a better uptake if it is prepared and monitored by a personal trainer or an exercise therapist rather than a practitioner. The most significant risk factors should be dealt with first and the exposures that are most easily modified should also be given priority. It is very easy to become overfocused on one particular aspect of the injury model, particularly in these times of increasing specialization. The psychologist might ignore the ergonomic factors, not fully appreciating the interplay between ergonomic and psychosocial exposure. The surgeon may focus on a particular aspect of the symptoms that are amenable to surgery and ignore the chronic aspect of the symptoms. Practitioners too often ignore the input cycle of overuse injuries and encourage symptomatic treatment. General practitioners frequently focus on pain relief at the expense of good management. The clinical ergonomics model stresses the big picture and the multifactorial nature of chronic symptoms. All chronic or recurrent injuries will have some psychosocial *and* some ergonomic *and* some personal issues. We owe it to our patients to explore these issues holistically to provide the optimum rehabilitation scenario. In some cases where there is no immediate danger of disability, the clinical ergonomics process can be carried out in a leisurely, educational-type process. In others where the person is off work, there is a large amount of expense involved and a real risk of disability, the process is much more urgent. The longer people are off work, the less likely it is that they will ever return to work. The physical and psychosocial barriers to overcome loom ever larger. Once a person has been off work 6 weeks with an injury, whether acute or chronic, the clinical ergonomics model should be given an urgent emphasis to facilitate a return to work in some capacity. I also use the clinical ergonomics model with staff training programmes to help prevent work-related injury and encourage employee awareness of the risk factors.

Managing ergonomic risk factors

The presenting symptoms, the case history and the response to treatment will usually give a fairly clear idea of any ergonomic factors that are responsible for symptoms or delayed recovery. The tension patterns involved give a clear idea of the muscles or tissues being overused. This in turn leads to discussion of the likely actions or postures that might lead to these musculoskeletal changes. This ability to identify tension patterns and link them into different postures provides therapists with valuable skills to assist with improving ergonomics. Once the ergonomic exposures are identified, the reduction of these is a logical corollary, with attempts to improve the posture and the forces generated in the posture, and to reduce or better manage the exposure period. Alternatively, there might be more efficient methods of managing the same tasks.

Some patients may be well aware of the causative exposure, others may have no idea there is one. It is usually up to the practitioner to introduce the possibility of poor posture as a contributing factor in causing the injury and to suggest likely exposures. For example, somebody suffering from chronic right shoulder elevator tension (levator scapula and trapezius) would probably be working with an elevated shoulder and arm, or working without sufficient arm support.

The possible methods of gaining information about possible ergonomic factors are:

- question and answer

- asking patients to provide photographs of their work postures
- site visit.

A complicated case that involves a risk of time off work or disability should have a site visit from a skilled ergonomic assessor. This will assist in identifying the ergonomic risk factors and making recommendations for the appropriate modifications. It has been my experience that the visit of an external assessor, debrief with appropriate management and the provision of a report including the key recommendations, plays a significant role in hastening the modifications to an unsatisfactory workplace. I like to carry out as many modifications as possible to the workplace while I am on-site to facilitate the process of change and to diminish the relevant exposures as soon as possible. I usually have a supply of the ergonomic aids I most commonly use (office chairs, wrist supports, copyholders, tilted workboards, ergonomic keyboards and mouse, etc.) that I leave on trial to facilitate the process of change and to use as educational aids.

I use a checklist system, which I have developed, to gain the relevant data, then take a photograph of the relevant work postures and 'score' the different body regions (good, average or poor) with the person involved. In the interests of efficiency I try and complete the recommendations and report with the relevant modifications while I am on-site. The average assessment takes 1–1.5 h. An assessment system should also take account of work organization, breaks, job satisfaction, stress levels, lighting, etc., and should have an educational component.

I believe that manual therapists are well placed to offer workplace assessment services because of their specialized knowledge of biomechanics and injury development. When they are familiar with a person's injury and the muscle tension patterns associated with it they can very often target the necessary ergonomic modifications very effectively. Ergonomic exposure is such a major part of cumulative and chronic injury that the extension of the skills of the manual therapist beyond the treatment room into the outside world can make a very real difference in many cases. There is a very real need of ergonomic improvements in the modern work environment and practitioners are well placed to recognize the importance of these and to facilitate the necessary changes. The clinical ergonomics approach to the issue of ergonomics in the workplace is a very person-focused approach as opposed to a management or systems approach. It highlights the individual nature of the problem.

Managing psychosocial risk factors

The role of psychosocial factors in the injury process has been covered in Chapter 6. It can be a significant factor in many injuries, and in particular the conversion of acute to chronic injuries.

The clinical priorities associated with managing psychosocial factors are:

- address fear and anxiety associated with the injury
- address any conflict associated with the injury
- look for psychosocial factors that may be related to the cause of the injury
- try and address psychosocial factors that might create a tendency toward disability or chronicity
- try and give tools that assist the person having control over the symptoms.

It is one thing to identify psychosocial factors that may be contributing to the build-up of an anxiety response and may be contributing to the injury, but modifying them may not be so easy. Although they can sometimes be modified relatively easily by resolving the conflicts, removing the fear of a more serious or terminal condition or sometimes by just listening, sometimes the stresses involved are not easy to modify. There may be an exaggerated or maladaptive response to essentially normal stresses, which require modification or relearning. There may be high levels of stress relating to factors that cannot easily be modified, which may require learning improved coping or management techniques.

Some of the stress management and modification techniques that can be useful are:

- exercise
- relaxation techniques
- diaphragmatic breathing
- yoga and meditation
- counselling
- biofeedback
- relaxation tapes
- cognitive behavioural modification
- reading – there is a great range of positive, self-help books available for every imaginable problem.

For an excellent review of relaxation techniques and their application see Keable (1997).

Chronic patients are often unhappy. This is not just associated with their injury but can also be with their jobs or their relationships. These can create stress and anxiety that can contribute to the stress–tension cycle. The injury can provide a focus for their negativity – they are able to avoid tackling the more difficult life issues. The practitioner must constantly maintain a positive outlook. Once you have developed a person's trust it can be worthwhile pointing out that the negative features in a person's life may be related to the pain patterns. Give patients the opportunity to talk about it and suggest tools to effect the appropriate changes.

Chronic patients can often feel that they are the unfortunate victims of circumstances, that despite their best efforts they have a problem that they can no longer control. This can lead to a progressive reduction in confidence that they can influence events and can result in depression and a learned helplessness. They can create a 'poor me' scenario where they are constantly seeking sympathy. This negative construct can be a recipe for chronicity. It is OK to feel bad for a while. This has to be understood and turned into a positive, forward-looking context. There are a number of tools that can help them regain a more positive view of life, and assist their ability to influence events. A clinical improvement and a sympathetic ear can provide a powerful incentive to start a new, more positive cycle of coping with difficulties and improving one's lot. The practitioner is in a real position to act as a catalyst for positive change. Regularly review patients' progress. Ensure that they have goals to work toward and positive events to look forward to.

A pessimistic outlook is a common characteristic of chronic patients. They have tried it all before and nothing seems to help. Indeed, most interventions seem to aggravate their condition. An increase in pain levels often suggests to them they are doing harm and that further decline of their condition is inevitable. This leads to pain avoidance behaviour, a gradual decline in normal activities and a progressive disability. This can make them feel out of control and demoralized. A poor therapeutic response or a limited therapeutic approach can hasten this process.

The patient may become hypervigilant for anything that accentuates the pain sensation. This 'catastrophizing' of pain sensations tends to magnify the consequences of injury and predispose toward disability.

Chronic patients can often be angry and hostile. This is unproductive behaviour, which alienates them and creates conflict in their work and home relationships. The reasons for the anger need to be addressed and the behaviour modified.

As practitioners, we have a responsibility to point out the links between these personality traits and chronicity but it is not necessarily our job to find the solutions. We can act as a catalyst for patients to seek their own solutions, to become empowered, and to achieve the best quality of life available to them.

A chronic pain problem can be the culmination of everything that went before it – if you always do what you have always done you will always get what you have always got.

People often need to understand the past that has created the present, make their peace with it, understand their feelings and move on, using new tools to change their patterns of thought and behaviour, to a positive future. This is not a process that can be hurried – the journey once begun can be quite exciting! People can use a chronic health problem to create major changes in their lives, to regain control over a life that seemed out of control.

Encourage patients to maintain their normal social networks. A problem can seem much worse if you become socially isolated. Encourage them to keep up the usual group activities. Work is a valuable part of our socialization and it is important to try and keep as much work contact as normal even if they are unable to cope with the prolonged ergonomic exposure.

Encourage them to have positive experiences. Have fun, try something new, explore new places. Distraction is a great form of pain normalization (Fig. 8.6).

Psychosocial management – a summary

- Stay positive – set goals.
- Minimize anxiety and distress.
- Review progress regularly.
- Keep active – avoid inactivity.
- Maintain work involvement.
- Structured exercise programme.
- Patient education and involvement.
- Pain management rather than avoidance.
- Check for psychosocial factors.
- Check for ergonomic exposures.
- Identify barriers to progress and seek solutions.

Managing personal risk factors

Personal risk factors intersect with psychosocial and ergonomic risk factors, which usually have a significant personal component. Personal factors also play an important part in the manual therapy model outlined, and some detail of the personal issues have been covered in the sections on ancillary treatment and plateau breakers. All treatment processes should have some ability to adapt to the injury, the situation and the needs of the individual. The manual therapy model takes as its priority the need to reduce pain, which is the most common reason for patient presentation. Personal factors are dealt with as they surface as barriers to recovery. The clinical ergonomics model involves a more systematic approach to personal factors, trying to ensure that the environment for recovery is optimized. The person has been identified as being at risk for chronicity or disability and we are expanding the treatment model and increasing the resources to try and circumvent the descent into chronicity, or to try and find a pathway out of the situation.

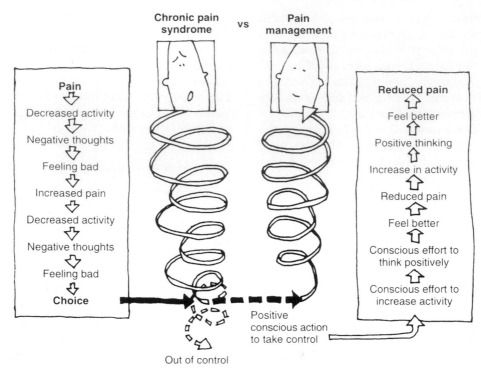

Chronic pain syndrome VS Pain management

Pain
⇩
Decreased activity
⇩
Negative thoughts
⇩
Feeling bad
⇩
Increased pain
⇩
Decreased activity
⇩
Negative thoughts
⇩
Feeling bad
⇩
Choice

Reduced pain
⇧
Feel better
⇧
Positive thinking
⇧
Increase in activity
⇧
Reduced pain
⇧
Feel better
⇧
Conscious effort to think positively
⇧
Conscious effort to increase activity

Positive conscious action to take control

Out of control

Figure 8.6 Chronic pain syndrome versus pain management. Reproduced with permission from Keable (1997).

Personal factors have particular relevance because they involve the person in the recovery process. They teach people that they are not a victim of circumstance but they are able to positively influence their situation by identifying factors they are able to modify. This requires a powerful educational and motivational component and it is important that practitioners who traditionally see their role as 'doing things' or providing a certain service start to value and appreciate their skills as facilitators of change.

Realistic prognosis

When assessing personal factors it is important to be realistic and to take into account the personal history of the problem and the desired activity levels of the patient to develop a realistic prognosis. It is realistic to expect that 70-year-olds with advanced degenerative change in the lumbar spine can become reasonably pain free. It is probably not realistic to expect that they will be able to tolerate the range and intensity of exposures they were able to do when they were 25-year-old manual workers. Patients can be taught to manage their exposures to minimize their disabilities. They can probably expect some symptoms from time to time and they can be taught to manage these so they do not progress. Human nature is such that people will often work to the maximum range of their capacity, and often only find their tolerance level by exceeding it occasionally. The hard-working, active, 70-year-old described may need assistance from time to time. If the person described has a degenerative spondylolisthesis with an unstable spinal segment, the symptoms will be much more easily provoked and the available activity levels will be much lower. However, if people are educated about avoiding flexion forces and lifting, they can still have an active and fulfilling life. There are still exercise programmes that they can do to help stabilize the spine, moderate their symptoms and increase their quality of life.

A full-time computer operator, who has worked in a difficult environment and developed grade 4 overuse injury of the upper limbs and cervical spine, is unlikely to be able to return to the same environment without substantial modifications to his or her job description and work environment. This requires good employer support as well as personal involvement by the patient. The failure of treatment to restore normality on grade 4 overuse is not the fault of the therapist but of the management of the problem long before the therapist became involved. The therapist's job is to optimize the situation as he or she finds it, not to perform miracles!

Establishing an appropriate prognosis for chronic patients requires good case history taking, good communication and some experience. Providing a realistic prognosis while remaining positive about improvement and function can save an awful lot of poorly directed time, money and frustration, all of which can contribute to chronicity.

Establishing a realistic prognosis makes the patient's role in the recovery process clear from the beginning.

Identifying risk factors

To optimize the recovery process it is important to identify the relevant risk factors:

● Personal factors that cannot be changed – the clinical history, age, sex, previous traumas, degree of degenerative change, anatomical characteristics.
● Personal factors that are easy to modify – exercise, fitness, smoking (easy to cut down, hard to give up), diet, body mass index, excessive use of stimulants or pain relief, domestic ergonomic exposure.
● Factors that may be hard to modify – work ergonomic exposures, some domestic exposures – child rearing, housework – some psychosocial exposures.

The factors that may be hard to modify are often key exposures involved in the injury process, such as work exposures and psychosocial environment. If these are identified as key exposures they should not be put in the too hard basket, but a programme of change instituted so that the patient can begin to tackle some of the more difficult issues with the support and motivation of the practitioner. Sometimes they genuinely are too difficult – an employer who is uncooperative and refuses to modify the work environment – or more commonly the situation where people suspect that their jobs would be under threat if they were perceived as a nuisance and would rather not approach their employer. The patient must be made aware that this can increase the risk of chronicity and there is a risk to accepting an unsatisfactory situation, particularly if there is a high level of symptoms or the condition seems to be deteriorating. Alternative employment might be the next best option. I have seen many cases that have had high levels of symptoms associated with a poor work environment that have responded successfully in an improved or different environment. However, the more chronic the symptoms become, the more difficult it can be to adapt to a new environment and the more likely there are to be some residual symptoms. There is not a job in existence that is worth becoming disabled for.

Although managing many of the personal risk factors is self-explanatory, such as smoking (don't!), high body mass index (lose it!) and exercise (do it!), the process of instituting change is often more difficult. A practitioner can motivate a patient but often a multidisciplinary approach and the assistance of other health professionals will help. Recovery processes often benefit from high levels of general health and good immune function. This will often require attention to other health issues and may also need the assistance of the person's GP and of other medical specialists. The orthodox medical system specializes in management of disease but, where optimizing health is the goal, other health practitioners such as naturopaths, homeopaths, herbalists or traditional acupuncturists may have a valuable role to play.

It is important to screen for domestic or personal ergonomic factors and to review these exposures. These are frequently hidden secondary factors that can have a major impact on the degree of exposure. A person will often identify the major work-related exposure and conveniently ignore the personal exposure. These exposures can often be eliminated or modified to reduce them. Somebody with chronic or recurrent back pain should not be spending hours at a time vacuuming or gardening. A person with chronic shoulder tendonitis should not be spending time with elevated arms such as window cleaning. A person with high daily exposure to computer work should not spend the evenings on the internet or in constrained postures such as sewing or craft work. Playing musical instruments often involves high degrees of musculoskeletal exposure. Personal time should aim to optimize recovery from the main ergonomic exposures while still trying to have a satisfying private life, function as a member of a family and a society. There are inevitably compromises involved but these should be as a result of awareness of the risk factors.

Starting an exercise programme

All injuries can benefit from appropriate exercises and a general exercise programme. Beginning exercise with a person suffering chronic musculoskeletal symptoms has to be done very carefully, with careful attention to the nature of the injury. Exercises to provide ease or reduce dysfunction, including muscle strengthening and stretching exercises, will be covered under the appropriate sections on regional injuries.

When advocating a general exercise programme to improve aerobic fitness and gain the myriad benefits of exercise, there are a number of guidelines to consider:

- Exercise should be rhythmic – it should involve contraction/relaxation cycles.
- It should involve active joint movements – no static contractions.
- It should start away from the injured segments, minimizing exposure to injured tissues.
- It should be non-weight-bearing to begin with.
- As exercise tolerance improves there can be a gradual increase in weight-bearing activity and a gradual phased introduction of the injured segments, emphasizing movement rather than force.
- Start very easy with long recovery periods and very gradually increase duration and intensity as symptoms allow. Avoid initial overenthusiasm!
- It is normal to have postexercise soreness, which can be exaggerated in a chronic pain scenario. This is OK. The exercise should not be repeated until the postexercise soreness is absent for at least 24 h. In this way, tolerance to the exercise increases. If the exercise is repeated too soon, tolerance decreases and pain is aggravated.
- If the postexercise soreness is severe, the intensity and duration of exercise is too great – do less.
- If exercising regularly, it is better to vary the type of exercise to provide relative rest and recovery to exposed tissues while still keeping up exercise levels.
- If the patient is having a bad spell, they should be told to reduce their exercise levels.

There is a fine line between exercising to improve function and overexposing sensitive tissues resulting in increased pain and sensitivity. Let your patients know it is OK to not always get it right. Encourage them to listen to their body and learn from their mistakes. Starting an exercise programme can result in temporary increase in pain levels but the long-term benefits are worthwhile. Exercise is the most effective method we know of reducing pain and sensitivity in chronic pain problems.

People with chronic upper limb problems might start with water-based exercise that minimized use of the arms, such as aqua jogging or aquarobics. They may alternate the two and gradually incorporate some arm activities in this relatively low gravity environment. They could progress to some land-based, relatively low gravity exercise such as exercycling. They could progress to stepping or another form of exercise machine that has some low arm position activity. They could further progress to fast walking or jogging. They could eventually do some light gym work emphasizing light weights and low arm positions, and/or swimming.

People with chronic low back pain might be best to start with swimming, moving onto aquarobics or water walking. They could then progress to land-based low gravity supported exercise such as exercycling or stepping. They could progress to walking, gradually increasing intensity, with some jogging. There would be some floor or gym exercises that could be incorporated depending on their level of symptoms and their injured tissues.

SUMMARY

- The case history and clinical examination provide important information about the type of injury, the tissues that have been compromised and the severity of the injury.
- Manual therapy is generally the most effective treatment for acute musculoskeletal injury. A large proportion of the effectiveness is due to good patient management and the enhanced placebo effect.

- Injuries can change in nature during the recovery process. The symptom picture can change and new issues may emerge. It is important to have management strategies for symptom plateaux or troughs.
- More chronic injuries will always have complications that require more comprehensive management. The clinical ergonomics approach screens for ergonomic, psychosocial and personal risk factors and uses these to reduce harmful exposures and create effective rehabilitation strategies.
- Rehabilitation strategies that involve people and enhance their coping strategies, such as exercise programmes or relaxation techniques, are more likely to be effective than passive modalities.

Low back pain

9

Epidemiology of low back pain

Low back pain (LBP) is a major problem, and now ranks as the most common medical complaint in developed economies. Despite the profusion of highly skilled therapists and increasing funds for therapy, despite new and sophisticated methods of imaging and despite a gradual reduction in the amount of heavy manual work, the reported incidence of injury and the time off work associated with back pain increased dramatically between 1970 and 1990. Most developed economies increased their expenditure on low back pain disability ten-fold in that period.

Why, in these days of many labour-saving devices and the best resources of modern medicine, are more and more people suffering the effects of LBP? Perhaps today's rapidly changing society is contributing various factors to the problem:

- Social attitude – the provision of generous benefits may encourage disability behaviour by back pain sufferers. The medical model perspective often encourages pathological labels for an essentially normal process.
- Changes in work practice – although there is less manual work, people spend more time in constrained and sitting postures, performing repetitive and monotonous tasks.
- Psychosocial – modern work practices can lead to increased stress and boredom and these have been associated with increased incidence of back injury claims. It can be difficult to diffuse stress with the reduced socialization and reduced activity levels of the modern workplace.

- Personal – the increasing size and weight of progressive generations, and the reduction in activity and fitness levels, lead to increased risk of musculoskeletal insult.

There are some signs that the progressive increase in LBP disability has stabilized (in the UK) since the early 1990s and reversed in other countries (USA and Sweden). This seems to be largely due to changes in benefit structures and stricter criteria of the claims acceptance, rather than to any reduction of injury. The incidence of back pain remains extraordinarily high; 70–80% of the working population suffer from LBP at some point in their lives. In any one year the incidence is about 40%, of these, 70% are thought to recover in 2 weeks and 90% to recover in 6 weeks; the remaining 10% will continue to have ongoing problems. This subgroup will utilize approximately 80% of expenditure related to back pain disability. It is in this area that practitioners must muster their resources to reduce morbidity and cost, to try and prevent these 10% of sufferers going on to become chronic.

A study in the UK (Croft et al 1998), based on two general medical practices in Manchester, followed 490 subjects complaining of LBP and found results that conflict with the statistics quoted above. Croft and colleagues tested the often-stated proposition that 90% of episodes of LBP that present to general practice have resolved within a month. Their key findings were:

- While 90% of subjects consulting general practice with LBP ceased to consult about the symptoms within 3 months, most still had substantial LBP and related disability.
- Only 25% of the patients had fully recovered 12 months later.

They went on to conclude that: 'Since most consulters continue to have long-term low back pain and disability, effective early treatment could reduce the burden of these symptoms and their social economic and medical impact'.

This study illustrates the importance of effective treatment and management programmes to produce a rapid recovery from a back pain episode and to minimize the risks of recurrence and chronicity.

Back pain is very common across all age groups in both sexes. LBP seems to be highest in the physically active years – in people aged 20–50. Acute LBP episodes reduce after age 50 but chronic low back pain can continue beyond this. Back pain in those under the age of 20 and over the age of 60 tends to be under-represented in statistics due to the reduced economic activities of these age groups and the reduced attendant costs. There is evidence that these groups have a high incidence of back pain discomfort in population surveys. There are many surveys that show a high rate of back pain among adolescents. A survey of 330 students aged 11–18 years showed that an astonishing 57% complained of LBP or ache in the previous 12 months (Wilson 1993). Other studies show incidences in the range of 30–40%. Balague et al (1988), in a large study of 1715 schoolchildren, found that the incidence dramatically increased over the age of 13, to 57% in males and 70% in females. Balague et al concluded that the prevalence was similar to adults. Fisk et al (1984) found a high incidence of Scheuermann's disease (SD) in a survey of 500 17- and 18-year-olds still in the education system. He found radiological evidence that 56% of males and 37% of females had the characteristic changes of SD and cited evidence that this was linked to increased prevalence of LBP in later life. It is a great concern that so many adolescents suffer LBP prior to entering the workforce and are already predisposed to further injury.

The majority of patients with back pain episodes are able to continue working. When mobility is substantially restricted, a short period of time away from work may be necessary. Individuals with a heavy workload may find it harder to continue work and find the transition back to work more difficult. The longer people are off work, the less likely it is that they will return to work. There are subtle psychosocial changes that take place when a person is off work. These include reduced self-confidence, reduced self-esteem and reduced socialization. There is also a gradual loss of work fitness. The return to work becomes a greater and greater hurdle as time passes and the lapse into disability can occur because these hurdles seem insurmountable.

This 5–10% of cases are inordinately expensive and go on to occupy 80% of costs relating to LBP, the vast majority of which is earnings-related compensation. The rate of disability due to back pain varies substantially with the social welfare provisions of each society. People take time off work due to LBP if there is financial provision for them to do so. Generally speaking, the more generous the earnings-related disability the higher the rate of disability due to back pain. In Sweden, following a reduction in the rate of sickness benefit, the annual prevalence of sick leave for back pain has fallen from 6.2% in 1992 to 3.9% in 1996. Compensation issues can create an adversarial climate, which can lead to increased stress and conflict and create a situation where LBP sufferers feel the need to 'prove' the extent of their injury, with an increased focus on their symptoms. Guest & Drummond (1992) compared a group of LBP compensation recipients with those whose claims had been finalized. They summarized:

Compensation recipients showed more signs of emotional distress, had greater difficulty coping with pain, and reported that pain disrupted various aspects of their life to a greater degree than subjects who had settled their claim. However, even after settlement there were clear signs of emotional distress.

The promise of a financial windfall on settlement of a claim could discourage workers from resuming employment after injury. Unfortunately, this course of action increases the risk of pain becoming chronic and of unemployment and hardship continuing. To prevent this potentially disastrous situation the compensation system should encourage workers to resume some type of employment as soon as possible after injury.

Recovery from back pain and avoidance of disability is promoted by trying to maintain physical activity levels and retain normal social relationships. The best way to provide these is to continue normal activities as much as possible. There is a very real need for employers and healthcare agencies to encourage a continued work role whenever possible and to provide opportunities for restricted workload or restricted hours when necessary. For workers who are still off work after 6 weeks, it is advisable to identify the barriers to recovery – ergonomic, psychosocial and personal – and to provide substantial resources to minimize these, with the aim of achieving some work involvement before disability becomes a behavioural habit.

If the injury is work related, a person should only return to work once the cause has been identified and the hazardous exposure modified. This may be an accident, a peak load or a cumulative load. The noted ergonomist, Mats Hagberg, stated 'It is unethical to send a worker back to work following a work related injury without a full workplace assessment' (Hagberg 1995).

A previous episode of back pain increases the risk of future episodes. The spinal structures often remain sensitized and react to a lower level of biomechanical exposure. This sensitivity can decrease with time and with appropriate manual therapy. Good management becomes important to reduce the incidence and severity of future episodes.

10

Risk factors for low back pain

HEAVY PHYSICAL WORK

It is clear that heavy physical work is *the* major risk factor for low back pain (LBP). The more time spent in flexed postures, the greater the risk of injury. If rotation is added, this increases the biomechanical load and risk of injury. The greater the force generated in these postures – pushing, pulling or lifting – the greater the risk of injury. Heavy work has been associated with increased incidence of injury, frequency of recurrence, relative chronicity and accelerated degenerative change. A manual worker with heavy physical workload will find it more difficult to return to work following a back injury. For a good review of the subject see NIOSH (1997b).

In a NIOSH analysis of National Health Interview survey data (NIOSH 1995), reported back pain lasting 1 week or longer due to repeated activities at work showed significantly higher odds ratios for those involved in strenuous physical activity. Lifting, pushing and pulling provided increased odds ratios of:

- 4.25 for more than 2 h exposure per day
- 9.25 for more than 8 h exposure per day.

With the addition of repeated bending and twisting odds ratios were:

- 5.79 for more than 2 h of exposure
- 14.48 for more than 8 h of exposure.

The injury can be caused by peak loading, repetition loading or by continuous poor posture. The risk of injury is modified by work management and personal factors. In general, the greater the biomechanical load, the longer the period of time spent in awkward postures and the higher the number of repetitions, the greater the risk of injury.

Personal modifying factors are: gender, age, personal dimensions, physical fitness and previous history of back problems. Job organizational factors such as work duration, breaks, work variety, temperature, unstable or awkward loads and the availability of lifting equipment can also influence the risk of injury in workplaces with high manual loading.

Risk factors for developing chronic LBP in heavy manual workers include high biomechanical load, high stress, low job satisfaction, low social support, uncooperative employer, smoking and high body mass index. These risk factors are well documented in the ergonomic literature and well supported by research. Heavy physical work consistently demonstrates the highest odds ratios when risk factors for LBP are studied. In a 2-year prospective study of blue-collar steel workers, Massett et al (1998) found an increased incidence of new cases of LBP in those who described their lifting efforts as moderate or heavy (odds ratio 2.3). Heavy manual work has been demonstrated as a risk factor for both peak loading and cumulative loading spinal injuries. This will be explored in more detail in Chapter 12.

SITTING

Whether sitting is a risk factor for LBP remains a subject of much debate. Some researchers find the research contradictory. Rhiihimaaki (1997) points out that the industries with a high risk of back injury in males are non-sedentary, with the exception of those involving driving. In females, some sedentary activities with high visual demands or repetitive movements are associated with a high risk of LBP, such as operating a sewing machine or cash register. However, most epidemiological research does not support prolonged sitting being a major risk factor for injury. It becomes difficult to disentangle the effects of sitting posture from subsequent peak loading and it may be that the effects of prolonged sitting

on spinal fatigue may predispose the spine to further injury from peak loading. The peak loading then becomes the obvious causative factor for recording purposes, while the effects of sitting can be underestimated. The relative peak loads while sitting are not as large as manual handling and it may be that seated workers are frequently able to continue to work while managing their injuries while heavy manual workers with LBP may be unable to work. Spinal fatigue from sitting postures is likely to be accelerated by:

- non-neutral spinal posture – reverse lumbar curve, increased thoracic curve
- unsupported body weight anterior to the spine – forward reaching and high visual demands
- repeated twisting or bending actions
- the length of time spent sitting
- poor quality seating or poor workstation design
- the amount of exercise taken when not sitting.

The rate of spinal fatigue during sitting postures may be positively modified by:

- the quality of the chair – the ability to maintain a good lumbar curve and minimize disc compression
- correct height of the work surface or VDU
- good visual angles and distance
- the ability to use an effective lumbar support
- work variety and breaks.

Clearly, whether sitting is a risk factor depends on the task performed while sitting, its duration and management, and how well the workplace is designed for the task. With an increasing trend towards sitting and other sedentary postures, and a continual reduction in activity levels, it is likely that sitting postures are going to be an increasingly important risk factor. Figure 10.1 shows how a poorly designed workstation can dramatically affect posture and increase spinal loading and accelerate spinal fatigue.

McGill (1997) describes the loading history prior to injury as being a vital consideration. In this context, sitting posture, with its lack of movement, reduction of fluid exchange in intervertebral disc (IVD) and muscles, and sustained

A

B

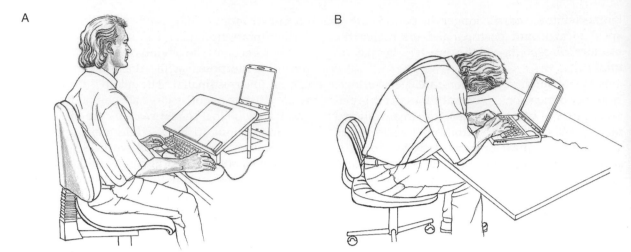

Figure 10.1 Sitting as a risk factor for low back pain depends on the task performed and how well the workplace is designed for the task. The figure shows A: a well designed workplace and B: a poorly designed workplace using the same subject for the same task.

loading on postural muscles and IVD, may prime the spine for increased risk of injury by exertion by lowering the injury threshold. In a study on cadaveric specimens in simulated sitting postures (Hedman & Fernie 1997), the escalation of forces was more severe in the flexed sitting postures, with large increase in tensile forces in the region of the posterior annulus. Prolonged sitting postures may also increase subsequent biomechanical loading as a result of habitual lack of exercise, hamstring tightness, abdominal muscle weakness and altered disc and muscle physiology. It is likely that the exposure periods are longer in sitting postures than in standing flexed postures and thus habitual sitting may be a more significant factor in the older age groups.

Prolonged sitting does not provide as obvious an association with LBP as manual handling and peak loading but it remains a significant factor in managing the incidence of LBP, its recurrence and chronicity.

DRIVING

Driving has been associated with increased risk of back pain disability. Porter & Gyl (1995) reported a six-fold increase in sickness absence due to back pain amongst drivers who drove

more than 4 h per day. The study showed that drivers were more uncomfortable if they:

- drove for long periods without stopping
- drove a car with a manual gearbox
- did not have an adjustable seat – seat height, cushion tilt and lumbar adjustment.

Other studies have found a high incidence of prolapsed discs and spinal degenerative changes in people who have occupations involving high mileage driving. In the USA, truck drivers consistently have the highest occupational incidence of back injuries that require time off work (Bureau of Labor Statistics 1999).

There is no doubt that driving is a demanding sitting posture. The exacting tasks required of arms and legs, and the high visual demands, offer little opportunity for postural variation. There is also significant stress associated with the rapid sensory input and the concentration required. Most researchers consider that the vibration of a motor vehicle is the most significant factor in accelerating spinal fatigue.

LACK OF EXERCISE/FITNESS

The role of exercise in injury prevention and injury recovery was discussed in Chapter 7. There is evidence that a lack of exercise can be an important predisposing factor to spinal injury. As the amount of physical activity people take is becoming less, with increasing reliance on mechanical devices for transport, work and even leisure, we are becoming less fit than previous generations. When we do exercise there are often sudden abrupt increases in workload on a poorly prepared musculoskeletal system. So we have a paradox – lack of exercise can predispose to back injury and sudden increases in activity levels can cause musculoskeletal insult. Regular moderate exercise will have a protective effect against these causative factors.

Leino (1993) followed 607 blue- and white-collar employees in the metal industry. He found that the men with low activity scores, when followed up 5 years later, showed a modest inverse association between physical activity and development of symptoms, and clinical findings in the low back. The effects were small but persisted when other factors such as age, social class, smoking and body mass index were controlled for. The same relationship was not found in women.

It has been proposed by a number of authors that exercise increases the activity of the trunk muscles and this increased activity would have a mechanically protective effect on the spine. Luoto et al (1995) examined 126 people who were free of back pain and followed them up 1 year later when 33 of them had developed LBP:

> The static back endurance test was found to be the only physical capacity measurement that indicated an increased risk for low-back pain. Adjusted for age, sex and occupation the odds ratio of a new low back pain in those with poor performance was 3.4 compared to those with medium or good performance.
>
> Luoto et al (1995)

Lee and his co-workers assessed and followed up 67 subjects who were free of back pain. After 5 years they found 18 new cases of LBP. The men who developed LBP were less involved in sport and both men and women who developed LBP showed a reduced trunk extension strength as compared with flexion strength. The authors conclude that an imbalance in trunk muscle strength might be a risk factor for LBP.

The spine requires muscular co-contraction to ensure spinal stability during everyday tasks. A weakness or an imbalance of the supporting

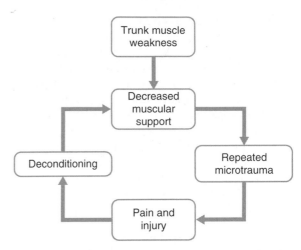

Figure 10.2 Trunk muscle weakness can lead to a chronic LBP cycle with reduced muscular support and increased microtrauma leading to pain and further deconditioning.

muscles of the spine will increase the risk of insult from the reactive forces resulting from normal activity. This can lead to repeated microtrauma or a fatigue failure of the neuromuscular system. Richardson et al (1999) have demonstrated a disorganized response of the abdominal muscles (notably transversus abdominis) in back-injured patients. Sihvonen et al (1997) report reduced multifidus activity and increased risk of segmental instability in subjects with chronic LBP. There is the opportunity for increasing chronicity with an initial trunk muscle weakness being exacerbated by microtrauma, deconditioning and increasing reduction in effective motor control of the trunk stabilizers (Fig. 10.2).

The understanding of the role of the trunk stabilizers in the aetiology of back pain and back pain chronicity is in its infancy. There is sufficient research to show that the subject is an important one and that improving strength and motor control of the trunk stabilizers is a vital part of managing LBP. We will explore this subject further in later sections.

VIBRATION

Whole body vibration (WBV) has been linked with increased incidence of back pain and development of chronicity. It is most significant when in the sitting position, where it accelerates disc, vertebral end-plate and muscle fatigue. It is mainly associated with driving and operating machinery. A NIOSH review of WBV (1997b) demonstrates positive associations between back disorders and vibration exposures with odds ratios of between 1.4 and 39.5, with many studies showing a dose–response relationship. Professions that demonstrated increased odds ratios for LBP were drivers of: buses, tractors, cranes, forklift trucks, earth-moving equipment, subway trains and cars. The highest odds ratios were for helicopter pilots.

Bonney (1995) describes the following recommendations to reduce the effects of vibration:

- reduce surface undulations
- good vehicle suspension and seat position
- reduce speed of travel, minimize exposure period, increase recovery time between exposures
- modify seat and controls to reduce awkward positions of the trunk. Use effective back support.

SMOKING

There is consistent evidence that LBP has been associated with smoking and that there is an increased likelihood of smokers developing chronic pain. Postulated mechanisms are:

- reduced circulation to tissues and delayed healing
- reduced disc oxygenation
- biomechanical strain of coughing.

The effects of smoking are not considered to be a major cause of back pain.

OBESITY

There is a consistent link between high body mass index and increased risk of back pain and back pain chronicity. There are obvious biomechanical reasons for this. The increased risk is considered to be minor.

PSYCHOSOCIAL FACTORS

There is evidence that psychosocial causes can be a factor influencing the incidence of LBP,

although their role appears to be a relatively minor one. In a much-quoted study of over 3000 Boeing aircraft workers, Bigos et al (1991) found that workers who 'hardly ever' enjoyed their tasks were 2.5 times more likely to report an injury than those who 'almost always' enjoyed their job tasks. This study caused a great deal of interest at the time, as job satisfaction was found to be the strongest factor for reporting a back injury. However, the Boeing study has been criticized for insufficient attention to personal physical workload (Krause et al 1998).

NIOSH (1997b) in a review of back disorders and psychosocial factors conclude:

- The studies reviewed suggest an association between back disorders and intensified workload as measured by indices of both perceived time pressure and workload. Four of the five studies found significant associations.
- Five of the seven studies that assess job satisfaction also found positive associations with back disorder.
- Limited support for an association with low back disorders and job control is also evident, while the evidence for a relationship between monotonous work and back disorders is mixed.
- These factors while statistically significant in some studies have only modest strength [risk ratios between 1.2 and 3.5].
- There remains a clear difficulty in separating the psychosocial effects from the biomechanical effects of these variables.

Many jobs are often physically demanding and monotonous or stressful, and it becomes difficult to separate the psychosocial stress from the ergonomic factors. People under stress tend to work longer periods in poorer postures with fewer breaks. Stress can also be the product of back injury, which can make people more likely to report a back pain episode or to give up work due to fear of exacerbation or reinjury.

In an award-winning paper that the authors claim to be 'the first prospective study of psychosocial job factors and reported spinal injuries with adequate control for current and past physical workload' (Krause et al 1998), the authors studied 1871 transit workers and concluded that:

Physical workload and psychosocial workload both independently predict spinal injury. Spinal injury was predicted by:

Psychological job demands – odds ratio (OR) 1.5

Job dissatisfaction – OR 1.56
Frequency of job problems – OR 1.52
Low supervisor support – OR 1.3.

These odds ratios were reasonably modest and were eclipsed by the physical workload odds ratios included in the study. In particular, working less than 30 h per week had a 2.7-times reduced injury risk compared to working full-time.

Psychosocial factors tend to be represented in the transition from acute to chronic incidence of LBP. Williams et al (1998) studied 82 males from a military medical centre suffering from first-episode LBP. They were assessed 2 months and 6 months after the initial episode, with the aim of assessing the extent to which job satisfaction predicts pain, psychological distress and disability at 6 months. The results showed that baseline job satisfaction scores significantly predicted outcome at 6 months beyond the variance expected by control factors. Williams et al (1998) concluded:

Satisfaction with one's job may protect against development of chronic pain and disability after

acute onset back pain and, alternatively, dissatisfaction may heighten risk of chronicity. Vocational factors should be considered in the rehabilitation of back pain.

When pain persists, nociceptive input becomes relatively less important as a cause of disability. There is a growing recognition that particular kinds of coping mechanisms and belief structures are important in predetermining psychological readjustments and the physical effects of chronic pain. It is thought that a patient's emotional and behavioural response to pain is determined by their appraisal of, and strategies for coping with, pain problems. Patients who believe they are able to control their pain, who avoid catastrophizing and who believe they are not severely disabled appear to function better than those who do not (Pfingsten et al 1997).

This subject of psychosocial aspects of musculoskeletal disorders and the mechanisms of musculoskeletal injury involved is more comprehensively reviewed in Chapter 6.

11

The type of injury

Not all back injuries are the same, nor should they be expected to recover at the same rate. Back injuries vary in type and severity, in the tissues affected, in the individual reaction to the injury and in the recovery environment. This is reflected in the presentation and the clinical history. Despite many years of research, there is still much that is unknown about the physiology of back injury. If an uncomplicated back injury was examined by six different practitioners one might diagnose a muscle strain, one might find a ligament injury, one might describe a spinal subluxation, one might diagnose a sacroiliac twist, one might take an X-ray and say there was nothing wrong, and the last might tell the patient they were somatasizing their psychosocial stress. They would all be looking at the injury from a particular viewpoint and all their diagnoses would contain an element of truth. There is no clear consensus on the injury process involved in the majority of cases of acute LBP. However, the majority of such cases are straightforward in clinical presentation, have no alarming symptoms and respond well to sensible treatment and management. The longer the period of active injury the more likely there are to be complications or barriers to recovery. The further down the referral network a practitioner is, the more likely that the more chronic and complex cases present. It is important to make a thorough and accurate assessment of a spinal injury, to monitor its recovery and continually to re-evaluate whether:

- recovery is reasonable for the injury
- there are any barriers to recovery
- anything can be done to enhance the recovery.

CAUSES OF BACK PAIN

Significant or unexpected load

This may be a heavy lift or trauma, providing a peak load in excess of the tissue capacity. In these cases there is likely to be some soft tissue damage – ligament and/or muscular injury – this should heal within a few weeks. Good management and appropriate manual therapy can accelerate the recovery phase and reduce the risk of recurrence or ongoing symptoms. If recovery is delayed there is likely to be a complicating factor (see Ch. 12) or a degree of secondary dysfunction, such as facet lock or soft tissue spasm with disturbance of normal joint mechanics and neurophysiological processes.

Cumulative load

Most spinal injuries are caused by loads that can normally be managed without injury. Repeated loading of the spine within its normal tolerance can lead to a reduction of the threshold for injury and subsequent development of symptoms. A sustained load on the spine, such as a long period of sitting, or stooping, may disturb good spinal mechanics and lead to a cumulative or minor trauma injury. The period of cumulative load can be a matter of minutes or it can be a cumulative period of many years. A cumulative loading injury will probably involve more joint dysfunction and degenerative change than a traumatic injury. The therapeutic and management approach will need to be more specific to address the dysfunction and the personal factors, and to modify the cumulative load.

Insidious onset

In many cases, patients cannot recall any significant exposures that may have caused their problem. This, of course, invites many further questions. Firstly, there is the possibility of a gradual pathological process. Secondly, there is the possibility of cumulative loading where there are no significant peak exposures that lead to a ready association with symptoms. Thirdly, there is more likely to be involvement of ergonomic, personal and psychosocial factors, which may contribute to the injury process. Successful management of this type of injury is likely to require specific attention to these individual factors.

It is in these latter two categories of cumulative load and insidious onset that there is more likely to be a transition from the acute to the chronic, ongoing case, and it is this area where the major improvements in case management are necessary.

RECOGNIZING CHRONIC LOW BACK PAIN

A small group of back pain sufferers do not respond readily to conservative management and manual medicine. For reasons that are not well understood they often go on to develop chronic pain and can become profoundly disabled. It is this small percentage that go on to provide the major expense in back-pain-related disability, and in particular the loss of wages and additional social security benefits associated with it.

Box 11.1 The author's experience

It was my misfortune to attract an inordinate number of these chronic back pain sufferers early in my career and I began looking for new models of management that might do more than provide short-term relief. In particular, I began to look at spinal loading history prior to injury – most of them seemed to be of insidious or minor trauma onset – and tried to reduce biomechanical load following injury, while using the classic therapy and rehabilitation approach to try and prevent relapse into dysfunction. I began to realize that chronic back pain was largely a cumulative problem and that early introduction of the appropriate biomechanical modifiers, combined with patient education and a willingness to adapt, could prevent chronicity. It also become clear to me that, to make an impact on chronic back pain disability, practitioners have to get out of their treatment rooms and into the real world where the injuries are happening. I have been teaching this approach to practitioners for some time and this book is a development of the clinical ergonomics courses I run. This approach and way of thinking about patients is not easy. It involves new parameters of thinking and getting out of the practitioner comfort zone, but it is exciting, challenging and rewarding.

I have found that 80–90% of acute low back pain sufferers will respond to traditional manual therapy.

continued

However, if the personal and environmental factors that created the problem continue, the injury is likely to be recurrent or chronic. Frequent recurrence can lead to chronicity. If the acute back pain has not returned to normal in 6–12 weeks (depending on the nature of the injury) it should be treated as a chronic back pain with a full ergonomic, psychosocial and personal review of risk factors.

I believe that therapists are the ideal people to undertake this review process:

● They have an understanding of musculoskeletal function and the injury process.
● They will have developed a relationship with the patient and an understanding of the nature of the injury.
● They have the opportunity to make an assessment of the injury and of the traumatized and dysfunctional tissues, and to relate these to the ergonomic exposures.
● They are in a position to pick-up the risk factors for the transition to chronicity at an early stage.
● They spend more time with their patients than the average GP.

Not all practitioners are happy to adopt this expanded role of their talents. Many are more comfortable working with the acute, clinic-based role. However, they should recognize the limitations of their approach and make early recommendations and appropriate referral to encourage early rehabilitation.

DIAGNOSTIC TRIAGE

The diagnostic triage has become an accepted method of categorizing LBP. It defines a spinal injury depending on the severity of symptoms and assists in providing appropriate resources depending on the type of injury. Most episodes of LBP will recover in a matter of days or weeks. This recovery can be accelerated by manual therapy, manipulation and appropriate management. The injury is likely to have recurrences of a similar nature. The process is predictable and readily managed and can be labelled simple back pain (see page 107).

Complex back pain

Failure to recover as expected or the presence of nerve root pain is likely to complicate the recovery process. This can be a pointer to degenerative or pathological complications such as disc pathology or spinal stenosis. These cases are also likely to recover with time but the recovery period may be longer and there are more likely to be ongoing symptoms. This category will require more active management and may require further investigations.

Back pain episodes lasting longer than 6 weeks are at greater risk of becoming chronic and developing into disability. These episodes are likely to be more complex with an increased risk of severe injury, degenerative change, disc pathology, nerve root involvement and psychosocial complications. It cannot be assumed that these cases will recover without more assertive management, hence the need for a more comprehensive treatment and management plan with greater resources. This category of patient – with complex back pain – is discussed in more detail in Chapter 12.

Red flags

There is always a risk that a person with back pain has a more serious medical condition. The risk of this is fairly small and there are usually clear clinical signals that indicate the risk. These are known as red flags. Waddell (1998) estimates that less than 1% are due to serious spinal disease, such as tumour or infection, and less than 1% are inflammatory, such as ankylosing spondylitis.

The presence of red flags does not mean that pathology is present but that there is an increased risk of pathology and this merits further investigation. Red flags associated with back pain include:

● features of the cauda equina syndrome – urinary retention, bilateral neurological symptoms and signs, saddle anaesthesia. These require urgent referral
● widespread or progressive neurological involvement
● significant weight loss
● history of cancer
● fever
● intravenous drug use
● prolonged steroid use
● first episode of pain over 50
● constant or progressive pain
● pain that is severe or unremitting with no relief.

For a thorough discussion of the use of clinical triage as a diagnostic and management tool, see Waddell (1998).

Simple back pain

Clinical findings

Despite large amounts of research and conjecture the precise nature of LBP is often difficult to ascertain. There are many sensitive structures within close proximity and attempts to isolate these and test them individually are difficult. Many areas of the spine are difficult to palpate or visualize with imaging. There are often a number of palpatory, mobility and positional findings and it can be difficult to decide which is the primary cause. There are frequently age-related or degenerative changes in the spine, and how much these are implicated in the injury process is a matter of considerable debate. Porterfield & DeRosa (1998) list the following as potential sources of pain:

- muscle – contusion, strain, overuse or spasm
- apophyseal joint – mechanical stress to cartilage or joint capsule and osteoarthrosis
- sacroiliac joint – mechanical stress to ligament or joint cartilage
- ligaments – trauma or mechanical strain
- spinal dura – compression by disc or inflammatory irritation
- intervertebral disc – the outer one-third of the disc is innervated and can be affected by mechanical or chemical stimuli
- dorsal root ganglion – mechanical pressure from osteophytes or disc bulge
- nerve root – compression or inflammatory irritation.

The disc, dura, dorsal root ganglion and nerve root are much more likely to be implicated in the more complex or chronic spinal problems than the uncomplicated back pain and will be dealt with in Chapter 12. Bogduk (1997) also describes vertebral bodies, periosteum, posterior elements and thoracolumbar fascia as possible sources of pain

Adams & Dolan (1995), who come from a more biomechanical background, summarize as follows:

Ligaments of the neural arch are most likely to be damaged by forward bending movements; the apophyseal joint surfaces by torsion and backwards bending; the vertebral body by compression and the disc by asymmetrical bending and compression, or following compressive damage to the vertebral body. The damage can occur during a single loading cycle simulating some accident such as a stumble or fall or in the process of fatigue failure where the forces remain below the level required for sudden failure.

On examination of simple LBP, there is remarkably poor diagnostic consensus. It may be that the main initiating injury becomes overtaken by subsequent events, such as a ligament/facet strain caused by repetitive flexion and twisting, and initiates a protective muscle spasm that causes muscular pain. The muscle spasm causes a secondary pelvic torsion and functional scoliosis, which leads to further mechanical strain and dysfunction. If this continues it is easy to see the sacroiliac ligaments becoming secondarily involved. Gradually, some neural sensitivity and even some disturbance in disc physiology complicate the picture further. Meanwhile, the initial soft tissue trauma may have resolved but the secondary dysfunction and deconditioning has become paramount.

It does seem that neuromuscular facilitation is an important part of the injury process but this may be secondary to other sources of nociceptive input. It seems that after a first back injury the spine is more sensitive to a repeat neuromuscular irritation. The threshold of neural reflex response is reduced and the nervous system retains a type of neural memory that more readily creates a reflex neuromuscular response at reduced levels of tissue irritation. Hence the increasing likelihood of recurrence of acute back pain at progressively lower levels of loading.

A prolonged period free of LBP seems gradually to reduce this neural sensitivity. However, this can be negated by subjects becoming more confident in their spinal mechanical loading! If only the conscious memory was as good as the neural memory.

Although the exact nature of the pathology remains uncertain, the patient with uncomplicated back pain will have a characteristic clinical picture. The pain will usually be in the central low back and sacral region. It may predominate on one side and spread into the pelvic or gluteal regions. The patient may describe some occasional referred pain or dull ache to one leg without a true nerve root compression. As the person improves, the pain usually becomes unilateral and more central. On standing examination the pelvis is elevated 1–3 cm on the painful side. The erector spinae and quadratus lumborum muscles will be tense and shortened on the painful side. There is often a functional scoliosis associated with the pelvic tilt, with a crowding in the lower lumbar region on the painful side causing a C-shaped scoliosis. Sometimes there is an attempt to lean away from the pain with the upper body, causing an S-shaped scoliosis. If sensitive neurological structures are involved, such as nerve roots or dura, there is often a lean forward and away from the painful side – the antalgic posture – with attempts to lean back to the midline exacerbating the pain. Sidebending towards the side of pain will further compress the facet joints, increasing pain. Backward bending towards the side of pain will further increase the pain. Sidebending away from the side of injury will usually ease the discomfort. Flexion and extension are usually painful at end range though in acute pain these may be very limited by pain and spasm (Fig. 11.1).

If there is a marked antalgic posture – leaning dramatically away from the side of pain – and attempts to lean back towards the midline cause acute pain, this is highly suggestive of a disc bulge or nerve root irritation. The antalgic lean is the body's natural mechanism to reduce the pressure on sensitive tissues such as the nerve root or dura on the injured side. These cases must be managed with care and every effort made to avoid increased disc or nerve root pressure – the disc is often unstable and in danger of prolapsing. Managed carefully these cases respond well, although the disc remains unstable for some weeks even after the pain has eased.

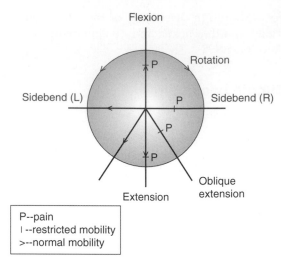

Figure 11.1 Recording of the typical mobility and pain pattern in an acute low back.

Supine examination. Hip and pelvic mobility and straight leg raising (SLR) test should be performed. Hip pathology is often confused with LBP and it should be tested for. Hip problems are a common cause of disturbed lumbopelvic rhythm and this should be tested for. The Fabere–Patrick test – a combination of flexion, abduction and external rotation – is the test of choice. Compare both sides. A positive test (limited mobility, with or without pain) is highly suggestive of hip joint degenerative change (Fig. 11.2).

Test hip rotation with the knee and hip flexed at 90 degrees. Test full hip flexion, flexion with circumduction and sacroiliac joint mobility while the hip is fully flexed. There may be some restriction of hip flexion and sacroiliac mobility on the painful side. In a subacute or chronic case there is usually shortening of the piriformis, tensor fascia lata and the deep hip rotator muscles, which can disturb the lumbopelvic rhythm.

On SLR, the hamstrings are usually reflexely shortened on the painful side. Tight hamstrings can limit hip flexion, sacroiliac mobility and lumbopelvic rhythm, which can be a risk factor for low back strain. On reaching the limit of easy leg raising, dorsiflexion of the foot stretches the sciatic nerve and markedly increased pain in the leg is indicative of nerve root involvement (Fig. 11.3). If there are positive nerve root signs

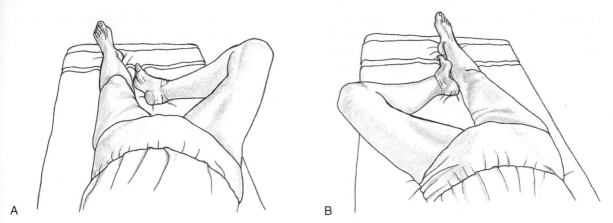

Figure 11.2 The Fabere–Patrick test is a reliable screen for hip pathology. The figure shows A: a positive test and B: a negative test in the same patient on the other side.

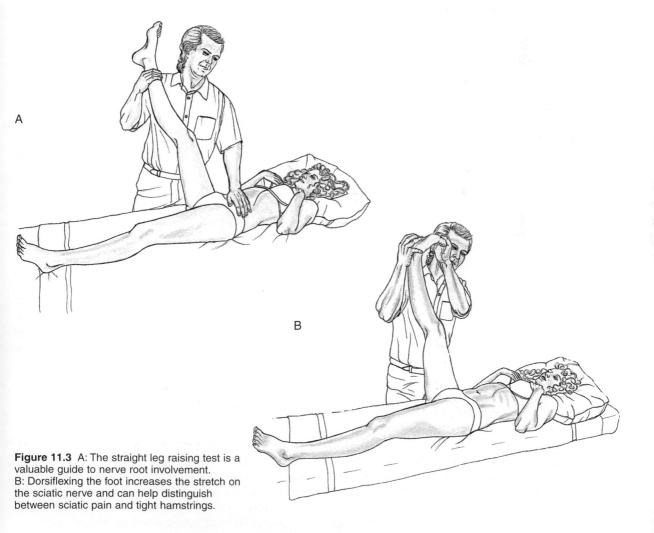

Figure 11.3 A: The straight leg raising test is a valuable guide to nerve root involvement. B: Dorsiflexing the foot increases the stretch on the sciatic nerve and can help distinguish between sciatic pain and tight hamstrings.

then test reflexes, resisted muscle strength and dermatome sensitivity (see Chapter 12). A reduced SLR test of 20 degrees or more, compared to the other side, suggests a more difficult prognosis (see Chapter 12).

With the patient lying prone, palpation will reveal much about the nature of the injury. Sometimes, lying an acute patient prone increases the facet joint compression which increases the muscle spasm, and they can have great difficulty getting off the treatment couch. This can be embarrassing! Placing the lumbopelvic region in a little flexion using a pillow underneath the lower abdomen avoids this problem. Palpation will reveal that the facilitated muscles – erector spinae, multifidus and quadratus lumborum – are usually worse on the affected side, with palpable trigger points at the level of injury. There will be tender interspinous ligaments, spinous processes and lumbar fascia at the site of the injury. The posterior superior iliac spine will be tender (insertion of iliocostalis and longissimus). If there is a significant pelvic torsion (it reduces in lying posture) there will be strain and tenderness through the sacroiliac ligaments, with some strain in the deep hip stabilizing muscles. Although the pathology is unclear, the injury probably involves one or more lumbar facet compressions with neuromuscular facilitation; 95% of these occur unilaterally at the L4–5–S1 joints. There may be some sacroiliac involvement and the thoracic spine can also be involved. In the absence of red flags, there is enough information to make a diagnosis and to begin therapy.

Management

Treatment should address the findings of the patient examination. This should include: soft tissue techniques to release the tight and shortened muscles; mobilization of the joint and its associated soft tissues; and restoration of normal joint function. Improved joint function will reduce the neuromuscular facilitation – the afferent barrage from the nociceptors and the mechanoreceptors which stimulate the splinting reflex which can be a significant cause of LBP. The vicious cycle starts to unwind.

Improving mobility will assist fluid dynamics and provide improved proprioceptive variation.

This assists in the recovery and desensitization of traumatized tissues. Manipulation can often produce a dramatic reduction in muscle spasm and an improvement in mobility. This can promptly restore pain-free mobility and normal pelvic balance in some cases. Manipulating an acute patient is tricky and requires great skill with sound clinical judgement. It should be used wisely by appropriately qualified practitioners.

Once the nature of the injury is understood the patient can be reassured as to its non-threatening nature and the appropriate management can be started. The patient is likely to make a prompt recovery, which will be facilitated by the addition of an enhanced placebo effect and an effective treatment. Patients should avoid bending and lifting and should minimize sitting postures. They should walk and remain active – not doing any one thing for too long as much as possible. They should avoid bed-rest and convalescence (the occasional 30-min rest excepted). All the available evidence shows that bed-rest delays, and activity enhances, recovery. Activity seems to improve circulation, stretch muscles and provides inproved proprioceptive functioning. Ice packs can reduce inflammation, provide pain relief and enhance recovery. Exercises are valuable to stretch the shortened and tense muscles, to restore joint mobility and to improve joint function. They also provide valuable biofeedback to a patient about the degree of muscle tension and help the person feel they have some control over the symptoms. Exercises should be specific to the person and the clinical findings. There is much debate as to the merits of gentle, rhythmic or ballistic stretches. They all have their uses and the type of exercise and the context are the key factors. In the acute stage exercises should be designed to:

- improve comfort, stretch and unload injured muscles
- improve function.

Improving comfort, stretching and unloading injured tissues usually involves movement to ease and reduce symptoms, emphasizing movements away from the sensitized tissues. This type of exercise will also encourage fluid flow and reduce sustained nociception or proprioception.

The most common helpful exercises that decrease load on the injured tissues are:

- Sidebending against a wall (Fig. 11.4). If there is a facet lock, muscle spasm or referred nerve root pain, sidebending with the painful side towards the wall will help to unload and stretch the tissues on the injured side. The exercise is performed standing an arm's length away from the wall, with the painful side towards the wall. The patient leans against the wall with the arm slightly bent at shoulder height; the other hand is placed on the pelvis. The pelvis is gently sidebent towards the wall while using a counterpressure with the other arm at shoulder height. This action is gently repeated about five times in a rhythmical rocking action. It should always feel comfortable and pain free (otherwise don't do it!). It should be done at least five times per day, or sometimes every hour – particularly if the person has to sit a lot. It can give considerable relief and reduces the tendency to relapse. In the acute stage it will ease the pain when performed with the painful side towards the wall and increase the pain if the painful side is away from the wall (it increases facet compression). It should be performed unilaterally on the side that reduces the pain. After 2 or 3 days it usually becomes possible to perform pain free both sides. Occasionally, in some cases of disc involvement, sidebending with the injured side towards the wall can increase the pain. It depends on the anatomical location of the disc bulge. In this case it is advisable to reverse the exercise to the painful side toward the wall only if it can be performed pain free.

- Bilateral knee hugging (Fig. 11.5) with knees to chest with a gentle rocking action will help unload the facet joints, stretch the spinal extensors and open the intervertebral foramen without creating significant shear force.

- Extension exercises can also be beneficial. The extension recovery position (Fig. 11.6) provides an effective method of relieving intervertebral disc pressure without creating too much compression on the posterior elements.

Exercises that improve function in subacute cases, or once the very acute symptoms are subsiding, try to restore normal joint and soft tissue mobility and improve biomechanical functioning. Helpful exercises are:

- Bilateral sidebending against a wall.
- Unilateral knee hugging (Fig. 11.7), which will stretch the gluteal muscle and mobilize the sacroiliac joint. Variations of these will also stretch the deep hip rotator muscles.

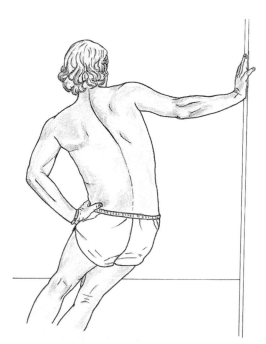

Figure 11.4 Sidebending against the wall is a very effective exercise to help unload and decompress the injured tissues on the side of injury.

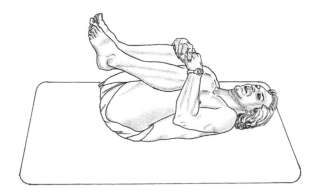

Figure 11.5 Bilateral knee hugging with a gentle rocking action releases the facet joints, opens the intervertebral foramina and stretches the spinal extensors. 30 s to 1 min regularly throughout day.

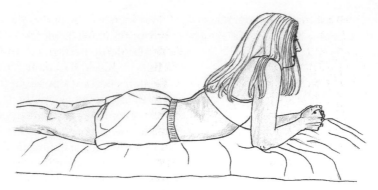

Figure 11.6 The extension recovery position can unload the intervertebral disc and assist disc nutrition and disc recovery. It should be performed for a few minutes at a time two to three times per day at lunchtime and after work, or following periods of disc compression. It is best performed on a carpet where some traction can be gained between the elbows and the lower limbs.

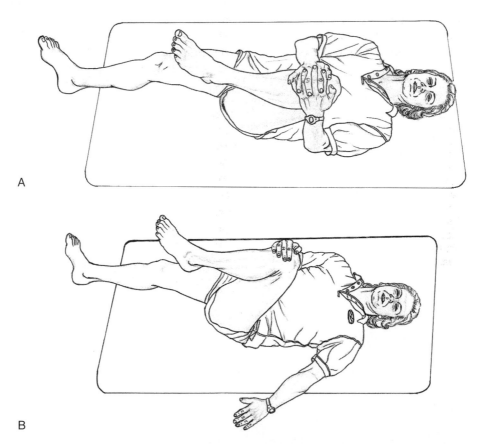

A

B

Figure 11.7 Knee hugging is a valuable exercise for pelvic and sacroiliac joint strain. It should be performed on the painful leg with the other leg fully extended. It should be held for 5 seconds and repeated 3–5 times in each position, approx three times per day. The figure shows A: full hip flexion, B: full hip flexion plus adduction and C: full hip flexion, adduction and external rotation.

Fig. 11.7C, see opposite.

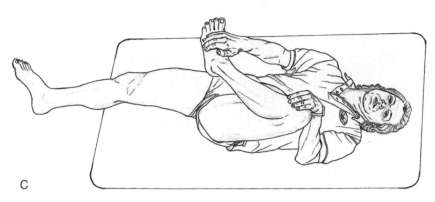

C

Figure 11.7 *continued*

- Rhythmic rotation – standing (Fig. 11.8) or sitting (Fig. 11.9), supine rotation.
- Extension exercises – (as advocated by McKenzie) must be done with care. Magnusson et al (1998) demonstrated that hyperextension significantly improved disc height recovery

compared with the prone posture, while Adams et al (1994) found peak compressive stress loading of the posterior annulus, and risk of injury of the neural arch, with hyperextended postures. Anything stronger than the extension recovery position must be done with

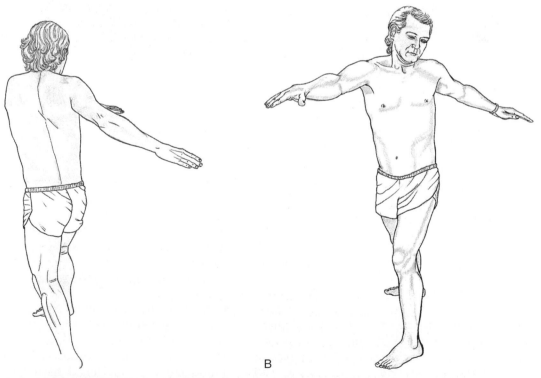

A   B

Figure 11.8 A, B: Active rotation in the standing position will help spinal rotation and coordination. The feet should be slightly turned in 30–50 cm apart. The weight of the arms can be used as levers for a rhythmic rotation action. Active rotation should be performed regularly throughout the day for 30 s to 1 min each time. In the rehabilitation stage small weights can be added to the hands to increase leverage which improves muscle strength and coordination.

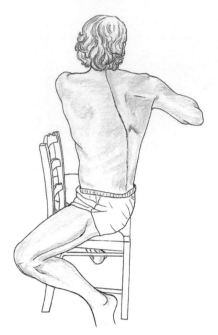

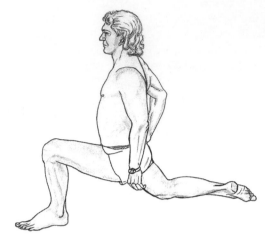

Figure 11.10 Pelvic extension stretch is useful for psoas spasm or anterior pelvic and thigh pain. The affected leg should be placed posterior to the body with the hand on the same side stabilizing the pelvis. Gently increasing flexion on the opposite knee with a rocking action completes the stretch. Perform regularly throughout the day for up to 30 s.

Figure 11.9 Rotation of the spine in the sitting position. A rhythmic rotation from side to side, with a double stretch at each limit of rotation. About ten times each side. This particularly targets upper lumbar and thoracic spine and can be done regularly throughout the day.

care and is not recommended if there is nerve root involvement.

- Hip and pelvic extension (Fig. 11.10) is very useful when there is psoas muscle spasm or referred femoral nerve symptoms.

The patient will usually respond promptly to this approach of manual therapy and exercise and should be much improved after two or three treatments. At this stage, any predisposing bio-mechanical factors that may have influenced the injury can start to be addressed. A hypermobile person who finds it relatively easy to move into extreme joint postures might be given inner-range resisted exercises to improve joint stability and coordination. A hypomobile person who has difficulty gaining range of movement might be given mobility exercises to improve this. Any muscle imbalances, such as weak abdominals or tight hamstrings, should be identified and addressed. Exercises should be shown and checked with the patient and some form of handout given as a reminder. Exercises work

very well if prescribed appropriately but the effect is fairly short-term – as long as the patient continues the exercises.

If the injury is thought to have been caused by overexposing the tissues to mechanical strain, this needs to be addressed. Frequency, duration and/or force of exposure should be reduced and the patient advised on proper lifting technique, sitting posture, etc. The occasional visit to a worksite is very beneficial for both patients and practitioners.

The nature of this category of LBP is that it is likely to be recurrent. The practitioner should aim at reducing the incidences of recurrence and the risk of developing chronicity. They should also try and educate the patient so they can manage some of their own risk factors.

Treatment summary for simple back pain

- Release tight or spasmed muscles.
- Mobilize compressed or stiff joints.
- Manipulation, if appropriate.
- Exercises to unload sensitive tissues, to stretch and mobilize shortened tissues or restricted joint movement.
- Encourage normal activity and postural vari-ation while avoiding extreme or sustained

joint postures. Limit forward bending, lifting and sitting postures.

- Be proactive about education, rehabilitation and ergonomic improvements.
- Low back pain sufferers are not a homogenous group and each patient should be carefully investigated and followed up to ensure an appropriate management regimen is prescribed.

The management of simple back pain is usually straightforward. Unless there are dramatic clinical signs, neurological symptoms or a failure to respond as expected, there is little point in undergoing extensive investigation or imaging, as this is not usually helpful in managing simple back pain. Most people will develop occasional episodes of LBP and most will recover with or without treatment. The role of the practitioner is to facilitate this recovery, to encourage early return to normal activities, to minimize pain and disability and to reduce risk of recurrence or relapse. Chapter 12 provides significantly more detail regarding the understanding of the LBP pathological process and the management techniques.

12

Complex low back pain

The more complex back pain episode may arise from a number of different scenarios:

- A significant trauma giving rise to a more severe or complex symptom picture.
- A simple back pain episode that fails to respond as expected and is still significant after 6 weeks – less than 50% recovery.
- The presence of nerve root involvement. This is more likely to have a structural cause, such as a disc pathology or degenerative change, and should always be treated more seriously.
- A chronic back pain that never really goes away, although it may wax and wane in severity. If a person's daily activities are modified or restricted due to back pain, or fear of back pain, the condition will be more complex than simple back pain.

A case that is defined as 'complex' will require a more active management approach than simple back pain – the natural healing process cannot be relied upon to effect a full recovery and there is an increased risk of chronicity or disability.

This type of injury justifies increased use of resources and a more comprehensive management strategy to try and avoid chronicity. The case history and physical examination will need to be more thorough with a neurological assessment of reflexes, muscle strength and dermatomes of the lower limb (Table 12.1, Fig. 12.1).

Gross mobility changes have been shown to have a poor relationship to disability or pain assessment. However, unilateral changes in mobility have shown better correlations.

Table 12.1 A summary of neurological tests and their relevant nerve roots

Test		Nerve root involvement
Reflexes	Quadriceps	L3–4
	Achilles	S1–2
Muscles	Hip flexors	L2–3
	Quadriceps	L3–4
	Anterior tibialis	L4
	Hamstrings	L4–5
	Extensor hallucis longus	L5
	Peroneals	S1–2
	Gastroc/soleus	S1–2
Sensory	Anterior thigh	L4
	Medial leg/foot	L4–5
	Lateral leg/foot	L5
	Sole	S1

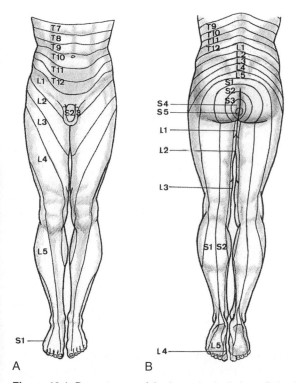

Figure 12.1 Dermatomes of the lower body. A: front; B: back.

Straight leg raising (SLR) tests side differences of greater than 20 degrees; pain in the leg or numbness/diminished sensitivity in the foot have been shown to be predictive of sick leave (Viikari-Juntura et al 1998).

The more severe sciatic symptoms with the SLR test below 30 degrees, a positive contralateral SLR test, pain on coughing or sneezing, with neurological deficit, is suggestive of extruded intervertebral disc prolapse (Jonsonn 1996).

Most cases of complex back pain should be given a standard anteroposterior (AP) and lateral X-ray. This will assist in ruling out pathology and provide some assessment of the degree of degenerative change and any anatomical variations such as scoliosis and sacralization. If there is profound neurological deficit, and if these are progressive or bilateral, a computerized tomography (CT) scan or magnetic resonance imaging (MRI) scan should be performed to provide more detail about the compromised nerve roots. It is not usually necessary to undertake CT or MRI scans with a nerve root entrapment that has a logical injury history and is making gradual progress.

The presence of nerve root signs does not necessarily mean that these are the entire explanation for the symptoms. Other tissues may have been injured and there is likely to be a significant level of joint dysfunction due to disturbed posture and muscle spasm. Manual therapy can address these changes and give considerable relief. Treatment should be directed at unloading the segment where the nerve root entrapment exists, opening the interverterbral foramen and stretching and mobilizing the affected segment to improve mobility and encourage fluid exchange. Manipulation can often be helpful, although it must be used with care and every effort made to avoid compression or torsion of the compromised disc and nerve root.

The treatment and management of the complex back pain is more demanding than that of simple back pain. The case history is usually more complex and clinical examination and investigation needs to be more thorough. The patient is often alarmed at the symptoms and sometimes depressed at the severity and apparent intractability of the problem. It is very important that the practitioner gives patients confidence so that they understand the nature of the injury and have the skills to treat and manage it appropriately. It is important to establish a realistic expectation of the duration of the recovery process. Where there is significant neurological involvement, patients should be advised to expect improvement of about 10% a week. In reality they usually respond more quickly initially (and are usually pleasantly surprised), and then more gradually. It is important to make patients realize early on that their cooperation can enhance recovery, and to provide them with the knowledge and the skills to optimize this. In the typical disc problem with nerve root impairment this will include:

- avoiding anterior spinal compression – bending and sitting
- frequent postural variation
- regular sidebending exercises
- neural stretching exercises
- some type of graduated general exercise such as walking or swimming as soon as symptoms allow.

If patients have to bend or twist as part of their work duties, use of a spinal brace can minimize lumbar flexion in the short term – use of these should not be prolonged. If patients have to sit for long periods in working postures they should be advised about seating that minimizes anterior spinal compression, such as kneeler chairs, forward tilt seats, lumbar support (see Chapter 13). Clinics can have chairs and appliances to loan to patients to help them with their recovery.

Once the treatment process has begun, the practitioner must pay attention to any possible factors that may be inhibiting progress or providing barriers to recovery. The LOAD model and the plateau philosophy (see Chapters 1–4) cover the importance of identifying the personal, psychosocial and ergonomic factors as part of the management. There is some urgency to gain a platform for recovery before the features of chronicity become dominant – the longer a person is off work, the more difficult it becomes to effect a return to work.

A simple back pain episode that has not been treated with manual therapy may well still have significant symptoms, with evidence of dysfunction, at 6 weeks. Manual therapy should be commenced forthwith and the likelihood

remains that it will respond uneventfully. Manual therapy is more likely to be successful early in the episode, before the physiological and psychosocial changes of chronicity become established.

A simple back pain episode that has responded slowly to manual therapy, but has improved at least 50% in pain and disability, is likely to continue to improve and may not need more concerted management, although further attention should be given to identify barriers to recovery. A back injury that has improved less than 50% in 6 weeks, despite good quality manual therapy, or where the patient is still unable to return to work, should be fully assessed. Every attempt should be made to identify barriers to recovery and to create a positive rehabilitation environment. Patients should be actively involved in the investigative process, so that they benefit from the educational process and learn tools for increased self-responsibility.

A patient with longstanding, chronic LBP without remittance is less likely to make a dramatic improvement with manual therapy and more likely to have ongoing symptoms. In such a case, the emphasis will be on management of the injury and improving the quality of life. The LOAD model here provides the framework of the management process. It is important to recognize these cases and to manage them appropriately, making a realistic prognosis and emphasizing patient cooperation and involvement. There are many features of a chronic pain problem that can be assisted and quality of life and degree of disability can be substantially improved.

It is important that the practitioner looks at the loading and injury history of patients with back pain. Patients with acute pain but without neurological pain complications generally recover very promptly; 80% of new patients with LBP require five treatments or less. Patients with neurological involvement are more likely to have complications and the recovery rate is often slower, usually requiring 5–10 visits.

By definition, complex back pain is more likely to have complicating factors that increase the complexity of treatment and management. It is important that the practitioner understands the nature of these complexities, and their physiological influences, and develops appropriate management strategies for dealing with them.

WORK STATUS

Return to work is a priority. Initially, this may be in a modified form, with reduced hours or light duties. It may require some rehabilitation equipment, such as a special chair or back support. If a work-related cause is suspected, or if there is a difficulty coping with a normal workload, a full work assessment should be carried out in an attempt to identify and minimize as many risk factors that contribute to the exposure as possible. For example, the frequency, weight and height of lifts could be reduced, work variety and breaks could be increased, lifting technique could be improved. All the research suggests that maintaining normal activity and socialization enhances recovery, and that convalescence and activity avoidance delays recovery. Some patients may become quite psychologically disturbed, with symptom magnification, if required to take time off work.

The above approach presupposes a cooperative employer who has some awareness of the recovery process. Unfortunately, an injury to an employee can sometimes create or exacerbate an existing difficult work environment. Injured workers, who are aware that they are not able to manage a normal workload, may lack the confidence to deal effectively with this. These situations can require great diplomacy from the practitioner or GP. The patient must be encouraged to be assertive and attempt to resolve the situation as soon as possible. The practitioner may be able to provide supporting letters and documentation.

A difficult psychosocial environment at work can be a major reason for delayed recovery, chronicity and failure to improve. The stress involved may delay or complicate recovery and the patient may seek to avoid the distressing prospect of returning to work by symptom magnification. Methods of circumventing these complications and encouraging an early return to work in some capacity are a priority.

DEGENERATIVE CHANGE

Age-related degenerative changes of the lumbar spine are a normal occurrence. The presence, if in keeping with the age of the subject, is not a sign of pathology, nor is it necessarily a cause of pain. However, the presence of degenerative change suggests that the spine is less able to loadbear efficiently, has a lower injury threshold and is of greater injury risk than the youthful spine. Degenerative changes of the spine can be accelerated by heavy work, trauma and mechanical disadvantage, such as asymmetry. Degenerative changes are more common at the lower two lumbar vertebrae, which have higher biomechanical exposure. The effects of age-related degenerative change are:

Intervertebral disc.
- Reduced synthesis of proteoglycans and reduced water binding capacity.
- Increase in collagen content of the nucleus and annulus, and reduction in elastin in the annulus. There is less distinction between the annulus and the nucleus.
- The disc becomes stiffer, with reduced ability to transmit and dissipate weight.
- The annulus takes a greater share of compressive load and becomes increasingly defibrillated.
- The discs change shape with increasing anterior/posterior diameter, some loss of height at the circumference, although this is partly compensated by increase in convexity at the upper and lower surfaces at the expense of the vertebral bodies.

Vertebral end plates. The end plates become thinner with occlusion of the vascular channels causing a decrease in perfusion of nutrients into the nucleus.

Vertebral body.
- There is a decrease in bone density and weakening of the trabeculae system, particularly at the centre of the vertebral body.
- The vertebral end plate can bow into the weakened vertebral body.
- Osteophytes project from the cortical bone to reinforce the annulus.

Facet joints.

- As the disc changes structure and function the facet joints receive an increasing proportion of load.
- The articular cartilage increases in thickness but progressively defibrillates in the zones of high stress.
- The subchondral bone becomes thinner.
- Osteophytes develop along the attachments of the joint capsule.

Bogduk (1997) describes these degenerative changes as:

A reactive and adaptive change that seeks to compensate for biomechanical aberrations. The process is active and purposeful and does not warrant the description of a degenerative process. ... The development of osteophytes is only a natural response to the altered mechanics of the lumbar spine in turn due to more fundamental biochemical changes in the intervertebral disc. Consequently spondylosis should not be viewed as a disease, but an expected morphological change with age.

There seems to be widespread support for this view. There seems to be no clear relationship between the existence of degenerative change and the presence of pain. The effect of ageing of the vertebral segment, with the gradual dehydration and stiffening of the disc, seems to protect against the likelihood of prolapsed discs, which occur most frequently in relatively young, well-hydrated discs. However, the difference between age-related changes and pathological changes is not clearly demarcated and the active and purposeful change can be remarkably imprecise, with osteophytic encroachment into the spinal canal or intervertebral foramen being a clear cause of symptoms. The degenerative change does suggest that the vertebral segment has been compromised and will be less efficient at dissipating mechanical strain – it will be more prone to trauma or overuse. An accelerated degenerative change, particularly if it is more advanced at one segment than neighbouring segments (a common finding), will suggest that there is a reason for this – previous injury, heavy workload or a combination of the two. Videman et al (1990), in a study of 86 cadaveric specimens,

found that a history of back injury was related to symmetric disc degeneration, annular ruptures and vertebral osteophytosis. He also found that these changes were related to the highest and lowest (sedentary work) degrees of physical loading, with the least pathology stemming from moderate or mixed loading.

While some age-related change is normal, it is also a signal of reduced loading capacity and predisposition to injury. If the changes remain uniform and symmetrical they can be regarded as normal. However, unilateral or uneven patterns of change should be regarded as an accelerated or pathological change. Asymmetrical disc degenerative change, i.e. delaminating and fissuring of the posterolateral annulus, and precocious disc degenerative change, can be major risk factors for chronic back pain. The relatively fluid disc with high peak disc pressures can breach the normally tough annular wall by either bulge or extrusion of nucleus pulposus. Repetitive loading of degenerated discs shows reduced fatigue resistance than normal discs. The risk for injury occurs at lower loads with fewer cycles. There seems little doubt that most of the severe and chronic back injuries are associated with disc pathology (Hofmann 1995).

Cumulative load

Figure 1.1 (p. 5) illustrates that the majority of cases of low back pain are insidious or are caused by a relatively minor event. The traumatically induced back pain is readily recognizable and does not usually represent a diagnostic challenge. The obvious traumatic injury, that represents perhaps 25% of back pain cases, does not provide a management challenge as the nature of the injury is obvious and the need to avoid the trauma or peak exposure that created it is largely common sense. However, the frequent occurrence of minor trauma and insidious injuries are a major concern. Even if effective therapeutic techniques are developed, without an understanding of the genesis of the injury, and the circumstances that created the injury process, the majority of back pain sufferers will be left in the dark, with little ability to manage their own risk.

This leads to a lack of confidence in their musculoskeletal system and is likely to lead to poor management and disability behaviour by LBP patients.

Chapters 1–4 dealt with the cumulative cause of injuries, including the muscle fatigue and the neurological sensitization process. These are equally true for LBP and the LOAD model can very profitably be used for management of chronic or recurrent back pain. However, the spine is a much more complex biomechanical structure than the peripheral joints and has a bewildering array of ligaments, muscles, nerves and joints. These are subject to much higher loads than the peripheral joints and the injury mechanisms are correspondingly more complex. The effect of repetitive loading on reducing muscular and neurological fatigue thresholds was discussed in Chapter 5. There is considerable evidence to suggest that repetitive cumulative loading can also alter intervertebral disc and vertebral end-plate integrity.

The spine is beautifully designed to cope with these stresses under normal biomechanical and physiological environment. However, in today's rapidly changing society the environment is frequently not normal, with added complications such as poor or constrained postures, vibrations, etc. These can lead to biomechanical and physiological alterations in the way our musculoskeletal structures cope, adapt and recover from different workloads. These altered processes can be injury promoting. Into this cocktail we must also add the effects of ageing and degenerative changes of the spine that can also alter spinal tolerance for musculoskeletal loading. Understanding these complex injury processes and managing the risk of injury will be the key to controlling the escalating incidence of back pain disability. In the words of Kumar (1990): 'This may be one of the reasons why injuries precipitate only after a combination of degeneration derangement and magnitude of load has been reached'.

Kumar investigated 161 institutional aides and found a point prevalence of back pain of 62%. There was no significant difference between the pain group and the no-pain group in age, body weight, height and recreational physical activity.

The main difference between the two groups was in cumulative biomechanical exposure:

- The cumulative spinal compressive load was significantly higher in the pain group.
- The mean duration of work prior to the onset of the first back pain episode was higher than the mean duration of work for the no-pain group.
- The cumulative load of the pain group was significantly higher than that of the no-pain group.

Kumar concluded: 'These observations clearly suggest that cumulative load exposure predisposes the spine to pain and/or injury and is therefore a risk factor'.

Kumar went on to suggest that the spine has a threshold level for injury precipitation and that it should be possible to identify the zone of cumulative load that predisposes the spine to injury.

Norman et al (1998) made a sophisticated analysis of spinal loading in automobile industry workers, comparing 104 LBP cases to 130 controls. They found four factors that separated cases from controls:

- peak spinal load
- cumulative spinal load
- peak flexion velocity
- usual hand force.

Workers who were in the top 25% for these risk factors were six times more likely to report LBP than those in the bottom 25%. Peak and cumulative loads emerged as independent risk factors.

The effects of cumulative loading are related to different types of loading and how these affect spinal physiology.

Punnett et al (1991) compared 95 cases of recorded back injuries in an automobile plant to 124 randomly selected workers free of back pain. Their jobs were analysed for posture and lifting requirements. The cases with recorded back injuries were related to the following work postures:

- mild trunk flexion (less than 45 degrees), odds ratio 4.9

- severe trunk flexion (more than 45 degrees), odds ratio 5.7
- trunk twist or lateral bend (more than 20 degrees), odds ratio 5.9.

The risk of back injury increased with exposure to multiple postures and with duration of exposure. Non-occupational factors such as gender, age, prior injury, medical history or recreational activities were not implicated. The effect of postural stress seemed to be greater than the effect of lifting.

The effect of mild flexed postures seemed to be surprisingly high compared to severe flexed postures, which biomechanical models would predict to show a greater increase in injury risk. Punnett suggests that this non-linear increase suggests that physiological effects of posture are important in addition to the biomechanical effects.

These well-designed studies show that it is the exposure to non-neutral postures and cumulative load that are key risk factors for back injury in manual work. They highlight that the loading history can alter the physiological processes that render the spine more susceptible to injury at lower thresholds of biomechanical loading.

The most chronic back problems are usually associated with disc disturbance. A study of 451 patients suffering from chronic low back pain (Hofmann et al 1995), with no history of previous surgery, were investigated using MRI or CT scan. In 77% one or more disc prolapses/protrusions were diagnosed, the majority at L4–5 or L5–S1. Significantly enhanced odds ratios were found for metal workers, mechanics, construction workers and nurses. Some studies have found evidence of a significant number of disc disorders in asymptomatic subjects in up to 35% of cases when examined by CT or MRI. Clearly, disc disorders do not always produce pain, there are other factors also involved. However, it is likely that a spine exhibiting disc disorders on imaging would be very prone to biomechanical overload.

In order to understand chronic spinal problems it is important to understand the effect of injury on the intervertebral disc and how the degenerative or ageing disc responds to biomechanical load. The difference between a symptomatic and an asymptomatic individual is often not the presence of degenerative change but the biomechanical loading that the compromised tissue has been subjected to.

Intervertebral disc injury

The disc has a daunting task. It combines the following roles:

- shock absorber, which accepts, dissipates and transfers loads onto neighbouring tissues
- ligamentous structure, which allows mobility but also limits mobility and creates spinal stability
- mobile container of a pressurized semi-fluid.

The intervertebral disc has a unique structure that allows it to perform these tasks with great efficiency under difficult circumstances. The nucleus is 70–85% water and also contains chondrocytes, proteoglycans and a loosely bound collagen network. The cell density is not uniform throughout the disc. It has highest concentrations at the end plate and near the periphery of the annulus where fluid diffusion is greatest. The function of the cells is to manufacture and maintain the collagen, proteoglycans and cell matrix. The proteoglycans have electrochemical properties that attract fluid and create a high internal osmotic pressure. This high pressure is resisted by muscular and ligamentous structures to create a preloaded state. Compressive pressure on the disc is dissipated by the fluid-like nucleus onto the surrounding structures (Fig. 12.2). Thus, the efficiency of the disc depends on the ability of the nucleus to maintain its internal milieu and the structural integrity of the container of the nucleus – the annulus and vertebral end plates.

The high internal pressure of the disc renders a normal arterial blood pressure ineffective. Disc nutrition is dependent on fluid exchange, predominantly through the ventral end plate and secondarily through the annulus. This fluid exchange is enhanced by loading and unloading compressive forces on the disc, creating a pumping effect as the fluid is squeezed out and then sucked in. Any fluid pressure less than the

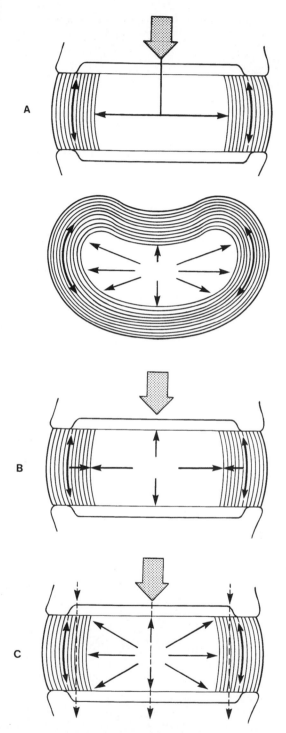

Figure 12.2 The fluid-like nucleus dissipates compressive forces over the outer structure of the disc – the annulus and the vertebral end plates. Reproduced with permission from Bogduk (1997).

standing erect posture tends to allow fluid to be drawn in, while any pressure greater than the standing posture, such as stooping, slouching or bending, tends to squeeze fluid out. Cyclic loading is therefore essential for the health of the disc and to facilitate the fluid exchange. Degenerative changes in the disc – reduced cell volume, reduced proteoglycans synthesis and dehydration of the disc – may be accentuated by the loading history and its influence on fluid dynamics and cell nutrition. Adams et al (1996) showed that when cadaveric discs were creep-loaded in flexion to simulate manual work or driving, the fluid loss from the nucleus caused a transfer of load from the nucleus to the annulus, with localized peaks of compressive stress appearing in the posterior annulus. They concluded that: 'Stress concentrations may lead to pain, structural disruption and alteration in chondrocyte metabolism. Disc mechanics depends on loading history as well as applied load'.

Degenerative changes in the disc start to interfere with the ability to dissipate compressive load. This inefficient loading of the disc allows accumulation of peak loads to portions of the disc that renders them more liable to injury.

The high internal pressure of the disc is one reason why there is an absence of nerve endings in the centre of the disc. Research has demonstrated the presence of nerve endings in the outer one-third of the annulus, although the role of these remains uncertain. The minimal neural representation may be a reason why there seems to be few warning signals from metabolic fatigue or mechanical dysfunction in the disc. Clinically, we often find that, despite the presence of a damaged disc, there are no symptoms until the outer layer of the annulus has been disrupted. Frequently, the most significant pain of a disc injury is in the affected tissues neighbouring the disc, such as the dura or the nerve root, rather than the disc itself. Muscles and ligaments tend to produce pain when they are fatigued or stretched but the discs do not seem to have a mechanism to provide us with these warning signs and this often results in injury-promoting postures. It is relatively common to find that the first sign of a back injury is a major disc disruption with an extruded disc, nerve root pain and neurological deficit – there has been minimal warning of premature disc disruption. This is a dramatic injury, which takes time to recover from, despite the best of treatment and management. The extruded nuclear material, with its affinity for attracting water, will swell to two or three times its size in the next 24–36 h, and will often cause nerve root compression at the next most caudal nerve root. In a large extrusion, multiple nerve root involvement is common.

Jonsson & Stromqvist (1996) examined 200 patients prior to spinal surgery and compared their symptoms to the type of disc protrusion seen at surgery. The types of disc herniation were classified as extrusion/sequestration, prolapse or focal. The focal and the prolapse were both contained, the focal being the least severe and the prolapse involving the disc material sequestered through the major part of the annulus fibrosus. Extruded and sequestered were defined as non-contained with the nucleus pulposus extruded through the entire annulus fibrosus and longitudinal ligament. They summarized their findings:

There was no significant difference concerning pain at rest or at night related to herniation. Pain on coughing was more common in extruded/ sequestered herniation. Use of analgesics as well as severe reduction in walking capacity was more common in patients with extrusion/sequestration. The highly restricted SLR test as well as the crossed positive SLR test were significantly more common in patients with extrusion/sequestration, and this was also true for the incidence of relevant reflex/extensor hallucis longus and sensory disturbance. In conclusion the clinical appearance of lumbar disc herniation was most aggressive in extruded and sequestered disc herniation. The symptoms and signs in disc protrusion were less severe whereas patients with prolapse had intermediate appearance concerning symptoms and signs.

Jonsson & Stromqvist (1996)

While the mechanical explanation of a disc protrusion causing nerve impingement has a nice logic to it, there is also evidence that a significant proportion of the pain of a disc injury comes from inflammatory reaction. Porterfield & DeRosa (1998) describe it succinctly:

Extruded nuclear material appears to be a noxious agent causing axonal degeneration and damage to the myelin-forming Schwann cells of the axons through complex biochemical reactions. In both instances, the biochemical milieu lowers the threshold for mechanical stimulation, especially in the pain-sensitive tissues within proximity of the herniated discal material, such as the posterior longitudinal ligament, outer aspect of the annulus, dural sheath of the nerve root, and epidural vasculature. Disc disruption obviously involves a disruption of the biochemical balance within the spinal canal.

In an animal study, Yabuki et al (1998) found that application of nucleus pulposus to nerve root increased endoneural fluid pressure and decreased blood flow in the dorsal root ganglia. The authors suggest that exposure of nerve roots to nucleus pulposus could establish a compartment syndrome in the dorsal root ganglia. This type of dramatic disc injury is more likely in the younger disc (aged 20–45), where the nucleus is more fluid. Older discs, aged over 50, have been almost impossible to prolapse in experimental conditions on cadaveric specimens. However, the older discs with the more viscous nucleus are less able to absorb compression forces, creating peak stresses on the posterolateral aspect of the annulus and leading to a progressive radial bulge (Fig. 12.3) when biomechanically challenged. This type of injury is more likely to respond to appropriate management without the inflammatory complications, but it is also more likely to recur.

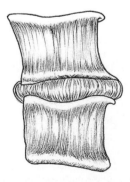

Figure 12.3 The more mature disc (over age 50) is less prone to nuclear extrusion but more likely to produce a radial bulge of the annular wall.

The low vascularity of the disc provides a poor environment for recovery of injury. Recovery will be enhanced by active rehabilitation and rhythmic exercise to maximize fluid transfer through the disc and spinal canal. There is evidence that a damaged disc never fully returns to its preinjury integrity. Once a disc has been compromised it becomes less efficient as a shock absorber and will tend to become progressively degenerative.

Gradual disc prolapse

In a series of experiments, Adams and colleagues have subjected cadaveric vertebral units to different combinations of loading, demonstrating that there are different types of disc prolapses under different biomechanical conditions. Adams & Hutton (1982) reproduced acute disc prolapse by a single high compressive load attached to a hyperflexed disc. Adams & Hutton (1985) subjected cadaveric discs to repetitive loading over a 5 h period and found that the discs went through a five-stage degenerative process (Fig. 12.4). Nearly all discs reached stage 2 – distortion of the lamellae of the annulus. Lower lumbar discs were more likely to reach stage 3 – radial fissure – and younger discs were more likely to progress to stage 4 – nuclear extrusion. They were unable to demonstrate leakage of nuclear material from discs over age 40, even in the presence of annular rupture. They concluded that this was due to the increased viscosity of the nucleus.

While it is possible to dispute that in vivo conditions can be replicated using cadaveric specimens, it is difficult to refute the broad thrust of the research by Adams and his co-workers: that disc integrity is linked to the type of loading to which the disc has been subjected, and that this in turn influences the disc mechanics, the rate of degenerative change and the risk of injury (Fig. 12.5).

Clearly, the key intervention in this vicious cycle is to modify the loading cycle of the intervertebral disc, to minimize biomechanical and physiological change and to reduce the injury risk.

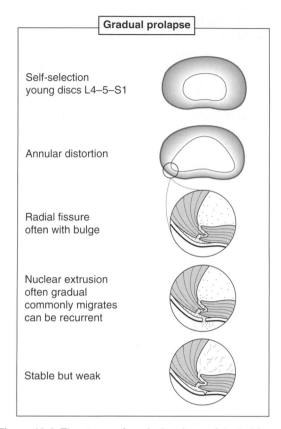

Figure 12.4 The stages of gradual prolapse. Adapted from Adams & Hutton (1985).

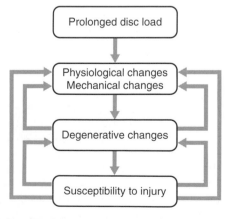

Figure 12.5 The biomechanical model for disc injury demonstrates how prolonged disc load can lead to degenerative change and increased risk of injury.

Internal disc disruption

Bogduk (1997) states that internal disc disruption is the: '... single most common cause of chronic low back pain that can be objectively demonstrated'. He proposes that the fundamental cause of internal disc disruption is vertebral end-plate fracture and describes how: 'Repetitive loading of the disc, in compression or in compression with flexion, can cause end plate failure at loads between 30–80% of ultimate failure strength'.

The fracture of the end plate interferes with the delicate metabolism of the nucleus, precipitating degradation of the matrix and an inefficient response to biomechanical loading (Fig. 12.6). Bogduk proposes that this may accelerate disc disruption and can lead to disc narrowing, annular fissuring and herniation as previously described.

In an award-winning paper, Adams et al (1994) report that, when the spine was subject to high load compression at varying angles of flexion, peak loads were found in the posterior annulus at 0 degrees and increasingly above 50 degrees. They concluded: 'the optimum stress distribution is achieved at about 50% of flexion'. This applies to dynamic loads and not to repetitive or sustained loads, where physiological disturbance becomes a more significant parameter of injury

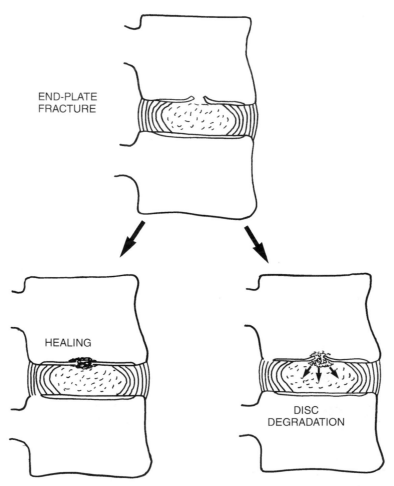

Figure 12.6 End-plate fracture can trigger degradation of the intervertebral disc. Reproduced with permission from Bogduk (1997).

risk. However, Adams' research does suggest that the intervertebral disc might be at more risk at both extremes of flexion range and the vertebral end plate at mid-range.

There is evidence that the juvenile spine is particularly vulnerable to vertebral end-plate damage. Scheuermann's disorder and Schmorl's nodes are relatively common examples of vertebral end-plate damage in the juvenile spine and the presence of these may be more significant than previously realized. Box 12.1 provides a summary of spinal loading.

Box 12.1 Summary: spinal loading

The available research suggests that the spine can be compromised in a number of ways by repetitive loading. There is evidence that muscles, intervertebral discs and intervertebral end plates can all have a reduced injury threshold by sustained or repetitive loading. This provides a clear picture of what type of advice practitioners should give to reduce the risk of injury and the severity of injury episodes:

- Avoid continuous or prolonged flexed postures – provide frequent postural variation with rhythmic and cyclic loading to enhance fluid dynamics and tissue recovery.
- Avoid repetitive loading such as lifting or short cycle production-line-type tasks.
- Where these postures exist, minimize musculoskeletal exposure by careful attention to good posture, minimal leverages, breaks and work variety.
- Pay careful attention to signs of musculoskeletal fatigue and take appropriate action.
- Encourage exercise and maintenance of musculoskeletal and cardiovascular fitness.

SCHEUERMANN'S DISORDER

Low back pain is remarkably common in adolescents, affecting up to 50% of individuals by age 15 (Burton et al 1996). In a 25-year prospective study of 640 adolescents, Harreby (1995) found that of the 11% who showed a history of LBP in adolescence, 84% showed a lifetime prevalence of LBP 25 years later, and that this was associated with increased morbidity and decreased work capacity. Salimen et al (1995) did a 3-year follow-up of 15-year-old schoolchildren with and without LBP, including MRI examination:

During follow up the occurrence of disc degeneration increased significantly more in the original group with low back pain than among asymptomatic subjects. Furthermore, disc degeneration at base line significantly predicted future frequent LBP.

CONCLUSION. After the rapid physical growth period, there seemed to be a causal relationship between the early evolution of the degenerative processes of the lower lumbar discs and frequent low back pain.

Scheuermann's disorder (SD) is a degenerative condition that affects the adolescent spine, causing disturbance in the vertebral end plates and usually affecting two or more vertebrae from T7 to L1. It is associated with the growth spurt and what is thought to be a relative osteoporosis at this time. The active period is 6 months to 1 year, following which the ventral end plate hardens and calcifies, showing characteristic and permanent changes on X-ray (Fig. 12.7).

A study by Fisk et al (1984), involving examination and X-ray of 500 17- and 18-year-old

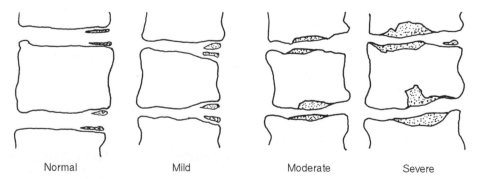

Normal   Mild   Moderate   Severe

Figure 12.7 The characteristic changes of Scheuermann's disorder can predispose toward lumbar disc degenerative change in adult life. Adapted from Wilson (1996).

students, found an incidence of SD, based on radiological diagnosis, of 56.3% in males and 30.3% in females. Fisk found that SD was significantly related to tight hamstrings, long periods of bed-rest and above average height in males (although this was not significant in females). There was no evidence of a link between increased risk of SD and dynamic loading such as heavy work, weight lifting or sport, although there was a nearly significant association between rowing and SD in males.

An earlier study (Stoddard & Osborne 1978) compared the X-rays of 925 patients suffering from backache with 853 controls and found evidence of SD in 42.6% of the back pain group compared to 13.1% of the controls. Stoddard concluded:

The incidence (of SD) in patients whose primary complaint was back ache was shown to be twice as high as the general population. There was also a significantly higher incidence of lower lumbar spondylosis in patients with previous SD ... SD is thereby shown to be an important etiological factor in spondylosis.

In his textbook of osteopathic practice Stoddard (1969) describes SD as a generalized condition affecting the whole spine, although worse at the lower thoracic region. He considered that SD patients were at increased risk of developing degenerative disc changes in the lumbar and cervical areas, with earlier onset of disc protrusions. This seems to concur with clinical findings with SD patients showing more chronic disc problems at an earlier age, and going on to have accelerated degenerative change. Fisk (1984) concludes: 'In the absence of possible dynamic stress factors it is suggested that prolonged sitting may be an important factor in the pathogenesis of endplate breakdown and thus SD'.

The demands of education mean that young people sit for long periods in poor postures (Fig. 12.8). This involves persistent anterior spinal compression, of the intervertebral disc and vertebral body, and it seems logical that this could interfere with the normal development of the spine at a vulnerable age.

This is supported by Wilson (1993), which showed that 71% of students with backache iden-

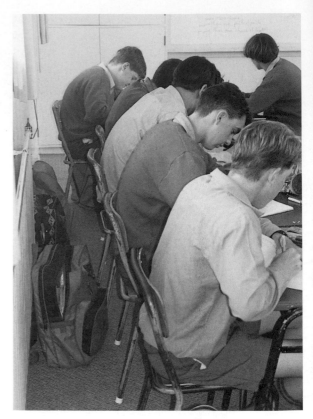

Figure 12.8 Long periods of poor sitting posture are linked to degenerative spinal problems in adolescents. Reproduced with permission from Wilson (1996).

tified sitting at school or at home doing homework as making their backache worse.

It seems that the demands of the education system, adolescent posture and adolescent back pain, increased incidence of SD, Schmorl's nodes and premature disc degenerative changes, and increasing adult back pain incidence and morbidity, are linked in some way. This does suggest that school furniture and student posture are subjects that should be taken much more seriously.

Meanwhile, successive generations of students are being exposed to injury-promoting postures (Fig. 12.9), the effects of which will be seen for years to come.

CONGENITAL ANOMALIES

Anomalies in the lumbar spine are relatively common occurrences, appearing to varying

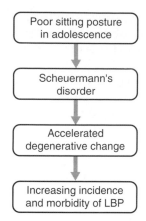

Figure 12.9 The link between poor posture in adolescents, degenerative change in the adolescent spine and increasing incidence and morbidity of back pain in adult life.

degrees in about 25% of LBP cases. They can place the affected or neighbouring segments at a mechanical disadvantage and can lead to increased likelihood of minor trauma, cumulative trauma or an accelerated degenerative process.

The fifth lumbar and first sacral vertebrae often can be incompletely formed, with a partial or complete sacralization of the fifth lumbar or a partial or complete lumbarization of the first sacral vertebra. Taylor et al (1989) found that 42% of patients with chronic LBP of more than 2 months' duration had a transitional vertebra with narrowing of the last mobile disc, compared to only 6% of controls. MacLean et al (1990) found a significantly increased incidence of lumbosacral transitional anomalies in patients with disc prolapse.

A number of mechanisms that may contribute to chronic pain:

- Accelerated degenerative change in joints formed by enlarged transverse process (TP) and sacrum, or enlarged TP and pelvis (Fig. 12.10).
- Incomplete formation of disc at affected segment.
- Accelerated degenerative change of facet joints and disc above sacralized segment due to increased loadbearing.
- Partially sacralized segment with reduced or disturbed mobility may reduce disc nutrition

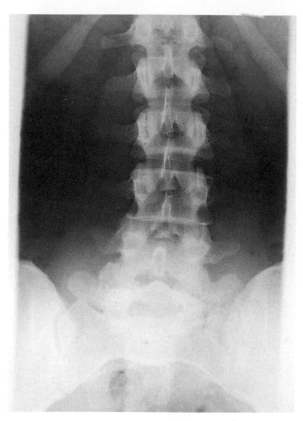

Figure 12.10 Lumbarization of the first sacral segment, with formation of a complete L6–S1 disc. Note the enlarged transverse processes with considerable overlap between the TP and the sacral alar on the left. This would certainly create aberrant movement patterns and may be a cause of the scoliosis shown. Note also the attempt at producing an extra rib at L1. The patient was a 22-year-old female with a 1-year history of constant, chronic back pain following a minor lifting incident. At the time of X-ray she was off work and the problem was proving difficult to manage conservatively. The radiologist's report made no mention of the anomalies seen.

and contribute to accelerated degenerative change.

For a thorough discussion of this subject see Grieve (1994).

The incidence of lumbar facet asymmetry is estimated to be 20–30%. Bogduk (1997) states:

Biomechanical studies have shown that asymmetrical zygopophysial joints do not equally resist postero-anterior shear stresses applied to the intervertebral joint. The unequal load-sharing causes the intervertebral joint to rotate whenever it is subject to sheer stress, as in weight bearing or flexion. The upper vertebra in the joint rotates toward the site of the more coronally orientated joint. Consequently the annulus fibrosus is subjected to innordinate stresses during weight bearing or flexion movements of the lumbar spine. Repeated insults sustained in this way could damage the annulus fibrosus.

Bogduk goes on to cite studies that both support and contradict this theory. Asymmetries in the articular components of the lumbar spine show a plausible relationship with cumulative trauma and degenerative change, although the relative significance remains controversial (Ko & Park 1997). This should be borne in mind when advising on prognosis, activity and exposure levels of the lumbar spine. The asymmetry is not the cause of injury – there are many people with asymmetries that remain symptom free – but they may contribute to the risk of spinal injury and subsequent chronicity.

SCOLIOSIS

Scoliosis of varying degrees is a common finding in back pain patients. It may be:

● structural, where it is secondary to malformation in the bony structure of the spine, such as a hemivertebra or fracture
● functional, where it is a response to pain or uneven mechanical forces such as muscle shortening or leg length difference.

A scoliosis that gradually increases over time is suggestive of pathology and should be investigated. A structural scoliosis will be consistently present in the standing, sitting and flexed postures. A functional scoliosis will be present in erect postures but tend to reduce in sitting or flexed postures (if pain allows). Scoliosis will often be exaggerated in the presence of LBP and it may be possible to reduce this towards normal with therapy and rehabilitation exercise. A functional scoliosis is a common finding in LBP and is usually secondary to the pain and its associated muscle tension. The most common finding is an elevated pelvis of 1–3 cm on the side of the pain with a lumbar concavity on this side and a secondary convexity in the thoracic region providing an S-shaped scoliosis. On the lumbar concavity there is usually muscle shortening and facet approximation with increased compressive forces. Mobility to this side is restricted and/or painful.

In the presence of a nerve root pain the pelvis will usually be high on the painful side but the spine will list away from the painful nerve root with efforts to move back toward the midline increasing the pain. In perhaps 10% of cases, theoretically where the disc bulge is medial to the nerve root, the pelvis will be elevated on the opposite side and the list toward the site of pain. This tends to push the disc bulge medially, providing less nerve root impingement. In the presence of nerve root pain the scoliosis is an effort to relieve pain and it is secondary to the problem.

Scoliosis is not necessarily painful. It is usually secondary to, and as a consequence of, pain and muscle tension. It is important to address the pain producing injury as the primary factor rather than the scoliosis.

The presence of scoliosis provides a mechanical disadvantage to the spine by increasing the torsion to which the vertebrae are subject. Twisted postures are a risk factor for LBP and the scoliotic spine will show higher degrees of vertebral rotation and sidebending than the normal spine. This will provide localized peak forces, particularly in flexed postures, which increase the risk of injury, complicate injury recovery and can increase the risk of chronicity. Hence the scoliotic patient will be at greater risk of injury and reinjury. Theoretically, minimizing scoliosis will provide better spinal mechanics.

A minor scoliosis is a very common finding and may be unrelated to the pain episode. There are many people with scoliosis who remain free of back pain. If the spine is pain free, with normal mobility and without muscle spasm or shortening, it is functionally normal. When a person with a minor scoliosis develops pain, the normal scoliosis usually exaggerates, but then returns to normal as the pain resolves. Masset et al (1998) found that where there is a frontal plane imbalance in the body (trunk or pelvis) of greater than 1 cm, then there is an increased risk of developing LBP (odds ratio 1.74).

> **Box 12.2** Summary: scoliosis
>
> Scoliosis is not usually the cause of back pain, although it is commonly associated with it. It is a background factor that influences the spinal loading and may be a predisposing factor to injury or chronicity. Where possible, it should be minimized by manual therapy and rehabilitation exercises.

LEG LENGTH INEQUALITY

Leg length inequality (LLI) is a very common cause of functional scoliosis. Opinion divides as to whether it is significantly related to LBP. Epidemiologists tend to say it is not significant whereas therapists tend to think it can be relevant. Some say it is not significant if it is less than 2 cm. It is perhaps best to assess its relevance on a case-by-case basis.

The above section on Scoliosis shows that there is a rational explanation for the presence of LLI increasing the amount of rotation, torsion and subsequent peak forces to which the spine is subjected. The increased loading may be a contributory factor for developing an injury, for injury recurrence or for chronicity. When a patient first presents there is frequently an apparent leg length difference due to the imbalanced pelvis and general spinal dysfunction. With treatment this will usually reduce and resolve. Most patients with a suspected LLI will recover as expected for their injury and have the occasional recurrence typical of an LBP history. It is not appropriate to intervene in these cases. A small percentage may have more frequent recurrences than expected or have some ongoing symptoms. In these cases, leg length may be modified if the LLI is felt to be having a significant input into the patient's ongoing dysfunction. This would probably be most likely if the patient needs to spend a substantial portion of the day in an erect posture.

Checking leg lengths

It is difficult to check leg lengths with any degree of accuracy. The often-recommended measurement of LLI in supine position, using a tape measure and reference points such as the anterior iliac spine or umbilicus, and the tibial malleoli, is very inaccurate. LLI is really only important if it creates a pelvic tilt in the standing posture. Even if there seems to be an apparent leg length difference when the patient is recumbent, this may be modified by any number of variables when erect, such as configuration of plantar arch, integrity of knee cartilages and pelvic balance or anomalies.

It is very difficult to assess leg lengths accurately when a patient is acute. A number of manual therapy sessions – to mobilize the lumbar spine and pelvis and to achieve normal balance – will be needed prior to making any interventions, which are usually then unnecessary; either the LLI has disappeared or the patient has recovered sufficiently and adapted to their idiosyncrasies.

Probably the most accurate way of assessing leg lengths is erect X-ray of the legs while standing in bare feet. Even so, some imbalances may creep in, depending on how the person is standing. The additional cost and exposure to radiation have to be considered.

It is reasonably accurate to measure leg lengths in the clinical situation with the patient standing erect by first palpating and comparing the height of the iliac crests, then palpating and assessing the greater trochanters while comparing one level to another (Fig. 12.11). If both of these are imbalanced to the same degree, a difference in leg length is likely.

Intervention

If the difference remains after a manual therapy session (including manipulation, which inhibits any aberrant muscle tension), a difference can be suspected. If the difference remains consistent over two or three sessions, despite manual therapy and exercises, and it is still justified by ongoing symptoms, an intervention can be made. The patient's shoes will wear faster on the side of the long leg, and this can be used to confirm the findings.

Adhesive heel wedges, placed inside the shoe, are cheap and easy to insert and remove. They are about 0.5 cm in diameter and one is usually

A

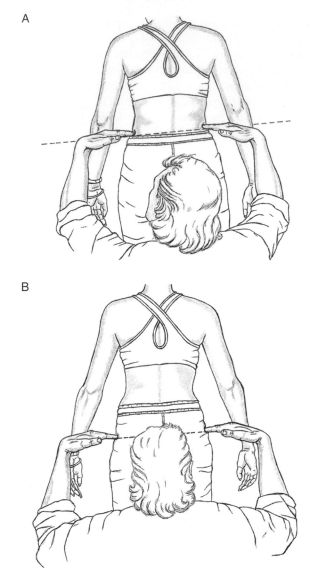

B

C

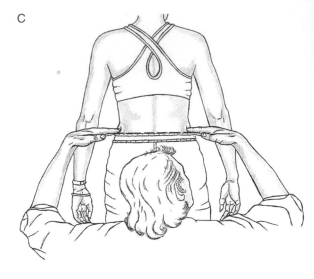

Figure 12.11 Measuring leg lengths in the clinical setting can be easy to do with a reasonable degree of accuracy once the patient is no longer acute. The figure shows
A: measurement of the iliac crests in erect posture.
B: measurement of the greater trochanters in erect position.
C: measurement of the iliac crests with addition of a 1 cm heel raise to the shoe.

sufficient. The aim should not be to remove the leg length inequality completely but to take away the worst effects to assist the body to adapt. Any intervention of more than 1 cm should be added to the sole of the shoe, modifying both the heel and forefoot.

HYPERMOBILITY

The presence of hypermobility implies that there is an increased range of movement at the joints.

Hypermobility can be an innate personal characteristic or it can be secondary to trauma or pregnancy/childbirth/lactation. It can be generalized or localized to one or more joints. Hypermobile people find it relatively easy to create large forces around joints without feeling soft tissue strain or proprioceptive feedback. This relative freedom and lack of warning can place them at risk of injury through peak loading, cumulative injury or degenerative change. Hypermobile people can often be attracted to activities that involve a lot of extreme joint postures, such as ballet, gymnastics and yoga, because they are naturally good at them. Extreme joint postures are at increased risk of injury and accelerated degenerative change.

Hypermobility is not a cause of LBP but can increase the risk of injurious activity. This can be counteracted by good education in the need to avoid loading joints in extreme postures such as hyperflexion or twisted actions of the lumbar spine. Inner range exercises to improve muscle tone can help improve joint stability in hypermobile individuals. Hypermobile individuals will be more likely to exhibit instability.

INSTABILITY

Ligaments are designed to ensure joint stability at the end-range of joint movement. As joints move progressively towards this end-range they become mechanically less efficient and tend to generate higher loads, being more liable to stress and strain. The spine has stabilizing muscles that assist the vertebrae in maintaining optimum or neutral joint position. These muscles link segmental levels and are situated deep and close to the centre of rotation of the vertebrae. Cholewicki & McGill (1996) found that, even when high forces were generated by the larger muscles of the trunk, the spine was unstable unless the local muscle system was coactivated. They suggested that a lack of deep muscle control can predispose to spinal injury. Sihvonen et al (1997) studied 100 chronic LBP sufferers without evidence of nerve root deficit using dynamic radiographs and found disturbed intervertebral movement in 51 of them, with 27% having L4 or L5 anterolisthetic hypermobility and 35% L3 or L4 retrolisthesis. They also found that abnormal EMG findings were associated with the instability, particularly in cases where symptoms included radiating symptoms (30 out of 39 cases), and conclude that:

To improve the functional support of the lumbar spine, rehabilitation should be directed to the medial back muscles because they provide the most effective support for intervertebral motion and because mild disturbances appear to be associated with their innervation in recurrent low back pain.

Sihvonen et al (1997)

In a thorough (and highly recommended) review of the stabilizing musculature of the lumbar spine, Richardson et al (1999) identified the lumbar multifidus (Fig. 12.12) and the transversus abdominis (Fig. 12.13) as being the key stabilizers of the lumbar spine. They both link in with the thoracolumbar fascia (Fig. 12.14) to provide the patient with what Richardson et al called: 'a natural, deep muscle corset to protect the back from injury'.

The multifidus is the largest and most medial of the lumbar back muscles. Its extensive attachments to the sacrum make it the major muscle mass between the pelvis and the sacrum, following the channels between the transverse and spinous processes. Its anterior direction provides an effective lever arm for it to resist flexion and shear forces and helps to control these movements during flexion. It has a high percentage of type 1 muscle fibres, suggesting an important stabilization function. The transversus abdominis acts to compress the abdominal contents and increase tension in the thoracolumbar and abdominal fascia. This effectively slightly flexes and stiffens the spine providing optimal loading for the vertebral unit and maintenance of lumbopelvic posture.

Richardson and co-workers found that patients with chronic LBP had delayed activation of the transversus abdominis when compared to normal subjects in response to spinal loading. The EMG studies showed a disorganized pattern of muscle contraction with short phasic bursts instead of a tonic response as in the uninjured subjects. This lack of effective motor control would increase the risk of further spinal insult. On ultrasound examination, the multifidus muscle showed marked reduction in size on the injured side and at the injured vertebral level when comparing LBP patients to controls. This has been associated with earlier fatigue and abnormal EMG response (Sihvonen et al 1997).

Richardson and co-workers developed an exercise regime designed to improve stability in the key stabilizers of the lumbar spine (see Chapter 13). LBP subjects utilizing this exercise approach show a return to normal size of multifidus compared to non-exercising LBP controls,

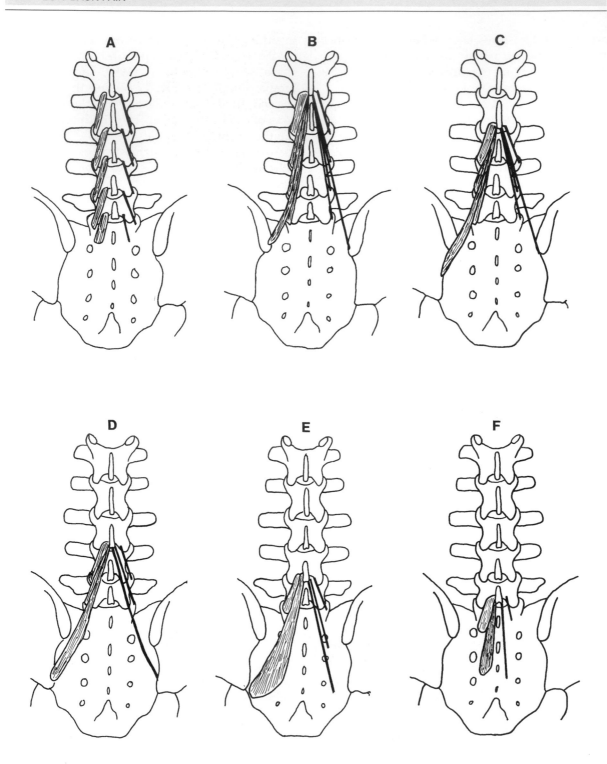

Figure 12.12 The component fascicles of the multifidus. A: The laminar fibres. B–F: fascicles from the L1–L5 spinous processes, respectively. Reproduced with permission from Bogduk (1997).

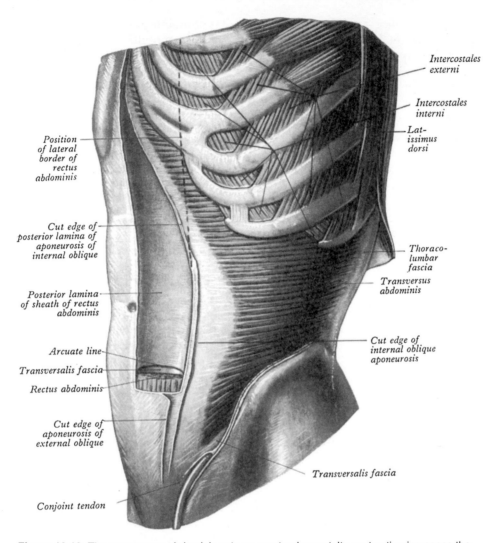

Intercostales externi

Intercostales interni

Latissimus dorsi

Position of lateral border of rectus abdominis

Cut edge of posterior lamina of aponeurosis of internal oblique

Posterior lamina of sheath of rectus abdominis

Thoracolumbar fascia

Transversus abdominis

Arcuate line

Transversalis fascia

Rectus abdominis

Cut edge of internal oblique aponeurosis

Cut edge of aponeurosis of external oblique

Transversalis fascia

Conjoint tendon

Figure 12.13 The transversus abdominis acts as a natural corset. Its contraction increases the abdominal pressure and, via the thoracolumbar fascia, it acts to stabilize the spine and minimize spinal mobility. Reproduced with permission from Williams et al (1995).

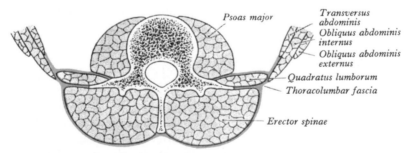

Psoas major

Transversus abdominis

Obliquus abdominis internus

Obliquus abdominis externus

Quadratus lumborum

Thoracolumbar fascia

Erector spinae

Figure 12.14 Transverse section though the posterior abdominal wall, showing the disposition of the thoracolumbar fascia. All other connective tissue strata have been omitted. Reproduced with permission from Williams et al (1995).

and a 30% injury recurrence rate compared to 80% for controls (Hides et al 1996). O'Sullivan et al (1997) used this approach on a group of chronic LBP patients with a radiological diagnosis of spondylolysis and spondylolisthesis. The exercise group showed a statistically significant reduction in pain intensity, pain descriptor scores and functional disability. These were maintained at the 30-month follow-up, while there was no significant change in the control group. This is an exciting development in the clinical management of spondylolysis and spondylolisthesis, which have, traditionally, been difficult to manage and have a high incidence of surgical intervention.

HYPOMOBILITY

Hypomobile individuals can also be at increased risk of injury. They often have to use large muscular forces to overcome soft tissue tension when reaching their limits of mobility. These limits may be reached relatively often in daily activities leading to peak loads and cumulation of loading. They may have a higher activation of nociceptors and proprioceptors, which can increase the incidence of reflex muscle spasm and can contribute to neuromuscular over-activity. Hypomobility can be a personal characteristic – some people seem to be born stiff – in which case it is usually generalized. A localized hypomobility is a very common sign of dysfunction in a joint secondary to strain or injury. This renders the joint less efficient and increasingly subject to strain.

The male pelvis and hamstrings seem to be stiffer than the female counterpart. Many men often find it difficult to sit in good sitting posture because their hips do not easily flex to 90 degrees. This posteriorly rotates the pelvis and pushes the lumbar spine into flexion, increasing the intervertebral disc compression and rendering the spine more susceptible to injury.

People with hip osteoarthritis and limited hip mobility often have to hyperflex the spine to perform simple tasks such as putting on shoes and socks, thereby increasing the risk of back problems.

Hypomobility can be countered by good lifting technique, mobilization and regular exercises to improve the range of movement in hamstrings, hips, pelvis and lumbar spine. Careful attention must be paid to sitting postures (see Chapter 13).

SUMMARY

- Effective management of complex or chronic LBP is a much more complex process than management of simple back pain. The practitioner cannot safely assume that the problem will readily respond to therapy. It becomes very important to understand the nature of the injury – its history, current symptoms, psychosocial and work environment and any personal or anatomical factors that may be complicating the injury picture.
- It is usually necessary to take images to help assess the degree of degenerative, structural or pathological changes. Injuries that include neurological involvement are generally slower to recover.
- Complex back pain is not homogenous and each case must be thoroughly understood and managed on its own merits. Some work involvement and normal socialization should be actively encouraged at the earliest opportunities. This can be difficult where the work involves high biomechanical exposure. Employer cooperation and workplace assessment to reduce biomechanical load are important.
- The intervertebral disc is frequently implicated in complex LBP. It is therefore important to understand the nature of disc injury and disc physiology so that the recovery process can be properly managed and the patient educated about effective management and a realistic timeframe for recovery.
- Effective management of complex back pain that both educates and empowers the patient will reduce the tendency to chronicity and disability. Effective management involves looking for barriers to recovery and providing effective management strategies that the patient can utilize based on the LOAD and the Plateau models. Effective management is an ongoing process.

13

Management of low back pain

Low back pain (LBP) is common to all populations. It is unrealistic to expect to prevent a major proportion of back pain. Despite the reduced dependence on manual work in Western societies, the reported incidence of LBP continues to grow. The focus is increasingly on reducing the social and economic consequences of LBP disability and providing work environments that are LBP friendly. There are many different approaches to LBP management and a vast literature relating to these approaches. There is a large body of research relating to the efficacy of LBP treatment, but many of these have questionable methodology and it becomes difficult to draw meaningful conclusions. LBP is a particularly difficult area to research:

1. It is variable in nature. It is very difficult to standardize diagnosis and treatment and in many cases accurate diagnosis is not possible. LBP injuries that appear similar can have a wide range of disability outcomes.

2. The high natural rate of recovery for most cases of LBP tends to flatter the success rate of interventions. Outcome studies require an adequate, matched control group so the intervention has a measurable comparison.

3. Some interventions may provide immediate relief but the high natural recurrence rate of LBP means that these effects may be quite short-lived.

4. It can be difficult to measure outcomes when there is no clear marker of recovery. Mobility and strength have not been shown to be good markers of recovery. Visual analogue pain

scales are probably as accurate as any measure but are highly subjective – they are true only at that moment and in that environment.

5. A well-designed study is difficult to perform in a clinical environment. Research methodology has been much criticized by epidemiologists for the following reasons:

- lack of control groups
- measurement of relevant outcomes
- inadequate follow-up
- operator bias – lack of blinding
- small study groups.

Studies that fulfil the strict criteria of epidemiologists are usually based on the measure of a single modality against a control group and often reduce the effective armoury of a skilled practitioner. Experienced practitioners are able to adapt their approach and treatment methods to the type and history of injury, the person injured, the resources available and the environment into which the person is being rehabilitated. It comes as no surprise that studies that do satisfy strict epidemiological criteria often find very little benefit from commonly used modalities. There are also quite often conflicting conclusions from epidemiologists when reviewing the same body of literature.

The researcher and the epidemiologists are population focused, attempting to measure outcomes applied to heterogenous groups. The practitioner's role is quite different – it is person-centred, trying to get the best outcome for the particular person. Practitioners soon realize that there are many routes to recovery and they work with the techniques they feel comfortable with, and can apply with confidence to achieve reasonable success rates. Recovery is the common outcome for LBP and practitioners are fortunate to work in this kind of positive environment where there is a natural recovery process. The role of the practitioner is to manage the recovery phase. This can include:

- enhancing the recovery process with treatment modalities
- minimizing disability during the recovery phase
- reducing the risk of recurrence and chronicity

- reassuring and educating the patient about appropriate behaviour
- screening for pathology or other complications.

6. Identifying the difficult case that may have a slow recovery or chronicity and attempting to remove the barriers to recovery requires a multifaceted approach, as outlined in previous chapters.

It is this last category of patient that is the real therapeutic challenge and the needs of this type of patient that created the motivation for this book. Many practitioners are very comfortable working with acute patients with whom they achieve very creditable results. If, after four or five treatments, the occasional patient has not recovered they often lose interest. Yet it is these occasional patients, the ones who slip through the therapeutic net, who represent the real therapeutic challenge; if they are not managed properly they will go on to utilize 80–90% of expenses relating to LBP.

The role of the practitioner is not slavishly to follow research-proven modalities. We have seen that research is still incomplete, inconsistent and frequently unsympathetic to clinical reality. The practitioner should be mindful of up-to-date research but should always be like a detective, filtering information and attempting to identify risk factors and remove barriers to recovery on a case-by-case basis. Where a treatment modality is 'unproven', if it has a logical basis to its modus operandi and a positive influence on known risk factors, there is a good justification for its use. Practitioners should be at the cutting edge, pointing the way for epidemiologists and researchers. Manipulation has been practised for thousands of years and has been part of the osteopathic and chiropractic profession for over 100 years. In this time it has been roundly condemned and criticized by orthodox medicine. However, since the mid-1990s the research consensus is that manipulation has a positive effect for acute LBP (less proven for chronic LBP) and manipulation has come in from the cold. Has manipulation always worked, or has it worked only since its efficacy has been identified?

REST

The overwhelming weight of evidence suggests that bed-rest is deleterious to recovery of LBP. Inactivity leads to a reduction in:

- strength
- endurance
- flexibility
- coordination
- fitness.

Inactivity encourages depression, social withdrawal and pain avoidance behaviour. These physical and psychosocial complications can prolong a case of simple back pain and may be an important factor for iatrogenic disability (Fig. 13.1).

Waddell (1998) has published a comprehensive review paper on the subject of bed-rest for acute back pain of up to 3 months' duration. After reviewing the 18 trials for bed-rest and activity, Waddell concluded:

There is no justification for actually prescribing bed rest for back pain. Advice to stay active and to continue ordinary activities as normally as possible is likely to result in faster recovery, faster return to work and less chronic disability. Most important, despite common fears about re-injury, it does not cause more recurrent problems. It actually leads to fewer recurrent problems and less sick leave over 1–2 years.

There has been a gradual move away from advocating bed-rest for all sorts of medical conditions and, somewhat belatedly, this is now being applied to LBP. Sir Richard Asher, who was a passionate critic of the prevailing advice of long periods of bed-rest for almost every ill, wrote in *The Dangers of Going to Bed* over 50 years ago:

Look at a patient lying long in bed, what a pathetic picture he makes. The blood clotting in his veins, the calcium draining from his bones, the faeces stacking up in his colon, the flesh rotting on his buttocks and the spirit evaporating from his soul!

This highly evocative description should be enough to get anyone on their feet! Despite Richard Asher's passionate plea, the orthopaedic profession has been slow to respond. As recently as 1993, a standard orthopaedic text recommended continuous bed-rest with traction for 2 weeks to reduce a prolapsed disc. Both treatments have shown to be ineffective.

Activity can be difficult for patients with acute disc injury or acute sciatica, who can find it very difficult to stand up in an erect posture. They will often be very antalgic – flexed and sidebent away from the nerve root pain – and often cannot maintain even this posture or be mobile for very long. However, they usually have maximum spasm and stiffness on rising, which then eases with walking and gradually releases with movement and exercise. They will often need to intersperse activity with short periods of resting. Patients who cannot stand easily could be advised to crawl on hands and knees to encourage early activity.

ACTIVITY

Activity assists recovery and early activity should be encouraged. We have seen that one of the most powerful effects of activity is to provide a vascular pump to pump the fluids and circulation so necessary for the homeostasis of the muscles, cartilage, intervertebral disc and nervous system. In the absence of muscular activity this circulatory pump is remarkably diminished. This facility is also diminished by

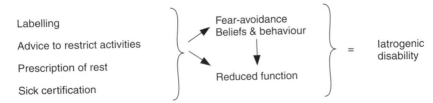

Figure 13.1 Healthcare for back pain can have a profound effect at all levels in a biopsychosocial model; it may also lead to iatrogenic disability. Reproduced with permission from Waddell (1998).

isometric muscle tension and muscle spasm – the activity must involve muscular contraction/relaxation cycles to provide the necessary fluid flow for maintenance of health and recovery.

Reducing activity levels can rapidly reduce task and psychosocial fitness. The sooner these can be recommenced the less the diminishment proceeds and the easier the transition to normal activities.

The proviso here is that the practitioner must make a clinical judgement that the activities will not exacerbate the injury. LBP is usually aggravated by bending and lifting, which create peak forces and a high degree of muscle tension – these should be avoided. Sitting in working postures also creates elevated disc pressures leading to disc creep – wedging of the intervertebral disc. Sitting and driving should be avoided as much as possible and, where they are necessary, frequent breaks and exercises recommended. If the LBP is of the cumulative or repetitive type the practitioner must try and isolate the cumulative factors and eliminate or modify these prior to resuming normal activities. For example, if there is a cumulative load from repeated stooping at a workbench of the wrong height, this exposure must be modified. If there is a problem with poor sitting posture at a desk then a work assessment should be carried out to provide improved ergonomics and reduced cumulative biomechanical load. There is evidence that the provision of modified work for injured workers, particularly in heavy manual work, can significantly improve outcomes.

Non-work activities are usually easier to manage, with swimming and walking being excellent rhythmic exercises that encourage the recovery process without significant biomechanical loading.

PSYCHOSOCIAL MANAGEMENT

Good psychosocial management of a tricky LBP case can be crucial to reducing the risk of chronicity and minimizing disability. Providing a supportive environment and realistic prognosis, and encouraging patient involvement in the recovery process is important. Helping the patient nego-

tiate the maze of medical information and services when they have an acute or chronic injury is one of the important roles of the practitioner. Removing fear of pain and disability can lead to a remarkable improvement in symptoms.

An episode of LBP may not necessarily be particularly severe to justify chronicity or work absence. People may feel overwhelmed with recurrent episodes of pain, or their coping strategies may be diminished by the increased physical or psychosocial demands of their environment. Practitioners can help put their symptoms in perspective and give them tools to cope with the new demands. They may be able to reduce the patient's disability and effect a return to work simply by providing a positive psychosocial environment. The key points for psychosocial management are:

- Maintain a positive outlook. Even the most acute back pain is likely to make a full recovery without the need for surgery. Give the patient positive messages about return to work and resumption of normal activities.
- Review progress regularly. Patients can be quite despondent if progress is slow or if they are having an exacerbation of symptoms. They tend to be very poor judges of their progression. Explain that episodes of exacerbation are common and are part of the recovery and learning process.
- Maintain work involvement and usual activities as much as possible.
- Avoid conflict. Try and keep a positive atmosphere with employer, health agencies and health professionals. Try and promote resolutions of work or relationship conflicts. Do not encourage a 'poor me' or victimhood scenario.
- Promote self-help, self-management and self-responsibility. Avoid the impression of a 'technofix' solution that leads to unrealistic expectations of recovery and avoids self-responsibility.
- Minimize and diffuse emotional distress. This leads to symptom magnification and other complications.
- Promote pain management rather than pain avoidance. Give advice and tools to promote

pain management such as hydrotherapy, exercises, distraction and relaxation.

- Identify barriers to recovery and seek solutions for these.
- Refer for help or for a second opinion if progress is not being made.
- Recognize chronic cases early and manage appropriately. Avoid recycling as acute cases.

John Clifford (1993), in a paper about successful management of chronic pain syndromes, identified the warning signs of psychosocial complications that may increase the risk of chronicity and require increased vigilance by the health professional:

- active conflict or hostility
- job dissatisfaction
- use of narcotics
- unusual treatment reaction
- dramatic expressions of pain or excessive pain behaviour
- multiple aids and orthoses
- victim or 'poor me' behaviour.

Good communication skills and sound psychosocial management are an often neglected part of patient care. They should be among the cornerstones of injury management.

There is an increasing realization that one of the most important determinants of the disability rate of low back injuries is related to the macrosocial environment. Those Western economies with high rates of disability tend to be those with generous financial provisions and a relatively easy transition from sick leave to long-term disability, with little financial penalty.

A dramatic turnaround has been seen in Sweden, which up until 1990 allowed 90% of income from day 1 for LBP work incapacity. Following a reduction in financial provisions in 1991 there has been a marked reduction in reported injuries, amount of sick leave and early retirement due to LBP. The total sick leave fell from 28 million days in 1987 to 19.2 million days in 1995. Other countries that have made long-term disability due to LBP less accessible are noticing similar but less dramatic trends. While these are highly cost-effective changes, it may be that some of the suffering and disability is driven underground. Changes such as these should be made only if there are adequate provisions for rehabilitation programmes and worksite support for early return-to-work programmes. Sweden has also been at the forefront of these initiatives.

Decisions regarding work status are often made by the patient's GP, and are often made without reference to functional or disability assessment. Early return to work can sometimes make life difficult in the short term, with employer understanding and work modification frequently required. GPs are often reluctant to make decisions that might be regarded as unpopular, or will make life difficult for the patient. However, long-term outcomes are much better for all concerned if early return to work is encouraged and accommodated. The evaluation of work status and disability is a specialist field and these decisions are best made by independent practitioners with adequate training in disability and functional assessment and who have no vested interest with the health agency or the patient concerned. Once a functional deficit has been identified it can be addressed as part of the rehabilitation programme.

MEDICATION

There does seem to be a consensus among researchers that the use of pain-relieving medication enhances recovery. It seems that pain blockade can reduce the spasm reflex associated with pain, thereby reducing dysfunction and disability, encouraging early activity and enhancing recovery.

The Royal College of General Practitioners *National low back-pain clinical guidelines* (RCGP 1996) recommends the following:

- Prescribe analgesics at regular intervals not p.r.n.
- Start with paracetamol. If inadequate substitute NSAIDs and then paracetamol-weak opioid compound. Finally consider adding a short course of muscle relaxants
- Avoid narcotics if possible

Evidence
- Paracetamol effectively reduces acute LBP**
- NSAIDs reduce acute LBP. Ibuprofen and diclofenac have lower risks of gastrointestinal complications***

- Paracetamol-weak opioid compounds are effective when NSAIDs or paracetamol alone are inadequate**
- Muscle relaxants effectively reduce acute LBP***

*** Generally consistent findings in a majority of acceptable studies.
** Either based on a single acceptable study or a weak or inconsistent finding in some of multiple acceptable studies.

There is no evidence that one NSAID is more effective than any other. NSAIDs tend to be less effective against sciatica than against simple back pain. Medication should be a part of good diagnosis and appropriate clinical management, and not a substitute for it. While pain relief can be used to encourage early activity it can also encourage inappropriate injury-promoting behaviour. Patients must be educated as to the nature of their injury and the appropriate or inappropriate activities.

MANUAL THERAPY

Recent research reviews have shown that manual therapy techniques tend to be more successful than passive modalities such as electrotherapy. Many factors contribute to this:

- increased time spent with the patient
- a relationship with therapeutic touch has powerful placebo effects
- opportunity for effective communication
- physical therapy tends to emphasize a more active participatory approach
- the effect of the physical therapy – improvement in mobility and circulation, changes in muscle tension, proprioception and pain levels.

There are different schools of manual therapy with subtly different emphases on technique and philosophy. Sometimes too much emphasis is placed on these subtle differences when, in reality, they have a great deal in common.

There are three categories of technique that provide an important part of manual therapy.

Soft tissue or myofascial techniques

Increased muscle tension is a very important cause of pain and dysfunction. Techniques to release tension in muscles and associated connective tissues, which are often contracted postinjury, are an important part of the practitioner's armoury. This can vary from deep massage or deep friction techniques, to trigger point therapies, or postisometric releases such as muscle energy techniques.

Mobilization or articulation

Mobilization techniques are designed to improve mobility and function in dysfunctional joints. Joints tend to exhibit dysfunction if they have altered soft tissue tone and proprioception following an injury. A dysfunctional joint may have a reduction in mobility, or an asymmetry that affects joint balance and rhythm. Mobilizations are usually performed at the functional limit to mobility. They are rhythmic, repetitive and provide a stretching to soft tissues. This improves mobility, encourages fluid exchange and reduces proprioceptive sensitivity.

Manipulation

Manipulation is also known as thrusting techniques or mobilization with impulse. It involves a thrusting technique where the dysfunctional joint is placed at one or more barriers of motion and the practitioner provides a force that moves the joint beyond the barrier. To achieve the best results with minimal application of force, the soft tissues should be released with myofascial and mobilization techniques prior to manipulation.

The following general principles (based on DiGiovanna (1991)) are important when using manipulation:

- Prepare the joint by relaxing soft tissues. Ensure patients are relaxed and have given their consent for the procedure.
- Place the joint in the barrier of motion – usually a combination of movements such as rotation/ sidebending and flexion or extension.
- The joint should be briefly held at this barrier, creating a 'physiological locking' prior to the thrust.
- The thrust should be specific, controlled, rapid, short duration and minimal distance

(usually described as high velocity, low amplitude). The thrust should be the minimum that is required to gap the joint. This is usually accompanied by an audible pop as the pressure changes in the joint cavity.

Manipulation can, in some cases, provide a remarkable reduction in symptoms, particularly in reduction of pain, release of muscle spasm and improvement in mobility. This is most likely to be mediated by neurological inhibition. In an acute case of relatively short duration, manipulation can be sufficient to effect recovery. In a more complex case where there is more likely to be underlying pathology or more complex biomechanical or psychosocial dysfunction, manipulation gains some short-term improvement but it will require a more comprehensive approach, based on identifying and minimizing the individual risk factors, to effect recovery. There are different theories advanced as to the efficacy of manipulation. These include: freeing of an entrapped meniscus, alteration in volume and viscosity of synovial fluid, release of endorphins. The modulation of nociceptor activity and inhibition of aberrant motor nerves responsible for muscle spasm remains the most attractive. In the words of Fisk (personal communication):

The obvious conclusion is that some sensory stimulation occurs during the manipulation which reflexly turns down the excitability of the related muscle alpha motor neurones, thus reducing the sensitivity of the muscle spindles to stretch.

Recent reviews of trials of manipulative therapy have highlighted the difficulties faced by researchers in this area. It is clearly difficult to provide adequate controls for a manual therapy with a large personal input into the therapeutic process, which can provide a significant placebo effect. Any attempt to control for this will also modify proprioceptive information and sensory awareness in the control subjects, thereby confusing the outcomes. This problem is highlighted with manipulative therapy, where there is a significant theatrical element to the intervention. Manual therapy does not involve the dispassionate application of a controlled manoeuvre irrespective of circumstance. Rather, the subjective application of a system of a therapy that is individualized according to the circumstances, performed by an operator with preconceptions and prejudices and received by an emotional being with a highly personal injury, an individualized history and a cocktail of risk factors. A great deal depends on the skills of the operator and the interaction between the operator and the patient. Attempts to control for these factors will reduce the essence of manual therapy and negate the skills of the operator. Little wonder that epidemiologists find this area difficult!

However, recent reviews of manipulative therapy have reached a consensus that manipulative therapy is: 'safe and effective for patients in the first month of acute low back pain without radiculopathy' (AHCPR 1994).

More recent reviews that have updated this review have reinforced this conclusion. After a review of the literature the Clinical Standards Advisory Group (CSAG 1994) came to the following conclusions:

Within the first 6 weeks of onset of acute or recurrent LBP, manipulation provides better short-term improvement in pain and activity levels and higher patient satisfaction than the treatments to which it has been compared. However there is no firm evidence that it is possible to select which patients will respond or what kind of manipulation is most effective.
  The evidence is inconclusive as to whether manipulation for low back pain of more than 6 weeks duration provides clinically significant improvements in outcome compared with other treatments. There is conflicting evidence from random controlled trials and systematic reviews on the effectiveness of manipulation in chronic LBP.

In a comprehensive review of the randomized clinical trials of manipulation, Koes et al (1996) state that, of the 36 randomized, controlled trials of manipulation, 19 report positive results and a further five report positive results in one or more subgroups. Koes was critical of the methodology used in most of the trials, concluding:

The efficacy of spinal manipulation for patients with acute or chronic low back pain has not been demonstrated with sound randomized clinical trials.

There are certainly indications that manipulation might be effective within some subgroups of patients with low back pain.

However, Koes also states: 'There is at least as much evidence in favour of manipulation for chronic low back pain as there is for acute low back pain'.

This would suggest that, where acute LBP is due to muscle spasm and joint dysfunction, manipulation can be effective in reducing this cycle of spasm, pain and dysfunction. In chronic or complex back pain where there is an increased likelihood of complications, manipulation performed in isolation is less likely to be effective, although it can be helpful if used in conjunction with other interventions that address the specific risk factors for chronicity.

Manipulation is not the possession of any one particular profession, although only some of them have the well-established infrastructure necessary for teaching safe and effective technique. It is a skill that needs to be learnt, developed and practised and this requires a structured programme with skilled teachers. It also requires a reasonable amount of coordination and dexterity – not everybody can be taught to be a good manipulator.

In skilled hands, with appropriate patient selection, manipulation is remarkably safe; probably safer than taking NSAID pain relief. Around 50% of patients report local discomfort or tiredness for 24 h. The incidence of serious complications in the lumbar spine – cauda equina syndrome – has been estimated at one in 100 million manipulations performed (Shekelle 1992).

EXERCISE

Exercise is an important part of rehabilitation from back injuries and is vital in the management of chronic or recurrent back pain. There are different types of exercise:

- exercise to improve comfort
- exercise to improve mobility
- exercise to improve muscle strength, stamina, stability and neuromuscular coordination
- aerobic exercise for general conditioning.

The recommended exercises for the first two categories are included in Chapter 12 and aerobic exercise was covered in Chapter 8. This section will cover the research findings for exercise as a therapeutic modality and provide some detail about exercises to improve spinal biomechanics. It will detail two separate but related philosophies for developing an exercise programme.

All patients should be given some exercises to aid recovery. There are many general benefits that arise from this in addition to the therapeutic aim of the exercise.

- placebo effect
- the feeling that patients are doing something to assist their recovery
- postural variation with improved circulation and proprioception
- biofeedback – improved body awareness assists in controlling body postures and muscle tension levels.

Exercises tend to be most beneficial when they are individualized to the patient's requirements, to the nature of the injury and the stage of the recovery. There is better uptake of the exercise prescription when the patient is able to do them, at least initially, under the supervision of the practitioner and when they are reinforced with a handout. An exercise programme is more likely to be beneficial when it is part of a coordinated treatment or rehabilitation programme – when it is supervised and modified if appropriate.

Blanket prescription of exercises without regard to the person and the nature of the injury are less likely to be successful and may aggravate an injury.

Research on exercise programmes for LBP

Koes et al (1991) published a review paper of randomized, controlled trails for patients with LBP. They concluded:

The quality of intervention research on physiotherapy exercises is disappointingly low. Despite its frequent application exercise therapy has not been shown to be more efficacious than other treatment modalities, nor has it been shown to be ineffective. There is little evidence in favour of a specific exercise regimen.

Faas (1996) updated this research with inclusion of 11 randomized trials published between 1991 and 1995: two trials of acute back pain with high method scores reported no efficacy of flexion or extension exercises:

Two trials of the McKenzie type of exercises reported positive results but had low method scores.

For subacute pain one trial reported positive results with a graded activity programme.

For chronic back pain three trials reported positive results with different types of exercises; two trials reported better results with intensive exercising compared with low grade exercising, but after 12 months this effect had disappeared.

The two trials of acute LBP that reported no efficacy had no preselection criteria for the exercise prescription, whereas the McKenzie trials that reported positive results both used preselection criteria. Anybody involved with clinical appraisal of acute LBP, its varying manifestations and the individual nature of each person and each injury, will appreciate the necessity for individual exercise prescription rather than blanket recommendations.

The intensive exercise trial showed short-term improvements (3–6 months), which disappeared after 12 months (compared with mild exercising). However, in the subgroup with high exercise compliance, positive results could be found after 12 months. This suggests that the beneficial effects of an exercise programme diminish as the exercises are curtailed. This is to be expected with a problem that has a tendency to be recurrent. It further suggests that finding an efficacious exercise programme is only part of the solution; it then needs to be presented in a structure that encourages compliance and permits reinclusion when this is appropriate.

Marshall et al (1997) followed 58 chronic LBP volunteers (at a minimum of 8 weeks postinjury) through an individually tailored, supervised, physical activity programme of at least 50 min, three times a week for 1 month. These were compared to controls for the 12 months following completion of the programme for lost time from work and utilization of medical services. The LBP cases had significantly less time off work but

no difference in utilization of medical services. However, 20% of cases dropped out before completion of the progamme, with some evidence that these were more chronic and more severe cases.

This study shows that an individualized exercise programme can be of benefit over a 12-month period, but there remains a difficulty of patient selection and compliance, particularly with the more difficult cases. An individualized exercise programme can be of benefit for chronic LBP cases but it will not suit everybody.

A review study of 16 papers on the prevention of LBP with exercise (Lahad et al 1995) showed a statistically significant short-term benefit from exercise intervention with fewer days off work and fewer days with pain than controls:

Of the available epidemiological studies seven observed significant associations between increased fitness or flexibility and decreased LBP, but four found no protective effect.

Together these studies suggest that exercise interventions may be mildly protective against back pain. Aerobic exercise appears to be as effective as exercises aimed at trunk muscles.

Exercise protocol

- Acute phase – exercises that increase comfort. These will be designed to unload, and to minimize the nociceptor activity of the injured tissues.
- Subacute phase – exercises that improve mobility, stretch soft tissues, encourage circulation and provide varied proprioception.
- Chronic and recurrent phase – exercises that improve muscle tone, joint stability, recovery and stamina. Aerobic exercise.

The acute, subacute and chronic categories are not necessarily based on time periods. They are based on the nature of the injuries and the relative priorities demanded by the symptom picture.

In an acute phase the priority is pain avoidance. This phase can be prolonged in a serious LBP with neurological symptoms. Some gradual onset cases do not have an acute phase. Some injuries can have a number of acute exacerbations. It is necessary for the practitioner or case manager to diagnose the injury, the current phase, the affected tissues and prescribe the appropriate exercises that tend to unload these tissues. They should create a feeling of relief. In the chronic or recurrent phase this should focus on optimizing function to enhance management of chronic pain and avoiding relapse or reinjury. The emphasis is on the psychosocial benefits of exercise, postural stability and postural stamina. Exercises should involve varied motions in more than one plane to encourage coordination, stabilization and stamina.

Exercise plan for spinal stabilization

The spinal stabilizing musculature is particularly important. Recent research suggests that fatigue or dysfunction in the spinal stabilizers (particularly multifidus and transversus abdominis) can be an important cause of back injury. For good reviews on the subject, see Richardson & Jull (1995) and Richardson et al (1999).

It is very important that the patient understands the concept of improving the muscular ability of the spinal stabilizers. It is a different concept from most exercises, where the aim is to improve muscle strength by rapid and vigorous repetitive contraction such as sit-ups. Instead, the aim is to improve the ability of a muscle group to maintain a contraction at low loads for long periods of time. This enables the spine to remain within its joint comfort zone despite dynamic activities or prolonged postures, and to minimize the accumulative stresses and strains of these activities.

A useful analogy for describing to a patient the role of the stabilizing muscles is a single sheet of paper. Any force applied to the paper will cause deformation and buckling. If the piece of paper is formed into a cylinder, which mimics the bracing or corset effect of the transversus abdominis and the multifidus, it is a much stronger structure, capable of withstanding load and maintaining its integrity. Chapter 12 detailed how spinal instability can be an important cause of back pain and highlighted the importance of reactivating the deep spinal stabilizers (notably the transversus abdominis and multifidus) following a spinal

injury. This following description of reactivating the deep spinal stabilizers borrows heavily from the pioneering work carried out by Richardson et al (1999).

Isolating the transversus abdominis

Put the patient into the four-point kneeling position, with the knees below the hips and the hands below the shoulders; the elbows should be relaxed. The spine should be in neutral and the abdomen should be relaxed. Ask patients to draw their lower abdomen up and in, without moving their spine and pelvis, while maintaining their normal breathing pattern (Fig. 13.2). Patients should hold this position for 10 s while

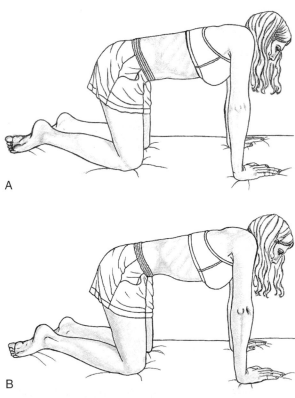

A

B

Figure 13.2 Isolating the transversus abdominis contraction in the four-point kneeling position (A) involves drawing in the lower abdomen below the navel (B) while maintaining neutral spine posture and normal abdominal breathing. The patient should aim to hold this contraction for 10 s and repeat it 10 times. Once the technique is mastered it should be incorporated into other postures such as sitting, standing and walking.

endeavouring to maintain normal abdominal breathing. They should try and avoid rapid or shallow chest breathing. The patient should try this a number of times with the emphasis on precision and control rather than strength, utilizing 20–30% of maximum contraction strength. Initially a person might fatigue quickly and be tempted to recruit larger muscles, which move the spine and pelvis. Signs of fatigue include fatigue, tremor and larger muscle substitution.

Successful performance of this manoeuvre can be tested in a prone patient using a pressure cuff under the abdomen inflated to 70 mmHg. According to Richardson et al (1999) a successful performance of the test should reduce the pressure 6–10 mmHg. The contraction should be held for 10 s (Fig. 13.3). Repeating the test ten times will

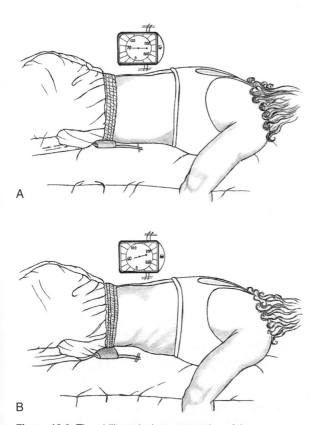

A

B

Figure 13.3 The ability to isolate contraction of the transversus abdominis can be tested in the prone position with a blood pressure cuff placed under the lower abdomen. This should be inflated to 70 mmHg (A) and, during the contraction phase, the pressure should reduce 6–10 mmHg (B). The patient should aim to sustain this for at least 10 s repeatedly.

test the endurance of the muscles. It is important to ensure that the patient has not tilted the pelvis or flexed the spine to achieve the result. If the pressure fails to reduce it is often due to the recruitment of other muscles and to the rectus abdominis increasing the pressure on the pressure cuff. Obese patients may find it impossible to perform the test in the prone position and could instead be tested in the standing or four-point kneeling position using visual and tactile feedback.

Multifidus

Assessment of the multifidus muscle begins with palpation in the prone position at each segment just adjacent to the spinous processes, with comparisons being made between different segments and side to side. The patient should be asked to gently swell the muscle below the practitioner's fingers while breathing normally. This will require co-contraction of the transversus abdominis. Patients will be tempted to extend the spine or use the thoracic portion of the erector spinae muscles – a much stronger, more lateral and more superficial contraction.

Richardson and co-workers report weakness in multifidus contraction with loss of bulk in acute and subacute patients specific to the level of the injury and the side involved. This manifests as a difficulty in activating multifidus at the affected level with jerky, poorly controlled movements. The patient should aim to be able to hold a controlled tonic contraction at each lumbar level, while the practitioner should feel for a deep sustained tonic contraction.

Testing lumbopelvic stability

This is tested in the supine position with knees and hips bent to 45 degrees. A pressure cuff is inflated to 40 mmHg and placed under the lumbar spine to detect changes in posture and loading. The patient is asked to flatten the tummy, activating the transversus abdominis, which should increase the pressure slightly. The patient should maintain this pressure reading while performing various leg movements reflecting stability in the lumbopelvic spine (Fig. 13.4).

A

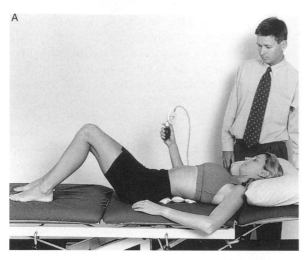

Figure 13.4 The progression of leg load in tests of control of lumbopelvic posture. A: Preparation for the test. The requirements of the test to keep the pressure as steady as possible and the importance of maintaining the deep muscle corset action during the test are explained to the patient. The patient is positioned in supine crook-lying, with the legs together, or the legs abducted to emphasize rotatory control. The pressure sensor is positioned longitudinally on the side of the spine and inflated to 40 mmHg. The patient watches the pressure dial and draws in the abdominal wall. The pressure will increase slightly. The patient is instructed to keep the pressure level steady throughout the test. B: Level 1: single leg slide, contralateral leg support. (Left) Leg slide with heel support to full extension and return. (Right) Unsupported leg slide: the heel is held approximately 5 cm from exercise surface. C: Level 2: single leg slide, contralateral leg unsupported. (Left) Leg slide with heel support to full extension and return. (Right) Unsupported leg slide: the heel is held approximately 5 cm from exercise surface. Reproduced with permission from Richardson et al (1998).

Bi

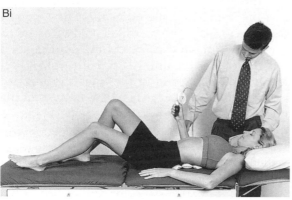

Bii

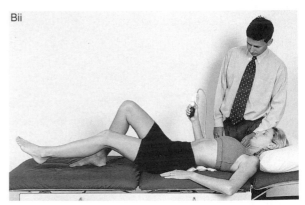

Ci

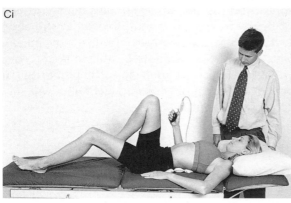

Cii

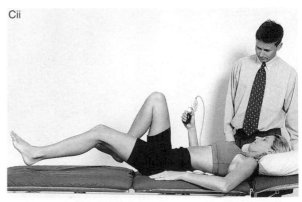

Any change in pressure suggests that the load has increased beyond the capacity of the muscle to stabilize the lumbopelvic spine. The pressure may increase or reduce, depending on the rotation of the spine or the move into flexion or extension. If this happens, the patient is usually unable to keep the abdomen drawn in and the abdominal wall bulges. This test is more effective in lower loads. In higher loads it is natural for more global muscles to be recruited to assist stability.

The therapeutic regimen of improving trunk stability via training of the deep lumbar muscles consists of three stages:

Stage 1. Motor skill training and development of strength and coordination of the deep muscles.
Stage 2. Incorporation of the skill into light tasks.
Stage 3. Progression into heavy functional tasks.

Isolating the deep muscles in low level contractions without introducing spinal, rib or pelvic movements while being able to maintain normal abdominal breathing is an essential prerequisite prior to moving on to Stage 2. When doing the exercises at home, the patient should check to see if they are recruiting the transversus abdominis properly by self-palpation. They should palpate with both hands just medial to the anterior superior iliac spine and ensure that they avoid pushing out against their fingers.

Once this has been achieved, the ability to sustain the contraction for longer periods is important and only then is it appropriate to use more dynamic actions. The next stage is to incorporate the skills into situations where gravity and postural muscles are also involved, such as sitting and standing, and then to incorporate movements of the limbs and trunk in these positions. The next phase should involve more dynamic movements. Walking is an important human posture where the ability to sustain the contraction can be learned with the opportunity of increasing speed and distance. Finally, the technique should be incorporated into tasks involving additional dynamic loads that utilize phasic contractions of the larger muscles. Initially this can be done in fixed postures but then can move onto more dynamic postures or situations where there is reduced stability, such as using an exercise ball.

Bridging from the prone position is another excellent exercise that can be quite challenging. The deep stabilizing muscles should be preloaded and the patient should form a bridge, focusing on gluteal contraction to extend the hips so the thighs are in line with the upper body, all the while maintaining a neutral spine position and maintaining normal breathing (Fig. 13.5A). This should be held for 5 s. The next stage is to incorporate a single leg extension with the emphasis

on keeping the trunk and pelvis steady and maintaining normal breathing (Fig. 13.5B). This should be held for 5 s on alternating sides. Once this is mastered, the exercise can be made more challenging by alternating rapidly from side to side.

The four-point kneeling position with extended arm and opposite leg is a challenging exercise that incorporates leverage and instability. The transversus abdominis should be preloaded and the leg lifted slowly until it is horizontal to the body, with the emphasis on maintaining lumbopelvic posture – not allowing the pelvis to dip or move into rotation or hyperextension. When this is achieved the opposite arm is raised (Fig. 13.6). The position is held for 5 s, alternating sides. Further challenge can be added by incorporating dynamic arm and leg movements, such as drawing shapes and extending the period.

The contraction of the transversus abdominis and the multifidus occurs synergistically with the diaphragm and the pelvic floor, thereby equalizing the pressure in the abdominal cylinder and tensioning the lumbar fascia for maximum spinal stability.

The motor control of these muscles is vital to good spinal stabilization. Injured patients show both lack of strength and poor motor control of these muscles (Richardson et al 1999). The exercises should be performed regularly throughout the day, in various postures, to encourage improved functioning of the muscle motor units and to improve strength, stamina and recovery. Care must be taken not to exercise the muscles to exhaustion, which will have the effect of reducing their ability to stabilize the spine.

Once the techniques of muscle stabilization are understood, and the skills to improve the muscle function and successfully stabilize the spine in a variety of loading situations without aggravation of symptoms have been developed, exercises can be introduced to strengthen the more global abdominal and trunk musculature. Richardson and co-workers have focused on the transversus abdominis and the multifidus as being particularly important to spinal stability. However, other trunk muscles also play an important role.

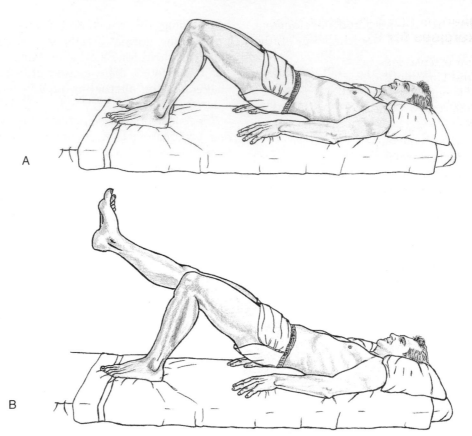

Figure 13.5 A: The bridge is an excellent exercise to develop the deep stabilizing muscles. From the supine position with the knees up, the stabilizing muscles should be preloaded. The pelvis should be raised utilizing the gluteal muscles so the thighs are parallel with the trunk, without inducing any spinal extension, and while maintaining abdominal breathing. This can be held for 5 s initially, building up to 10 s, and repeated up to 10 times. B: From the bridge position this exercise can be made more challenging by extending each leg alternately, or by holding the extended leg for a few seconds.

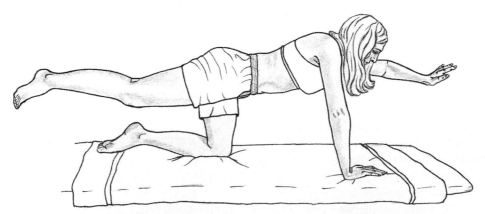

Figure 13.6 Extending the leg and the opposite arm from the four-point kneeling position incorporates both leverage and instability. This posture should be held for 5–10 s, alternating sides, while holding the pelvis and trunk stable without allowing a dip into rotation or hyperextension. An advanced stage of the exercise includes drawing shapes with the arms and leg to make the task more dynamic.

High challenge–low biomechanical stress exercises for trunk muscles

Following an extensive series of biomechanical studies at the University of Waterloo, Ontario, Stuart McGill published a review paper on the type of exercises most suitable for rehabilitation of spinal injury (McGill 1998). The aim is to provide significant challenge for the muscles and enhance their performance while minimizing loading of the spine to reduce the risk of exacerbation. McGill includes the following recommendations for designing an exercise programme:

- There is some evidence that exercises are most beneficial when performed daily.
- No pain, no gain, does not apply to low back exercises, particularly when the activities are repetitive.
- Aerobic exercise has been shown to be effective for injury prevention and for rehabilitation of LBP.
- High intervertebral disc pressure on waking suggests that it is unwise to perform full range activities in the early morning, particularly involving flexion.
- Improving muscle endurance has more protective value than improving strength.
- The type and duration of exercises should be selected to suit the person concerned, the presenting injury and the stage of recovery. There is no such thing as a set of ideal exercises to suit all people.
- Persevere with the exercise programme; improvements can take up to 3 months.

McGill proposes a series of exercises that are suitable for the early stages of rehabilitation:

The cat stretch. This flexion/extension cycle reduces joint stiffness and relaxes joint structures, resulting in lower loads while the spine remains supported (Fig. 13.7).

Hip and knee exercises. These exercises should emphasize mobility and coordination in the hip and knee joints so they can be effectively used in flexed postures to substitute for a flexed spine (Fig. 13.8).

The curl-up. Curl-ups provide a high challenge to the abdominal muscles while maintaining rel-

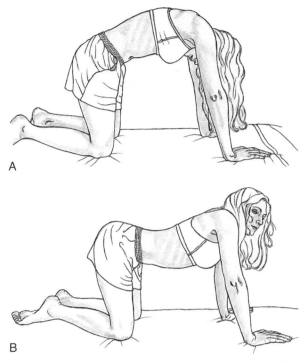

Figure 13.7 The cat stretch is performed in the four-point kneeling position with slow cycling from full extension (A) to full flexion (B) emphasizing mobility rather than force.

atively low loads on the spine (Axler & McGill 1997). The straight curl-up (Fig. 13.9A) provides a high challenge to the rectus abdominis while the oblique curl-up (Fig. 13.9B) provides a high challenge to the abdominal obliques. A variation of this – the single leg curl-up with the other leg extended and slightly raised (Fig. 13.9C) – also challenges the lumbar stabilizers in a relatively neutral spinal posture. The rectus abdominis and the abdominal obliques provide important links to the thoracolumbar and abdominal fascias and enhance their role in stabilization of the spine.

The horizontal side support. This is an effective exercise for activating the quadratus lumborum and oblique abdominal while maintaining a neutral spine (Fig. 13.10). It does place high loads on the weight-bearing shoulder.

The four-point kneeling position with extended leg. McGill recommends using the leg extension first, progressing to extended arm and leg (see Fig. 13.6), which produces higher spinal compression.

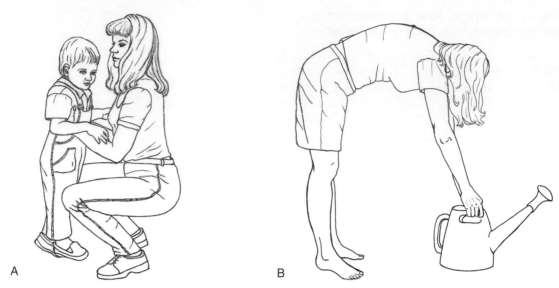

Figure 13.8 Good flexibility and strength in the hip and knee joints (A) helps avoid flexed spinal postures (B).

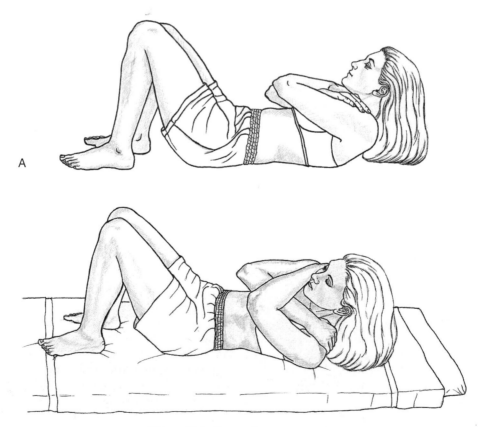

Figure 13.9 *For caption, see opposite.*

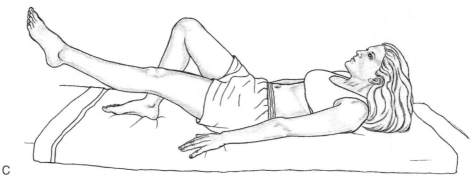

C

Figure 13.9 Curl-ups are an effective method of challenging the abdominal muscles with minimal spinal loading. A: The straight curl-up should be performed with the knees bent, the arms at the side, or folded across the chest. The neck and shoulders should be raised so the scapulae are just off the floor without excessive neck flexion – keep the eyes gazing at the ceiling. This can be held for 5 s, increasing to 10 s and repeated up to 10 times. B: The oblique curl-up is performed in the same position, with the arms across the chest and the elbow pointing towards the opposite knee (some distance away from contact). This can be held 3–5 s, alternating sides, up to 10 times each side. C: The single leg curl-up with one knee extended is an effective method of incorporating the spinal stabilizers. Initially this can be done with the hands underneath the pelvis, progressing to hands by side and then across the chest.

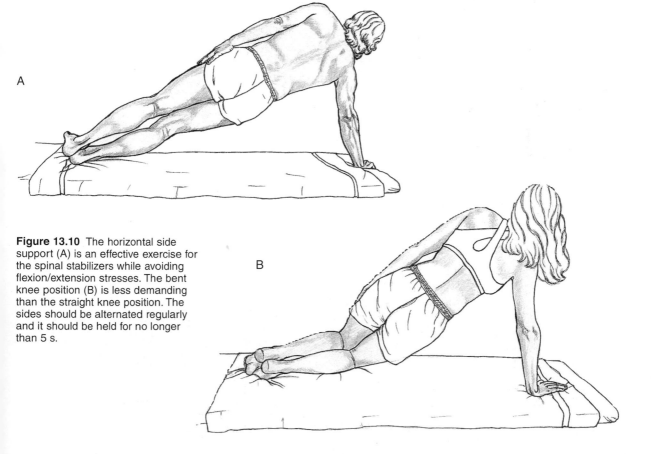

A

B

Figure 13.10 The horizontal side support (A) is an effective exercise for the spinal stabilizers while avoiding flexion/extension stresses. The bent knee position (B) is less demanding than the straight knee position. The sides should be alternated regularly and it should be held for no longer than 5 s.

Exercises to avoid

Exercises recommended for LBP patients that should be avoided because of high biomechanical stress are: supine leg exercises, pelvic tilts and sit-ups (knees bent or straight) (Axler & McGill 1997, McGill 1998).

People tend to be motivated to do exercise by the presence of pain and an enthusiastic therapist. Once the pain levels diminish, the motivation to exercise frequently disappears. Continued exercise can be encouraged by the use of group dynamics – exercise classes or an established routine. Unfortunately, the effect of exercises diminishes rapidly once they are curtailed, although the psychosocial response to future pain is improved, with reduced feelings of helplessness and disability.

ERGONOMIC EXPOSURE

In the absence of significant trauma, LBP is most likely to be caused by what a person does most often. For most people this is work, but it can also be domestic or recreational activities. Clues to this can often be in the pain patterns – worse during the working week or worse after a session of house cleaning. In cases of recurrent or chronic back pain, these activities should be reviewed and an effort made to improve postures and reduce biomechanical exposure.

Manual handling

The application of different lifting techniques is often difficult to incorporate into the practical demands of the workplace. There is no evidence that one type of lifting technique is superior to another. The key features with any lifting technique are to reduce leverages on the lumbar spine, to avoid fully flexed and rotated postures, and, in particular, to avoid a combination of the two.

Key lifting guidelines

- Keep the weight as close to your body as possible.

- Avoid fully flexed postures.
- Avoid twisted postures.
- Preload the spinal stabilizing muscles by sucking in the lower abdomen.
- Lift symmetrically.
- Avoid jerky movements.

Heavy manual work, lifting, and peak biomechanical loading are the most common readily identified causes of back pain. Reducing peak load and cumulative exposure can reduce the incidence of injury and its attendant morbidity. There are many before-and-after studies of ergonomic interventions reducing biomechanical loading and in turn reducing LBP incidence and morbidity. Although these are often criticized for their lack of randomized controls and lack of analysis of confounding factors, waiting for irrefutable scientific evidence of reduction in incidence of LBP from ergonomic interventions would be a disservice to workers in industries with known high biomechanical loads.

Good ergonomics involves good job design – reducing peak loads; avoiding stooped, bent and awkward postures; reducing total exposure in time and to weight lifted; ensuring correct height of workbenches and making available lifting equipment. It also requires management support for such things as task structure, work variety, job organization, maintenance programmes and availability of light duties.

Ergonomic analysis can be a highly technical process with sophisticated computer and video analysis, but significant improvements can be made by practitioners applying their musculoskeletal knowledge in a practical situation and providing a sound dose of common sense! It is

---

Box 13.1 The author's case history

I was becoming quite miserable when my own back was becoming quite chronic after a 6-month history of LBP following an acute injury. A small intervention in my treatment room – providing a table for the pillows I use when treating patients, instead of picking them up from the floor 30 times a day – produced a rapid resolution of symptoms. The bending action of picking up the pillows had never caused me pain but the cumulative load was hindering my ability to recover.

quite amazing how much difference a small intervention can make, such as oiling the wheels of a trolley or suggesting that objects are stored on benches rather than on the floor.

Standing

Long periods of standing increase compressive forces on the lower limbs, the lumbar spine and pelvis. Lumbar facet joints often do not like long periods of compression from standing. The lumbar curve and the facet joint stress can be reduced by resting one foot on a footrest, and alternating legs as appropriate. Standing on hard floors can accelerate fatigue. The use of cushioned shoes and shaped insoles helps to dissipate these forces and spread the load over a greater contact area. These interventions tend to be more cost-effective than providing antifatigue floor coverings.

Standing for long periods is fatiguing and it is preferable to alternate between standing and sitting, without prolonged periods in either posture. The sit/stand posture, with use of a forward-tilting stool and the weight distribution shared between the feet and the bottom, is excellent for this purpose (Fig. 13.11). If a more conventional chair is used it will need to be extra high, which can make it awkward to get on and off. This tends to discourage postural variety. The work surface can be adjustable in height to cater for standing and sitting postures, but it needs to have a simple mechanism, which is quick to adjust from either position, or it will not be used.

Slightly stooped spinal postures provide a long leverage on the lumbar spine with a high degree of compressive force. A significant degree of muscle tension is required to maintain this posture. Punnett et al (1991) have found the risk ratio of back disorders from mild trunk flexion to be similar to fully flexed postures. Clearly, standing workstations must be designed to minimize stooping-type postures. Careful attention should be given to workbench height and the trade-off between good standing posture and visual demands. This is covered in more detail in Chapter 14. Where more than one person is working at a workplace designed for standing it

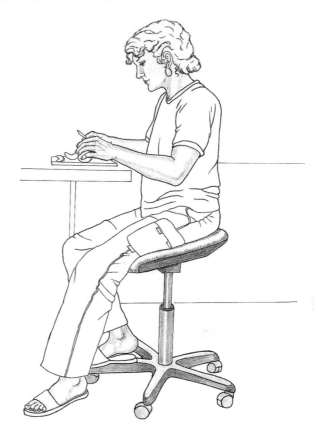

Figure 13.11 The sit/stand seat is ideal for use at a workstation designed for standing.

should be adjustable to suit their individual needs. It is not uncommon to find a man over 6 feet tall working at a workstation designed for the average-height woman, and suffering from recurrent, acute chronic back pain.

Sitting

Epidemiologists generally remain unconvinced as to whether sitting is a significant risk factor for back injury. The studies are conflicting (NIOSH 1997b, Riihimaki 1997). Kelsey (1975) found that of workers who sat for over 50% of the time, those aged under 35 had a risk ratio of 0.81 compared to controls, while those over 35 had a risk ratio of 2.4, suggesting a long cumulative loading period. People who sit for long periods in poor postures are thus at significant risk of developing spinal injuries from relatively minor trauma following periods of sitting. The issue is not so much whether they sit, but in what postures they sit, what furniture they use, what tasks they perform while sitting and how long they sit for. People who spend a large proportion of the week in an unsupported sitting posture, with a reverse lumbar curve and relatively low levels of physical activity, will not only accumulate physiological fatigue but will be at increased risk of injury to any sudden increases in loading. It may well be that the prolonged sitting in poor postures predisposes the spine to injury while the increase in loading becomes the culprit.

Most people with low back injuries are very sensitive to sitting postures – they are frequently unable to sit or find that periods of sitting aggravate their symptoms. This can frequently be a cause of delayed return to productive activity for patients whose work requires sitting for a majority of the day. Proving a good sitting posture should be a priority for patients who are required to sit for long periods.

Human beings are well adapted to the upright three-curve spinal posture. When we sit, a number of changes occur that affect spinal balance, strength and physiology:

- Single curve structure – the lumbar lordosis reverses, the thoracic curve exaggerates, the cervical curve frequently reverses – depending on visual demands.
- Intervertebral disc – there is increased pressure with dehydration, reduced fluid flow and nutrition, disc creep.
- Muscle – general inactivity of major muscle groups can weaken and shorten the abdominals, hamstrings and psoas. This can lead to biomechanical imbalance and inefficiency. Spinal postural muscles can be overused.
- Bone – relative osteoporosis for non-weight-bearing bones.
- Sclerosis – a gradual compensatory degenerative process for bone that has sustained pressure – vertebral end plates and facet joints.
- Ligaments – anterior laxity, posterior tension and ligament creep.

Sitting has become a major feature of modern life and, while postural variation is important, it is often impractical to advise people not to sit. Hence the importance of optimizing sitting posture. To produce optimum sitting postures, the above-listed effects of sitting should be minimized – to try to create a three-curve sitting posture.

Advice on sitting often assumes that good sitting posture is merely a matter of 'sit up straight'. In reality this can be difficult to do for long periods of time – it is very fatiguing on the spinal extensors. Good sitting posture requires the right tools and good task design.

It is usually assumed that good sitting posture requires a 90 degree angle at the hip joint with thighs parallel to the ground, and this continues to be recommended by many sitting guides. In reality, many people, particularly males, find it difficult to maintain a 90 degree angle at the hip joint and still maintain a reasonable lumbar lordosis. In most people, when hip flexion reaches 60 degrees the pelvis starts to rotate posteriorly and the lumbar curve starts to reverse and, in order to maintain a 90 degree angle between the trunk and thighs, there is 20–30 degrees of lumbar flexion. These ideas have been well-developed by Keegan (1953), Mandal (1981, 1985), Bendix & Biering-Sorensen (1983), Bendix & Hagberg (1984), Bendix & Bloch (1986) and Wilson (1994).

A schematic representation of this theme illustrates that in order to keep an erect lumbar spine we should look at limiting hip flexion to 60 degrees (Fig. 13.12). Tasks that demand an upright sitting posture – desk- and computer-based tasks – require a seat that allows a forward slope of the thighs of 20–30 degrees. Seating that has a fixed or adjustable forward tilt seat will provide this forward slope and, while this is important in cases of back injury, given the cumulative and widespread nature of back problems, can also be used to provide an optimal sitting posture for young people with no apparent injury. A good quality, fully adjustable chair (including seat tilt) is to be recommended for everyone who sits for prolonged working periods, on the basis that even if they do not have a current problem they will most probably develop an injury by middle age. This is a cost-effective intervention to avoid the cumulative effect of spinal injury produced by poor sitting posture.

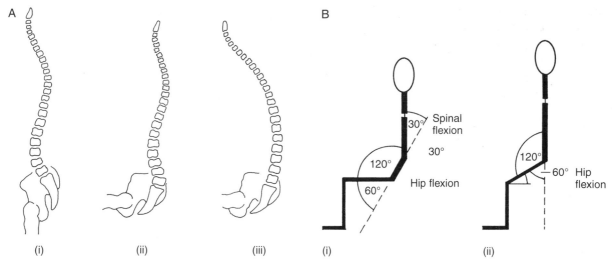

Figure 13.12 A (i) The normal standing posture, (ii) the idealized sitting posture, (iii) the actual sitting posture usually adopted with a reverse lumbar curve. B: Schematic comparison between (i) the traditional sitting position (note the 30 degrees of spinal flexion) and (ii) the balanced sitting posture (note the erect spine). Reproduced with permission from Wilson (1996).

A forward slope of the thighs will help maintain erect spinal posture (Bendix 1984). This can be achieved by providing a forward tilt seat or a well-designed seat with a waterfall front (Fig. 13.13).

Backrest

The backrest is an important component for reducing disc pressure and lowering EMG readings in spinal postural muscles (Andersson &

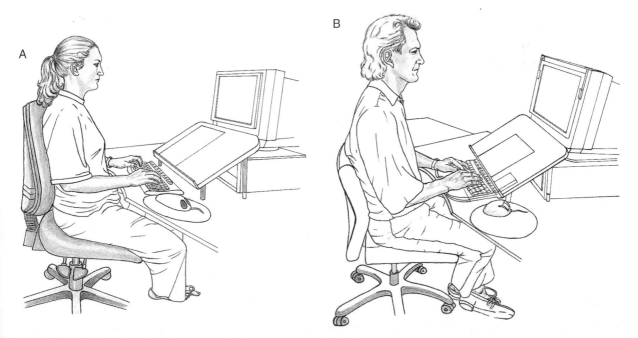

Figure 13.13 Different chair designs using the forward sloping thigh principle.

Ortegren 1974). This increases comfort, reduces postural fatigue and allows postural variation. A well-designed backrest can:

- help maintain a lumbar curve by lowering disc pressure and spinal extensor EMG readings (Andersson & Ortegren 1974)
- unload some of the weight of the trunk
- allow some postural variation – a more reclined sitting posture for client interviews, meetings or telephone calls (Fig. 13.14).

A backrest should provide good pelvic and lumbar support to avoid backward rotation of the pelvis and to maintain a lumbar curve. It should also be high enough to support the mid-back. It should be easily adjustable from the sitting position.

Postural variation

An unvaried posture of any type is unphysiological and sitting is no exception, even when the sitting posture is well-designed. Variations of posture should be encouraged – a mixture of sitting, standing and walking is ideal. A person should have a break from sitting for at least 10 min per hour or, better still, every 30 min.

Variations of posture while sitting are beneficial for musculoskeletal physiology. A chair that allows continuously variable adjustment will facilitate postural variation. A number of mechanisms allow change in sitting postures, to reflect the tasks being performed, without the use of levers.

Providing a good quality chair is not enough! People must be educated in good spinal posture, the importance of variation and how to adjust or manage their workstation. Recent research shows that most people rarely adjust their chairs and often have no idea what the knobs on their chair are for, or have them adjusted in such a way that makes their posture even worse! People generally feel most comfortable in positions that feel familiar – subjective comfort ratings are very unreliable and do not reflect biomechanical loading. There are many studies to show that people are unaware of increased levels of muscle tension and higher EMG readings. They

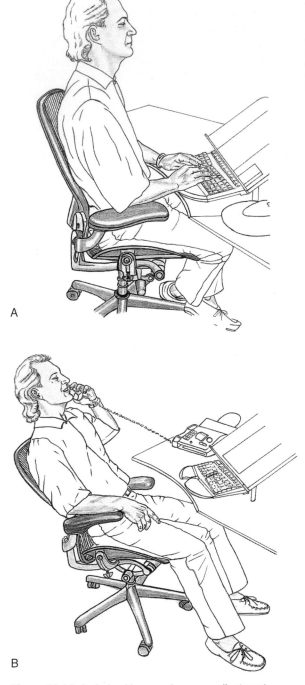

A

B

Figure 13.14 A chair with a synchronous adjustment mechanism can change postures as the demands of the task change from the forward tilting posture for computer work (A) to the reclined posture for telephone work or meetings (B). This allows maximal postural variation with minimum effort or thought required to effect postural change.

sometimes take a few days to get used to a new sitting posture, until it becomes familiar.

With increasing forward inclination of a seat, the spine becomes more upright and the lumbar spine becomes more neutral or moves toward lordosis (Bendix 1984). This is biomechanically advantageous. However, as the seat inclines there is increased tendency to forward slippage of the person on the seat. This can be influenced by different variables such as: seat contour, degree of upholstery friction, and user's clothing. Finding a comfortable seat inclination is often a trade-off between these two variables (Fig. 13.15).

There are a number of ingenious chair designs that allow upright spinal postures with forward sloping thighs that help maintain a lumbar lordosis, which prevent forward slippage. These can be a variation of the horse riding position as in a saddle seat, or with a kneeling pad.

Kneeler chair

The kneeler chair was developed to provide optimum forward tilt while providing a platform to prevent forward slip (Fig. 13.16).

The kneeler chair will never replace conventional seating, although it can provide an important role in rehabilitation and management of back injuries. Ergonomic researchers have generally not supported the use of kneeler chairs (Drury & Francher 1985, Lander et al 1987) while Bendix et al (1988) concludes that 'it may be a good alternative for some seated periods and special tasks'. However, the research has mainly been done with normal subjects at conventional tasks for very short periods. The kneeler chair comes into its own with back-injured patients, who frequently have difficulty with sitting. The kneeler chair, with its upright posture, is likely to minimize disc

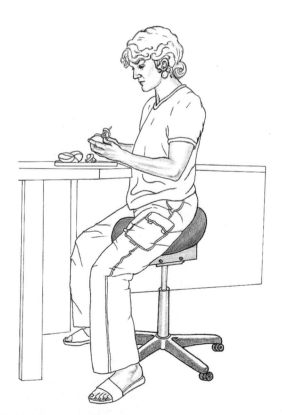

Figure 13.15 Example of a chair design that allows a good spinal posture, with forward sloping thighs, that prevents forward slippage.

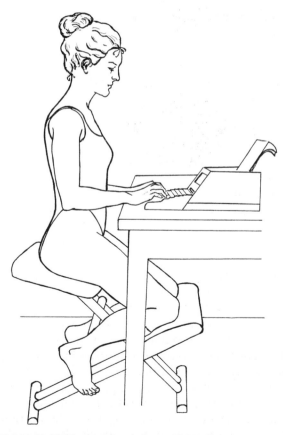

Figure 13.16 The kneeler chair provides optimum trunk–thigh angle while preventing forward slippage.

pressure while sharing the load with the facet joints. Frequently, a patient with a lumbar disc injury will be able to tolerate the use of a kneeler for short periods of sitting when they cannot tolerate sitting at a conventional chair. The use of a kneeler chair can assist in return to productive activity in acute disc injuries and in chronic back pain. However, the kneeler chair is not without its disadvantages:

- pressure points on knees and shins become progressively uncomfortable
- increased knee angle can affect circulation to lower legs
- awkward to get on and off
- it provides a fixed posture with little opportunity for postural variation – it becomes increasingly fatiguing with use
- it is difficult to use foot pedals
- it is socially unconventional.

In summary, the kneeler chair will never replace conventional seating but it can have a significant role to play in rehabilitation when sitting for shorter periods of up to 2 h. When given a choice between using a kneeler chair and using an adjustable tilt conventional for rehabilitation, most people choose the latter.

The backward-tilt chair

During the 1970s and 1980s, following the classic series of disc pressure studies during sitting (summarized in Andersson 1985) prevailing ergonomic wisdom decreed that the ideal sitting posture involved the use of a backrest as the most important feature of providing a lordosis and reducing disc pressure. In order to maximize the use of the backrest, a flat or reverse tilt seat with a backward leaning posture was recommended (Grandjean & Hunting 1977, Grandjean et al 1984, Grandjean 1988). While this type of seating may be good for the reclined posture where the backrest is used, it is positively dangerous for work postures that require an upright or forward-leaning posture. The forward-leaning postures commonly used for reading/writing and computer tasks make it difficult to effectively use a backrest (Fig. 13.17). The use of a reverse tilt seat

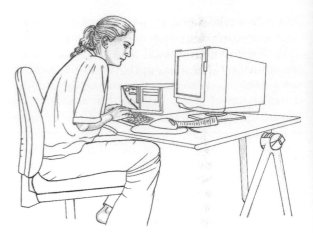

Figure 13.17 The reverse tilt chair represents a hazard to people who have to work at desk or computer-tasks.

in these circumstances further increases the lower lumbar disc compression. These types of chairs are still commonplace and should be avoided. Most ergonomic textbooks and sitting guides still recommend the 90 degree trunk to thigh angle, and many chair designs still feature the reverse tilt seat. In these days of increasing amounts of time spent sitting for work, pleasure, relaxation and transport this could be a reason why back pain disability continues to escalate in Western societies. It may not be possible to stop people sitting but practitioners should at least attempt to optimize sitting postures.

Designing a good sitting posture is important but is of limited value if the workstation is poorly arranged. Good visual angles are important to maintain a well-balanced and supported spinal posture (this will be dealt with in Chapter 14). Working with the weight of the arms unsupported anterior to the body (as in typing or using a keyboard) also places a load on the lumbar spine (Aaras et al 1997, Aaras & Ro 1998) (this will be covered in Chapter 16).

Car seat

Driving is a well-documented risk factor for LBP and the type of seat can have a bearing on the degree of discomfort (Porter & Gyl 1995). Porter found a protective effect from increasing adjustability of the seat and an automatic gearbox.

More modern cars with more efficient suspension systems are likely to protect against vibration. A higher car seat can ease the biomechanical strain of getting in and out and provide a more upright spinal posture.

Udo et al (1997) reviewed the literature for design of car seating and designed a seat with the following features:

- a lumbar support of 30 mm to retain lordosis and reduce disc pressure
- lateral support to keep the spine stable and supported in the upright position
- a firm cushion at the ischial tuberosities to provide stability and ease of postural change
- a softer cushion at the front of the seat with a waterfall edge
- an adjustable head rest
- a rubber mat under the seat to reduce vibration.

Thirty male subjects complaining of back pain used the seats for 6 months and were compared to 30 controls in a standard car seat. The subjects using the new seat showed improved mobility, reduced tenderness, improved Lasegue's test and significantly improved subjective evaluation.

SLEEPING POSTURE

Many back pain sufferers complain of pain at night and aggravation of symptoms on rising. Clearly, the type and quality of bed used and the sleeping posture adopted is an important factor.

It is normal for an injured person to be more aware of the discomfort when first going to bed. The removal of other sensory distractions such as light and sound increase the perception of any pre-existing sensation of pain. The sleeping posture should allow relaxation of neuromuscular tissues and this discomfort should gradually diminish.

Most people choose a sleeping posture where their muscles and joints are balanced in the mid-range of joint mobility (see Fig. 5.1). This is usually the sidelying position with a neutral lumbar spine and the hips and knees flexed to the middle third of their mobility range. Moving slightly off the sidelying position, more into the recovery position, helps reduce the width of shoulders and hips and assists in keeping the spine in neutral. Having one knee slightly more flexed increases the surface area of contact, reducing pressure points. This is the most common sleeping posture and is created in the search for comfort. Lying flat on the stomach or flat on the back with legs extended creates too much extension for many people, causing facet joint compression and reducing the size of intervertebral foramen. This can be relieved by flexing the knees and hips.

It is also necessary to keep the spine in neutral in the lateral profile. This requires a reasonably firm bed that does not bow or sag. However, a firm bed must have a soft top that allows the heavier and more curvaceous areas of the body (hips and shoulders) to bed down into the surface, assisting the neutrality of the spine and avoiding pressure points. This upper layer needs to provide some cushioning and recoil such as latex or foam rubber. Wool and cotton tend to bed down and become too firm.

Pressure points over the shoulder and hip are common and are the reason why people tend to toss and turn at night in the hunt for comfort. This will be exacerbated, and can become a cause of dysfunction in the shoulder and hip muscle stabilizers, in a hard bed. People with pain often wake up during a shift in posture; a comfortable bed helps avoid these manoeuvres. A comfortable bed always helps maximize muscle recovery from fatigue and assists the healing process.

It is probably not a complete coincidence that the peak age for chronic and recurrent low back pain (40–45) coincides with the ageing of the marital bed! It is pertinent to review the type and age of bed with back pain patients and to recommend an inner sprung or slat bed with a well-cushioned top. If there is a significant difference in size of sleeping partners, each side should be individually framed and supported.

During the 1980s in New Zealand, there was a mass consumer exodus into waterbeds, which at first impression seem seductively comfortable. However, there has since been a mass exodus out of them. The alteration in sleeping posture from an overly soft surface seems to contribute to chronic morning pain in the long term. There are also concerns about the electromagnetic radiation from the heater required to keep the water warm and its possible effect on neuromuscular sensitivity and other delicate homeostatic processes. Waterbeds are not to be recommended.

Muscles shorten over night and, as the normal age-related effect of loss of tissue elasticity takes hold, morning stiffness becomes more common. This is usually remedied by some gentle stretching exercises and a warm shower. However, to wake up with muscle spasm suggests something is amiss. Muscles and joints should recover over night rather than become fatigued and sensitized. Patients should be advised to avoid full lumbar flexion the first hour of the day. The intervertebral disc is superhydrated the first hour of the day and there is an increased risk of injury.

EDUCATION PROGRAMMES

Few would dispute the importance of education for LBP sufferers and those at risk from back injury. The importance of avoiding peak loading, poor postures and risk behaviours are self-evident. The value of explaining the recovery process, active rehabilitation and appropriate exercises, are an established part of good management of LBP.

It comes as something of a surprise that formal education programmes to teach lifting techniques and more general low back schools have often been of limited value in reducing incidence and morbidity of LBP.

Back schools

A back school is a structured educational process about back care. It usually incorporates a series of discussions about anatomy, biomechanics, lifting, posture and exercise. These programmes can vary widely in application, in subjects – preventative or targeted at those with a history of back pain; and in their target audience – employers, industry or independent.

A major review paper by Koes et al (1992) found 16 randomized clinical trials reporting the efficacy of back school programmes. Seven studies reported positive results compared to the reference treatment while seven reported results no better or worse. The four best methodological studies took place in an occupational setting and all showed positive results, which tended to diminish with time.

The results indicate that back schools may be effective for patients in occupational settings in acute, recurrent and chronic conditions. Most of the successful interventions consist of a modification of the Swedish back school and were quite intensive (3–5 weeks stay in a specialised centre).

The two best studies reported no differences in the study groups after 1-year and 2.5-year follow-up respectively. So far, the reported benefits of back schools were usually of a short duration.

Despite reported success in reducing incidence and recurrence of LBP with some subgroups, the lack of consistency has concerned researchers. In a review of four studies on the efficacy of back school with acute LBP subjects, using return to work as a measure, Scheer et al (1995) found only one with positive results with return to work, but even that did not demonstrate prevention of LBP in the following year. They concluded:

Although an ergonomic education programme for recently injured workers makes inherent sense, there is not incontrovertible published evidence that back school is more efficacious than placebo for acute LBP.

The efficacy of back schools and other educational programmes will always show mixed results because of the wide variability of subjects, settings and applications. Well-motivated subjects, keen to learn and apply information, are likely to benefit from an educational programme, particularly if they have the ongoing support of their employer.

LUMBAR/ABDOMINAL BELTS

Before-and-after studies have found a reduction in LBP incidence when back belts have been used in manual handling jobs. In a large study, Kraus et al (1996) found the incidence of low back injury reduced by 34% between 1989 and 1994. This study has been criticized for lack of a control group, and because a number of other interventions that affected the workers over the same period were not controlled for (McGill 1999).

Laboratory biomechanical studies have not been able to demonstrate reduced EMG readings or reduced biomechanical loading in the lumbar spine when a lumbar belt is used. Miyamoto et al (1999) found that wearing an abdominal belt raised the intramuscular pressure of the erector spinae and proposed that this would stiffen the trunk and stabilize the lumbar spine. Thoumie et al (1998) found a 20% reduction in mobility and a 4 degree reduction in the lumbar curve. Wolstad & Sherman (1998) found reduced axial twist in belt users. A number of researchers have noted an increase in systolic blood pressure and heart rate when using back belts and advise caution in recommending them. Other writers have talked about the danger of physical and psychological dependence on back belts and the increased injury risk when they are not used.

The reduction of lumbar mobility may help in avoiding peak loads. This may also reduce fluid flow and recovery processes in fatigued tissues. Review papers of the available research generally find the evidence unconvincing:

NIOSH believes that well-designed studies to assess the potential benefits and disadvantages of using back belts are still needed. Because of design flaws, the limited studies that have analyzed workplace use of back belts cannot be used to either support or refute the effectiveness of back belts in injury reduction.
NIOSH still believes that evidence for the effectiveness of back belts is inconclusive.
NIOSH (1997a)

McGill (1999) makes the point that the use of belts is not a quick fix and should not be a substitute for education and ergonomic appraisal. Richardson et al (1999) describe the transversus abdominis as the: 'patient's own natural deep muscle corset that surrounds the abdomen in the same way as an external corset to protect the back from injury' and recommends a range of exercises to strengthen it.

This is one of those areas where the more you read the more murky the whole area seems to become! Perhaps the best approach is to allow the use of back belts (on patient request) for acute LBP to facilitate the return to work while providing a proprioceptive reminder of the necessity to

be careful and to help avoid biomechanically stressful postures. It is important to stress the need to use the belt only when biomechanically loading and to spend increasing periods of the day without it.

REHABILITATION PROGRAMMES

A number of rehabilitation programmes that incorporate exercise programmes have increasingly been used for the management of chronic LBP, with encouraging results. These have a number of different formats but they usually include educational, psychological and social components along with supervised and structured therapeutic exercise aimed at improving musculoskeletal strength, endurance and flexibility in a group setting. It is very difficult to compare the results of the different studies directly because they differ markedly. Patient selection, content of the programme, assessment procedures, period of follow-up, type of control group and the financial and social incentives for recovery (or disability) can vary widely. However, it is worthwhile investigating some of these approaches to try and find what the successful formats involve, which components are beneficial for the management of chronic LBP and who is most likely to benefit.

Mayer et al (1987) assigned 116 patients to a 3-week intensive functional restoration programme and compared them to a group of 72 patients denied funding for the programme by the insurance carrier and with 11 patients who dropped out without completing the programme. The programme was 57 h per week and included exercises to enhance spinal mobility and strength, training in functional tasks, education, work simulation and hardening and an intensive psychological programme; 85% of both groups were contacted for follow-up. At the 1- and 2-year follow-up, 85% and 87%, respectively, of the treatment group were working actively, as opposed to 41% of the non-treatment group. The reinjury rate, spinal surgery rate and use of additional treatments were lower in the treatment group. The drop-out group fared worst of all, with only one out of the nine people contacted at work. This study showed a very impressive outcome for the patients who completed the programme, although the exclusion of drop-outs from the final data does flatter the statistics somewhat. There is some question as to whether the control group is a valid comparison because it was based on lack of funding for the programme rather than random selection.

Hazard et al (1989) reported on a similar programme that had an 81% return to work rate for graduates of the programme compared to 29% for the controls (who were also denied funding for the programme). The programme graduates showed significant improvement in pain levels, disability, depression and functional evaluations.

Torstensen et al (1998) randomly assigned 208 chronic LBP patients to exercise therapy, physiotherapy or a self-exercise walking programme. The exercise group (36 × 1 h) had an individually designed programme designed to improve mobility and improve muscular stability in supervised groups of five. The physiotherapy group received 36 sessions of a combination of treatments (e.g. massage, stretching, electrotherapy, exercises) based on what the physiotherapist thought would be most appropriate. The walking group was advised about the benefit of exercise and instructed to walk for 1 h three times a week in their own time. There was a 15% drop-out rate. Return to work rates were approximately equal for all groups (57.7% for the exercise group, 62.7% for the physiotherapy group and 57.1% in the walking group). The exercise and physiotherapy groups showed improved outcomes compared to the walking group including reduced pain, increased activity, increased satisfaction, less sick leave and substantial cost savings. There were no significant differences between the exercise group and the physiotherapy group in any outcome variable. This study suggests that skilled therapists with a range of tools at their disposal can achieve results similar to a structured rehabilitation programme. Therapists are well placed to intervene in the transition from acute to chronic pain and the deconditioning that accompanies it.

Bendix et al (1998a) compared the effects of an intensive functional restoration (IFR) programme with a control group (project A) and an IFR programme with two less intensive programmes (project B). The intensive programme consisted of a 3-week full-time programme followed-up by 3 weeks of 1 day per week. The programme had an intensive exercise component with additional psychological and educational components. The first less intensive programme consisted of 6 weeks of a 1.5 h exercise programme twice a week for 6 weeks plus 6 h of back school education. The second programme consisted of 45 min exercise and 75 min psychological training twice a week for 6 weeks. The intensive programme was a total of 135 h; the less intensive programmes were both 24 h. The control group was free to receive their normal care, of which 80% reported seeking treatment, including 61% traditional physiotherapy and 35% chiropractic manipulation.

At the 4-month follow-up, the results of the IFR group were outstanding compared with the control group and the two less intensive groups. At the 1-year follow-up a significant effect in favour of IFR was noted in both studies, although this was much stronger in project B. At the 2-year follow-up only those in project B showed significant improvement in most of the variables. In both groups there were fewer days of sick leave and fewer contacts with healthcare professionals than with the control group.

Lonn et al (1999) investigated the effect of an active back school programme on the recurrence rate of LBP. They randomized 43 patients to the programme consisting of 20 lessons over a 13-week period and compared them to 38 controls. The active back programme consisted of ergonomic instruction and lifting training followed by strengthening of the leg and trunk musculature and stretching exercises. Each participant was given individual instruction and encouraged to do home exercises. The control group was given no further instruction or treatment. Both groups were free to follow their own physical activities or treatments. At 12 months follow-up the active back school group had reduced LBP episodes and sickness absence, with significantly improved low back function and quality of life. The 12-month mean number of LBP episodes reduced from a mean of 1.6 to 0.4 episodes in the treatment group compared to 1.7 to 1.1 in the control group.

Keel et al (1998) reported on a multicentre Swiss study. 243 patients were assigned to an experimental 4-week inpatient programme, consisting of general exercise, strength training for trunk muscles, educational group sessions and individual therapy or counselling if required. These were compared with 168 patients who were undergoing a traditional treatment programme of 20 days' inpatient care comprising mostly individual therapy such as massage, hydrotherapy and physiotherapy. The drop-out rate was 31.1% with no significant difference between the two groups. After 1 year the return to work rate was 78.9% with no difference between the groups. The experimental group reported 23% less work incapacity compared to controls and worked an average of 1.4 h per day more. There were better long-term outcomes in the experimental group.

The subgroup of patients who improved the most were generally younger and most often housewives. The subgroup who deteriorated generally had a lower educational level with less professional training and described difficult environmental influences at work.

Kankaanpaa et al (1999) randomly assigned 59 chronic LBP patients to a 12-week (24 × 1.5 h) active rehabilitation programme or a control treatment of thermal therapy or massage for 1 month (1 × week). The active rehabilitation programme included behavioural support, ergonomic advice, stretching and relaxation exercises and a graduated exercise programme designed to improve mobility, coordination, strength and endurance of the trunk muscles. The results showed that the rehabilitation programme was effective in reducing back pain intensity, improving functional capacity and increasing lumbar paraspinal muscle endurance. The lumbar endurance tended to diminish at the 1-year follow-up, while the improvements in function and disability became more significant at the 6-month and 1-year follow-ups.

Friedrich et al (1998) compared a group undergoing an exercise programme and normal therapy to one undergoing the same programme with the addition of a motivational programme designed to assist exercise compliance. The combined exercise and motivation group was found to have better compliance and attendance with the programme, with significantly reduced levels of disability and pain. However, there was no greater adherence to a home exercise programme in the long term.

Frost et al (1998) compared two groups of chronic LBP patients. Both groups were taught specific exercises to be done at home and referred to a 3-h back school for an education programme. In addition, the intervention group attended eight 1-h supervised exercise sessions. When assessed 2 years later, the intervention group showed significantly reduced disability.

In a large study of 816 patients with chronic LBP disability at the Copenhagen Back Centre, Bendix et al (1998b) attempted to develop a profile of which patients were most likely to benefit from a functional restoration rehabilitation programme and which patients were least likely to benefit. Younger people were more likely to benefit while older people were more likely to seek a disability pension. Women were more likely to return to work than men. Longer periods of time away from work and severity of pain before entering the programme were indicative of a poor outcome. Smoking and exposure to vibration were associated with reduced likelihood of returning to work. Good isometric back endurance prior to the programme correlated with a good outcome.

The patients who were more likely to withdraw from the programme had a high number of sick leave days and longer periods with inability to work. There are no great surprises here, the results are consistent with previous research. It may reflect that those least likely to benefit have the most severe symptoms and the most difficulty in rehabilitating. It also suggests that there is an optimum time to place an individual on a rehabilitation programme – when the acute symptoms have subsided and the patient is capable of rehabilitation, before disability becomes a behavioural habit and while there is an accessible job. It reinforces the need for active management over the transition from acute to chronic LBP.

In a Scandinavian study of LBP patients off work for 8–12 weeks who took part in a light mobilization programme, Haldorsen et al (1998) studied the subjects who failed to return to work after 1 year and compared them with those who returned to work. The non-returners showed more restricted flexion and lateral mobility, impaired left Achilles tendon reflex, more previous X-rays, were older, had more children, had more children at home, had been less physically active, had a longer history of back pain, reported a higher physical workload and reduced ability to continue work, had been in one job for a longer period and had a low Internal Health Locus of Control score. The findings are consistent with the previous papers – the non-returners tended to be more chronic with greater physical deconditioning, found it more difficult to return to a physically demanding job and had reduced ability to adapt to a new one.

Pfingsten et al (1997), in a study of 90 chronic LBP sufferers attending an intensive 8-week programme of education, exercise and psychological intervention, reported a return to work rate of 63% of those out of work when the programme began. The changes in physical parameters such as mobility, strength and muscle endurance demonstrated little correlation with return to work. The factors that affected a person's return to work were:

- Pension – those who had applied for a pension, or who were already receiving one, were unlikely to return to their jobs.
- Length of time off work – the longer patients were off work, the less likely they were to return.
- Outlook – the patients who had a positive outlook regarding their return to work tended to return. A return to work did not occur in 70% of those who believed prior to treatment that it would not be possible.

A discriminative analysis showed that return-to-work outcome is most likely if the treatment reduces the perception of disability and reduces depression.

There is now a significant body of literature to demonstrate the success of active rehabilitation and functional restoration programmes. These seem to be effective in improving spinal function, reducing pain and disability, and improving return-to-work rates in chronic LBP sufferers.

Among the features that are found in the most effective programmes are:

- A graduated exercise programme designed to restore mobility, muscle strength and duration.
- An educational component to give ergonomic advice, improve knowledge base and control over symptoms.
- A psychosocial component to improve confidence and remove any negative beliefs or psychosocial factors that may be barriers to recovery.
- Exercises that are individualized, supervised and graduated. They should be performed 2–3 times per week for a minimum of 6–8 weeks. Adherence to the exercise regimen is likely to drop off as soon as the structured process is complete and the symptoms improve.

A successful outcome is less likely when there is prolonged time off work, advanced physical and psychosocial deconditioning, no job to return to, a physically demanding job, a poor psychosocial environment or compensation issues.

The Sherbrooke model (Loisel et al 1997) proposes a three-stage, integrated intervention to assist both the worker and the work environment:

Stage 1 – on the sixth week of absence from work an occupational practitioner examines the patient and makes appropriate recommendations to the medical personnel. An ergonomist visits the worksite to collaborate with the injured worker and management to suggest improvements to the work tasks aimed at earlier, safe and stable return to work.

Stage 2 – after 8 weeks of absence, examination by a medical back pain specialist to exclude serious pathology, and attendance at a back school programme lasting 20 h spread over 4 weeks.

Stage 3 – after 12 weeks, if a return to work has not been effected and there is a serious risk of chronicity, a multidisciplinary functional rehabilitation programme is instituted, followed by a progressive return to the worksite.

This model successfully combines the advantages of an ergonomic initiative to try and facilitate the return to work and, if this fails uses an education and functional rehabilitation programme. In a study based on the Sherbrooke model (Loisel et al 1997), 130 back-injured workers absent from work for at least 4 weeks were randomized into four groups:

- usual care
- clinical intervention
- occupational intervention
- full intervention (clinical and occupational).

The full intervention group returned to work 2.4 times faster than the usual care group (a mean of 84 days and 174.5 days, respectively) with the specific effect of the occupational intervention accounting for most of the improvement. The advantage of this programme is its filtering system, which attempts an ergonomic intervention with the cooperation of the employer prior to the rehabilitation programme.

In an ideal world, a group of therapists with the skills to recognize the more serious cases that are in danger of become chronic, and the physical and social deconditioning that accompanies chronicity, would have the tools to work with these patients to provide the appropriate management and treatment regimens (including manual therapy, ergonomic interventions and conditioning exercises) with the goal of reducing the morbidity of back pain and preventing the increasing personal and financial costs that LBP disability incurs.

EPIDURAL STEROID INJECTIONS

The rationale of epidural steroid injections is based on the anti-inflammatory actions of the drug on inflammatory processes such as disc prolapse and nerve root compression. Epidural injection can provide a local dose of the drug with less systemic side-effects.

A review paper by Koes et al (1995) reported on 12 randomized clinical trials on epidural injections for LBP and sciatica:

Overall, 6 studies indicated that the epidural steroid was more effective than the reference treatment and six reported it to be no better or worse than the reference treatment. ...
The best results show inconsistent results of epidural steroid injections. The efficacy of epidural injections has not been established. The benefits of epidural steroid injections, if any, seem to be of short duration only.

SURGERY

Surgery is a considerably overused treatment for LBP when one takes into account its cost, potential complications and the lack of evidence of long-term benefit. The rate of surgery varies substantially from one country to another, the highest rate being in the USA, where approximately five times the number of operations are performed than in the UK.

However, surgery does have a role to play in certain circumstances:

Cauda equina syndrome requires emergency surgical decompression.

Disc prolapse with severe, unremitting sciatica and profound neurological deficit that shows little sign of improvement in 4–6 weeks, can be considered for surgery. There is some evidence that outcomes can be improved at 1 year with severe prolapses if they are operated on early. However, there is no difference in outcome between surgery and non-surgery cases at 2 and 5 years. Most disc prolapses, even when severe, will make a full recovery without surgical intervention. Jonsson & Stromqvist (1996) found that extruded or sequestered disc prolapses had significantly better outcomes following surgery than contained disc herniations. The extruded/sequestered discs demonstrated an excellent outcome for sciatic symptoms at 12 months, with 90% showing improvement, compared to 79% for prolapse and 60% for focal protrusion. For LBP symptoms, the 12-month results were 84%, 67% and 50%, respectively. The extruded/sequestered discs had a much shorter period of morbidity prior to their surgery and had obviously been referred more quickly. It is probable that the symptoms were much more likely to be due to the effects of the disc extrusion while the contained disc injuries had a much longer period of morbidity and were more likely to have chronic pain complications. Graver et al (1998) followed 122 patients who had surgery for a herniated lumbar disc, of whom 73% returned to work, and concluded:

Female sex, low stature, long duration of sickness absence and strenuous work activities were shown to be related to lower frequency of return to work. These factors should be taken into consideration when selecting patients for surgery.

Other studies have shown that a support programme that encourages postoperative patients to resume activity, and which promotes early rehabilitation and physical activity, can improve outcomes (Donceel et al 1999).

Instability. An unstable vertebral segment, most commonly seen with spondylolysis, can produce a progressive forward slip of the vertebral body (usually L5). This places a shear force on the intervertebral discs, which can prolapse or herniate, and can cause significant neurological symptoms. If the shift of the vertebral body seems to be increasing and/or the neurological symptoms become pronounced, surgical fusion can be of benefit. However, not all spondylolysis is progressive and patients can frequently stabilize without surgical intervention (O'Sullivan et al 1997). Strengthening of spinal extensors, particularly multifidus and deep abdominals, can assist resistance of anterior shear forces.

Stenosis. Osteophytic encroachment of the spinal canal or vertebral canal can cause spinal stenosis. This can be from advanced degenerative change, congenital narrowing of the spinal canal or degenerative spondylolisthesis. The symptoms are usually found in patients aged over 50 who complain of aching, heaviness or paraesthesia in one or both legs when standing or walking for certain periods. Symptoms are eased by sitting or flexion. The patient usually has a history of previous back problems, and the symptom history is often gradually progressive. These cases can often be managed conservatively if the patient can accept some disability and can manage this effectively. Often, the condition can remain stable for long periods of time. Where the condition is severe and unremitting, or progressive, surgical decompression will usually relieve neurological symptoms, but it will remain a chronic degenerative spine.

The decision to operate should always be based on appropriate imaging, definitive diagnosis, patient consent and a clear idea of what procedure is being performed and what it aims to achieve. In most cases, conservative therapies should be trialled before proceeding. Surgery is expensive, creates biomechanical changes and carries risks, it should be used wisely.

As long as the decision whether to operate is made by orthopaedic surgeons who have a vested interest in the provision of the service, there will continue to be overuse of this modality. Decisions about surgery should be made by independent and knowledgeable rehabilitation specialists, not by surgeons.

OTHER MODALITIES

Other modalities that have no proven efficacy and are falling from favour include bedrest with traction, plasterbracing, TENS, and ultrasound.

SUMMARY

There are many different LBP subjects, with different loading histories, different traumas and different pathologies, trying to be rehabilitated into different workplaces and different psychosocial environments. With this myriad of influences it is little wonder that the treatment of LBP is so difficult to research. With the multitude of factors involved there will always be only limited commonality. Research of single interventions on multiple populations will always struggle to find a common denominator. Application of multiple interventions on complex LBP will have a much stronger likelihood of reducing symptom levels below the threshold required for recovery. Individual case management by skilled practitioners will help identify appropriate interventions in a far more efficient way than blanket prescriptions. There is enough information to show that there are effective interventions to reduce the incidence of transition from acute to chronic LBP, and to reduce the effects of chronic LBP. However, best practice requires:

- a base of well-resourced and skilled practitioners
- a good knowledge of the appropriate risk factors
- effective screening based on the type of injury, the person and the circumstances
- the opportunity to make timely interventions
- cooperative employers and healthcare agencies.

LBP disability is very costly to Western society. LBP interventions can also be costly but, if used wisely when appropriate, and based on individual needs, they can be highly cost effective.

Guide to appropriate interventions

1. Acute LBP mild – less than 2 weeks' duration:
   - analgesics or NSAIDs
   - normal activities
2. Acute LBP mild – more than 2 weeks:
   - analgesics
   - manual therapy/manipulation
   - avoid sustained or peak loads
3. Acute LBP – moderate:
   - analgesics
   - manual therapy/manipulation
   - exercises for pain avoidance and functional improvement
   - maintain normal activity levels as much as possible
   - minimize injury-related disability – light duties
4. Moderate LBP – longer than 1 month with poor progress:
   - as above
   - psychosocial assessment
   - ergonomic assessment to assist return to normal work activities
   - review exercises to include conditioning exercises
5. LBP – severe or with acute neuralgia:
   - analgesia
   - manual therapy
   - exercises for pain avoidance
   - minimize bending and sitting
   - light activity only
   - minimize rest as pain allows
   - frequent episodes of light activity

   - ice packs or heat/cold treatment
   - return to light duties or modified activities as soon as practical
   - ergonomic assessment to enhance return to normal activities
   - reassurance, education and avoidance of anxiety
   - recovery may be slow (particularly with neurological deficits or suspected disc extrusion). If no signs of ease in 2–4 weeks, image and refer as appropriate
6. Acute LBP with frequent recurrence:
   - analgesia and manual therapy as necessary
   - ergonomic analysis
   - education programme
   - exercise programme to improve muscle strength and stamina
   - aerobic exercise
7. Chronic LBP:
   - Analgesia only when necessary – acute episodes
   - manual therapy
   - education programme
   - exercise programme to improve muscle strength and stamina, aerobic exercise
   - ergonomic analysis
   - identify barriers to recovery – personal, psychosocial and ergonomic
   - psychosocial assessment
   - minimize conflict and anxiety
   - emphasize self-responsibility, management skills and identifying and managing barriers to improvement.
   - refer as appropriate if improvement ceases.

These categories are a guide only. They should be modified as appropriate depending on the individual case characteristics and the resources available.

Neck, shoulder and upper limb pain

14

Neck pain

Neck pain is remarkably common. Population-based questionnaires show a range in incidence ranging from 20 to 50% over the preceding 12 months; depending on the definition of neck pain, the design of the questionnaire and the population studied. Higher incidences are found in females, in the 40–60 year age groups, and in occupations that involve physically strenuous arm movements or have exacting visual requirements. Most neck pain is episodic but some 10–20% of people report chronic neck pain. Neck pain is often associated with shoulder pain. There is frequently referred pain to the medial and upper scapula region and many of the muscles that influence the neck, such as the trapezius and levator scapula also affect the shoulder region. Many researchers combine neck and shoulder pain into one category. Here the upper and medial regions of the scapula are included in neck pain and there is a clear distinction between neck pain and true shoulder (glenohumeral) joint pain.

The neck has a structure reminiscent of the lumbar spine, with a tripod 3-joint structure linking most of the vertebrae, and it is often assumed the injury mechanisms are similar. The considerable amount of research completed on the lumbar spine is often loosely applied to the cervical spine. However, in keeping with its quite different role, the structure, function and injury characteristics of the cervical spine have important differences:

● The cervical spine is designed for mobility – to provide a flexible stalk to allow optimal use of our senses, particularly vision. This mobility is at the expense of structural stability.

- The osteoligamentous structure of the cervical spine is relatively slight to allow functional mobility. It has a greater reliance on muscle tension to provide stability.
- The cervical spine is not primarily designed for work, manipulating tools or lifting weights. It does not have the structural or muscular capacity for these tasks.
- The weight of the head at the top of the cervical spine acts as a magnifier for joint stress and muscle tension. In neutral postures these are minimal, in off-neutral postures these can be dramatically magnified.
- The exposures to cervical structures are primarily postural. There is very little opportunity to substitute other joints to replace poor neck posture in the way that hip and knee flexion can substitute for lumbar flexion.
- The relatively unstable cervical spine is prone to injury from sudden increases in loading as in whiplash-type injuries or impact to the head.

RISK FACTORS

In a major review of the literature based on over 40 epidemiological studies relating the physical workplace environment and neck musculoskeletal disorders (NIOSH 1997b) the researchers concluded that there was:

- Strong evidence that working groups with high levels of static contraction, prolonged static loads or extreme working postures involving the neck/shoulder muscles are at increased risk for neck/shoulder musculoskeletal disorders (MSD). Twenty seven out of 31 studies found a statistically significant positive association between posture and neck/shoulder MSD. A consistently high odds ratio was found (12 statistically significant studies with odds ratios over 3) providing evidence linking tension neck syndrome with static posture or static loads.
- Evidence for a causal relationship between highly repetitive work of the arm and hand and neck/shoulder MSD. Twelve studies

showed statistically significant increase in risk with odds ratios greater than 3. Two studies measuring repetitive head and neck movements (frequency and duration) showed strong associations with neck/shoulder MSD.
- Evidence of forceful exertion involving the arm or hand and neck MSD. Of the 17 studies identified, 11 found a significantly positive association and six others had non-significant findings. Six showed a statistically significant increase but did not derive odds ratios; two found odds ratios greater than 3; seven found odds ratios of between 1 and 3, and two were less than 1.
- Insufficient evidence to provide support for the relationship between vibration and neck disorders.

Prospective studies that have included interventions to reduce repetitive work and improve postures have shown a reduction in symptoms and a decreased incidence of neck MSD, providing additional evidence of the link between workplace exposures and injury risk.

A substantial literature review (Hagberg 1995) found high prevalences in groups of workers exposed to static contraction of the shoulder and neck muscles and/or use of force and repetition. The prevalence ranged from 14 to 61% of workers with odd ratios ranging from 2 to 7. Reported rates were higher in women.

Occupations identified with increased risk include: operating a supermarket checkout, operating a sewing machine, poultry processing, data entry, assembly-line work, industrial work, dentistry, orchard workers, letter carriers, teachers, nurses, carpenters.

Risk factors linked with increased risk include: increasing time spent on the telephone, neck in greater than 15 degrees flexion, upper arm abduction greater than 60 degrees, increasing time spent data processing, bifocal use in data processing, working with hands above shoulder height.

ANATOMICAL CONSIDERATIONS

The atlanto-occipital articulation is atypical for the cervical region. The atlas has two ovoid, concave, medial facing surfaces that articulate with the occipital condyles. This structure has less stability than the typical 3-joint structure and permits a greater range of motion. There are 15–20 degrees of flexion/extension, 4 degrees of lateral flexion and 5 degrees of rotation.

The atlanto-axial articulation (C1–C2) is also atypical, with two lateral facets and a medial joint formed by an upwards conical projection of the axis between the anterior arch of the atlas and the transverse atlas ligament. This structure permits a much higher degree of rotation than a typical cervical vertebra, while still retaining stability in other planes. The range of rotation is 30–50 degrees, and represents 50% of the total cervical rotation. There is about 10 degrees flexion/extension.

The third to the seventh cervical vertebrae have the more typical vertebral structure, with 2 facet joints and an intervertebral disc separating each level. The superior surfaces of the vertebral bodies are saddle shaped, with prominent lips at the lateral aspect of the vertebral body. These are known as the uncinate processes and they articulate with the adjacent uncinate processes forming the uncovertebral joints. The saddle shape helps provide stability against anteroposterior shear forces, and the uncovertebral joints provide stability in the lateral plane (Fig. 14.1).

The cervical facet joints are orientated in a plane of 45 degrees in the frontal plane, which helps resist shear forces in flexion.

The third to the seventh cervical vertebrae work as a functional unit and allow a moderate degree of mobility, in the range of 10–20 degrees of flexion at each level, and 8–12 degrees of flexion and sidebending. Mobility is maximum at C5–C6. During flexion/extension movements a small amount of anterior/posterior translation occurs, estimated at 2–3 mm.

It has been assumed by many writers that the cervical intervertebral disc is of a similar structure to lumbar discs, and that the type of disc derangements are similar. However, the anatomical studies of cervical discs suggest that this view is erroneous. The role of the cervical disc is quite different, with increased ability to tolerate mobility and reduced need for compressive

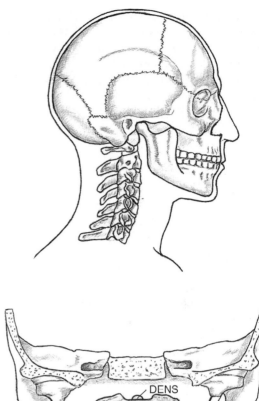

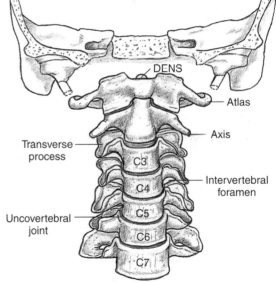

Figure 14.1 The structure of the cervical spine.

strength. The cervical nucleus pulposus shows evidence of fibrosis by mid teens and complete fibrosis by early adulthood.

The adult nucleus pulposus is better described as a fibrocartilaginous core penetrated to a greater or lesser extent by the uncovertebral clefts and surrounded by a discontinuous annulus fibrosus.

Mercer & Jull (1996)

Cervical disc protrusions are less common than lumbar disc protrusions but should be suspected with pronounced neuralgic upper limb pain. They occur most commonly at C5–6–7 in the 35–55 age group. They have also been reported on MRI at 10–15% incidence in the asymptomatic population.

Musculature

The cervical spine musculature is particularly at risk from neuromuscular fatigue and the cumulative strain of neuromuscular tension for the following reasons:

- The primary role of the cervical spine is postural. Suboptimal postures are often held for long periods of time, particularly for maintenance of vision.
- The high degree of mobility of the cervical spine can generate high loads and create localized peak stresses.
- The weight of the head, particularly in non-neutral postures, acts as a magnifier for load.
- There are few large muscles available for managing loads.
- There is little opportunity to recruit other joints or muscles to assist in maintaining posture.
- Modern work practices involve longer periods of sustained postures with less variation – fewer EMG gaps – than more traditional tasks.
- Forceful arm movements create significant asymmetrical loads on the cervical spine, particularly via the scapular stabilizers that attach to the cervical spine – the trapezius and levator scapula.

Scapular stabilizers

Trapezius. This has a broad region of attachment: medially at the occiput, ligamentum nuchae and thoracic spinous processes; and laterally to the spine of the scapula, acromion and lateral one-third of the clavicle. The trapezius is often cited as the most common site for trigger points (Fig. 14.2).

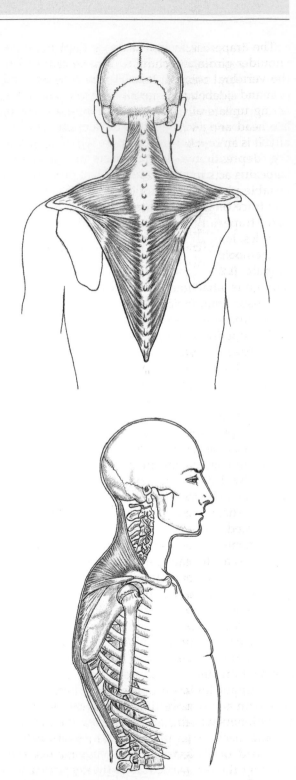

Figure 14.2 The trapezius muscle is primarily a muscle of the shoulder girdle but can be a significant cause of neck pain.

The trapezius is primarily a muscle of the shoulder girdle, attaching the shoulder girdle to the vertebral column. Its action provides a rotation and sidebending moment to the spine when acting unilaterally and an extension moment to the head and cervical spine when used bilaterally. It is an important muscle for carrying, resisting depression of the shoulder girdle. The trapezius acts to stabilize the scapula, providing a stable platform for moving the shoulder joint. The force on the neck during the stabilizing role of the trapezius is resisted by the anterior cervical muscles, longus capitis and longus colli.

Rhomboid (R) major and minor, and levator scapula (LS). These muscles typically have a tendinous attachment at the thoracic spinous processes (rhomboids), and the cervical transverse processes C1–4 (LS), with the LS attaching to the superior angle of the scapula, the R minor to the base of the spine of the scapula, and the R major to the medial border of the scapula. The LS travels more anteriorly to attach to the cervical transverse processes (Fig. 14.3). The LS has a number of actions – it elevates and stabilizes the scapula, provides a sidebending and rotation moment to the cervical spine when acting unilaterally, and an extension moment when acting bilaterally. This last action is particularly important in flexed neck postures, where it resists the anterior shear force.

The medial border of the scapula has no bony attachments and these three muscles (with the trapezius) act to stabilize (and rotate) the scapula to provide a stable platform for use of the upper limb. When the upper limb is being used these muscles act continuously and generate considerable muscular tension, much of which can be transferred to the attachments at the base of the occiput, the cervical transverse processes and the ligamentum nuchae. Via these muscles, actions of the upper limb can be an important cause of neck pain and dysfunction. It pays dividends for practitioners who have patients with insidious or chronic neck pain patients to investigate the workload of the upper limb and find ways of reducing the tension in the scapula stabilizers – improving the postures, reducing the forces and unloading the weight of the arm.

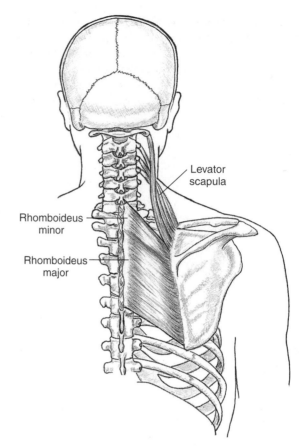

Figure 14.3 The rhomboids and levator scapula are important scapula stabilizers. They act to transfer load to the cervical and thoracic spines and can be important contributors of stress to these regions.

Cervical extensors

Splenius muscles. The splenius capitis and cervicis are large flat muscles that course from the ligamentum nuchae, the cervical and thoracic spinous processes (SPs), to the superior nuchal line, the mastoid process on the occiput, and the posterior tubercles of the cervical transverse processes (TPs) (Fig. 14.4). Acting unilaterally, they provide a strong rotation action to the cervical spine, and working bilaterally they have a powerful extensor action. The extensor action provides control of flexed neck postures when sitting and standing.

The semispinalis cervicis and capitis. The semispinalis cervicis arises from the TPs of the upper thoracic vertebrae and courses anteriorly and to

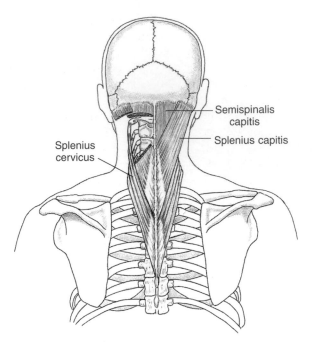

Figure 14.4 The splenius muscles play an important role in controlling cervical flexion.

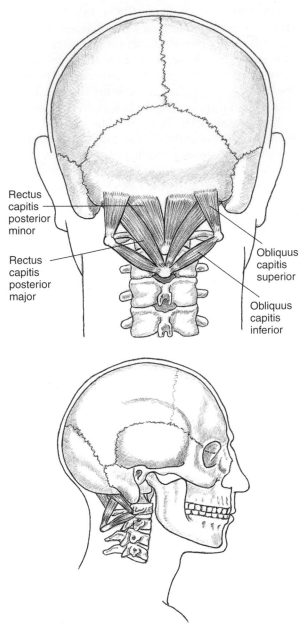

Figure 14.5 The suboccipital muscles provide control of head position.

attaches to the tips of the cervical SPs C2–5 (especially C2). The semispinalis capitis nearly covers the semispinalis cervicis, arising from the TPs of the upper thoracic and lower cervical vertebrae and the articular processes of the lower cervical spine having strong attachments to the occiput. They have a strong extension moment and are considered the prime muscles for increasing and dynamically maintaining the cervical lordosis, in the same way that multifidus acts in the lumbar spine.

Suboccipital muscles

Four pairs of muscles provide the deep muscular control of the upper cervical region. There are two paired groups of muscles in the midline – the rectus capitis posterior major and minor. The minor muscle ascends from the posterior arch of the atlas and ascends to the occiput; the major muscle is just lateral to this and ascends from the spine of the atlas to the occiput (Fig. 14.5).

The inferior oblique has a broad attachment from the SP of the axis to the TP of the atlas. The superior oblique attaches from the TP of the atlas ascending superiorly and medially to the occiput.

These muscles provide control of position of the upper cervical unit and head independently from the remainder of the cervical spine. This effectively fine-tunes the head position for optimum use of senses. The suboccipital muscles have an important proprioceptive function and become increasingly active as the head moves from neutral posture.

Lateral muscles

Scalene muscles. The scalenes all attach to the transverse processes of the cervical vertebrae and, descending down, the anterior and middle scalenes attach to the first rib, while the posterior scalene attaches to the second rib (Fig. 14.6A). The scalene muscles provide stabilization of the cervical spine in lateral movements while the anterior scalene can flex the cervical spine – or resist extension. The scalenes are intimately related to the neurovascular outflow as it traverses the thoracic outlet with the lower branches of the brachial plexus and the subclavian artery finding a path between the anterior and middle scalenes. The scalenes are often involved in whiplash injuries. Any neurological or vascular symptoms in the upper limbs may involve the scalenes. The scalenes often become overactive and taut in breathing disorders.

Sternocleidomastoid (SCM). The SCM passes obliquely across the side of the neck attaching superiorly at the mastoid process and inferiorly at the sternum and medial clavicle (Fig. 14.6B). It has many functions, acting as a guy rope to the cervical spine in both flexed and extended postures and acting to initiate and stabilize rotation and sidebending postures. It is often involved in whiplash injuries, torticollis, dizziness and temporomandibular joint (TMJ) problems.

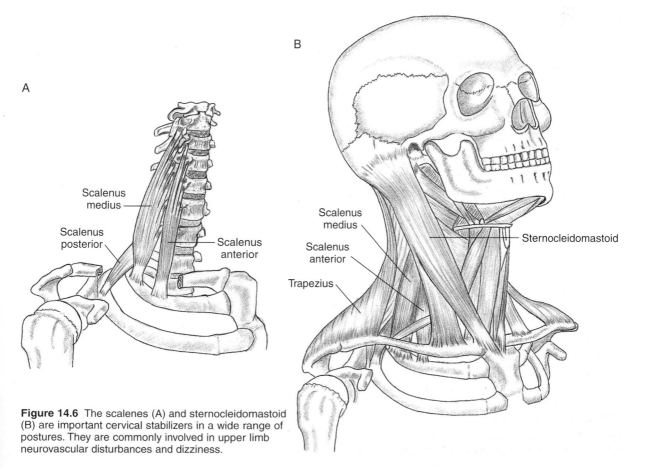

Figure 14.6 The scalenes (A) and sternocleidomastoid (B) are important cervical stabilizers in a wide range of postures. They are commonly involved in upper limb neurovascular disturbances and dizziness.

Cervical flexors

Longus colli and longus capitis. The longus colli has extensive attachments between the atlas and the thoracic vertebrae. The longus capitis travels from the anterior tubercles of the cervical TPs to the occiput (Fig. 14.7). They provide a flexion force to the neck and when acting bilaterally they create compression.

Rectus capitis anterior and rectus capitis lateralis. The rectus capitis anterior and lateralis have a flexion moment with attachments between the atlas and the occiput. They have an important stabilizing and proprioceptive function for fine-tuning head postures.

The cross-sectional area of the cervical flexors is much less than the extensors. Flexion in the upright posture is largely controlled by the extensors acting against gravity. The flexors' role is more for stabilization, control of extension, and flexion from the prone position. This lack of flexor strength can leave the cervical spine vulnerable in whiplash injuries.

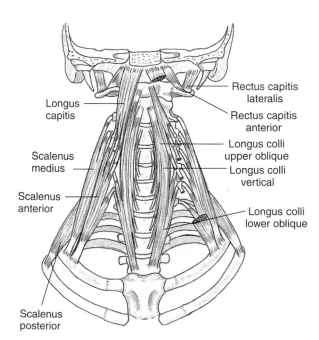

Longus capitis
Scalenus medius
Scalenus anterior
Scalenus posterior
Rectus capitis lateralis
Rectus capitis anterior
Longus colli upper oblique
Longus colli vertical
Longus colli lower oblique

Figure 14.7 The longus capitis and longus colli are important flexors and stabilizers of the cervical spine.

Neuromuscular control

The cervical muscles have complex interrelationships to maintain stability and to fine-tune posture and movement. Movements are often complex and multiplanar. With the additional needs of stabilizing a highly mobile region, there is often a high degree of muscular activity in upright postures and a need for continual feedback to facilitate the continual adjustments to posture. This feedback comes from specialized cells known as muscle spindles. The muscle spindles monitor the contractual state of the muscle and register any changes in contraction or velocity and relay the information to spinal, cerebellar, extra-pyramidal and cortical centres of the brain. There is evidence that the cervical muscles are richly endowed with muscle spindles, reflecting the important stabilizing function of the muscle fibres. Spindle density of 200–500 per gram can be found in the deeper muscles of the cervical spine, compared to 50 per gram in a large muscle such as the rectus femoris. Sympathetic nerve endings have recently been described in muscle spindle cells and this provides a possible mechanism for the change in sensitivity and increased levels of muscle tension when subject to stress. The cervical musculature seems to be particularly prone to the effects of stress and can display an inability to relax during periods available for rest.

The mechanisms of muscle fatigue were reviewed in Chapter 4. There has been more research carried out on the trapezius muscle than other muscle groups due to the widespread myalgia associated with this muscle, its important role as a stabilizer for both neck and scapular and its ready access for study. Research has consistently demonstrated morphological change in this muscle with subjects suffering from myalgia. These changes include:

● increased size of type 1 muscle fibres
● reduced blood flow and reduced levels of high energy phosphates
● increased number of red-ragged fibres with mitochondrial disorganization.

More recently, Kadi and co-workers (1998) investigated 21 women with work-related myalgia of the neck and shoulder region for at least 1 year. They found increased size and area of type 1 fibres, irregular mitochondrial patterns and an increased proportion of cytochrome-c-oxidase (COX) negative fibres. COX deficiency is indicative of an energy crisis in the muscles. Kadi et al (1998) conclude:

These changes provide additional evidence for a disturbance of the microvascular circulation.
  In conclusion, static work associated with the inadequate capillary supply and the presence of fibres bioenergetically deficient are presumed to be key factors involved in trapezius myalgia.

Larsonn et al (1998) also found lowered microcirculation in the trapezius on the affected side in 71 patients suffering from chronic neck pain who had been diagnosed with cervicobrachial syndrome. They also report similar findings of disturbed regulation of microcirculation in the trapezius muscle in patients with chronic neck pain due to a previous whiplash car accident: 'Many of the patients were found to develop chronic trapezius myalgia which might maintain the 'whiplash' pain'.

Altered trapezius circulation with secondary morphological change appears to be a common pathway for neck injuries of varying aetiology, including overuse and traumatic injuries. Studies of patients with trapezius myalgia have shown that patients use their muscles at a higher static level and have fewer EMG gaps compared to healthy subjects (Veierstad et al 1993).

The reduced capacity of the muscles to tolerate stress, the reduction in circulation and the earlier onset of muscle fatigue under loading must be taken into account when designing treatment and rehabilitation programmes for chronic neck patients.

ERGONOMIC CONSIDERATIONS

A good understanding of the cervical musculature helps appreciate the muscle loading that takes place in different postures. When designing rehabilitation programmes for injured patients it is important to keep muscle loading to a minimum for work postures and to try and create dynamically varying work environments. A significant body of ergonomic literature is concerned with the loading in different postures and the relative risk of injury.

Computer work

Villanueva et al (1997) measured neck flexion angles and EMG readings in ten healthy subjects performing a mouse-driven VDU task that required constant visual attention to the screen. They measured three different screen heights of 80 cm, 100 cm and 120 cm to the centre of the screen (desk height was 67 cm). The postural analysis showed that neck posture became more erect at higher screen heights, and this correlated with significantly decreased EMG readings of the cervical extensors. Thoracic curvature was significantly reduced with increasing screen height, with greater use of reclined postures (presumably making greater use of the backrest). Six subjects showed reduced EMG readings of the descending portion of trapezius with reducing thoracic curvature, while two subjects showed increasing levels of trapezius EMG – with reclined postures – forward-reaching to the mouse.

Turville et al (1998) compared VDU positions with visual angles of 15 and 40 degrees. They found significantly reduced head tilt angles at 15 degrees, with six of the ten measured muscles exhibiting half of the EMG readings compared to 40 degrees. The average EMG readings increased from 3% MVC at 15 degrees to 6% MVC for the 40 degree angle. Jaschinski et al (1999) gave 38 computer operators freely adjustable VDU screens and allowed them to adjust them as they found most comfortable. The screens were preset at low and high monitor positions and distances of 66 cm and 98 cm, with each subject having the opportunity to try each position. There were no source documents. The preferred mean gaze inclination was −10 degrees and a mean visual distance of 90 cm. Shorter distances were associated with increased eye strain.

Hamilton (1996) measured levels of neck extensor and sternocleidomastoid muscle tension, head position and mechanical load at C7, in reading and typing tasks with source documents in six different positions:

1. flat on table left of keyboard
2. document stand left of keyboard
3. low centre between monitor and keyboard
4. high centre in place of monitor (monitor shifted to right)
5. flat on table right of keyboard
6. document stand right of keyboard.

The results showed that the orientation of the head and the muscle tension generated was related to the position of the source document. Highest loads were generated in flexed and rotated positions, followed by rotated positions. Lowest loads were developed in central positions with a significant advantage to the high centre position. Higher loads were produced in typing as opposed to reading. Neck flexion was found to be the critical factor in production of neck extensor tension. Hamilton concludes:

The placement of the source documents in a computer workstation significantly affected the level of tension that existed in the neck extensor muscles. An increase in either vertical or horizontal displacement from centre produced an increase in neck tension. Typing increased neck muscle extension significantly more than reading.

These studies clearly demonstrated the importance of the visual source in determining head position, joint forces and muscle tension. For subjects who primarily use the VDU, a high, central VDU position is beneficial for neck and thoracic postures with reduced levels of muscle tension in the cervical extensors and the descending fibres of trapezius. For subjects who make extensive use of source documents in addition to the VDU, increasing priority must be given to a high central location for a document holder. However, caution must be advised in the degree of backrest inclination as reclined postures seem to activate the trapezius fibres due to overreaching. Ergonomists generally recommend trying to maintain visual angles in the 0–30 degree below horizontal range to avoid neck flexion. Pheasant (1997) regards this as the preferred display zone; Kroemer & Grandjean (1997) regard +5 degrees to 30 degrees below horizontal as the 'cone of easy eye rotation'. In many computerized workstations both the VDU and copyholder will compete for this space

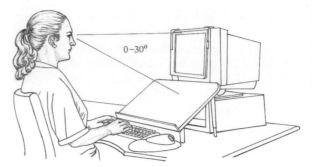

Figure 14.8 A high central location for VDU and document holders, with an upright spinal posture, appears to optimize neck and thoracic postures while minimizing muscular activity of the neck and scapular muscles. Priority should be given to the 0–30 degrees viewing zone.

and the relative position of the two depends on the amount of use of each, the size of the screen, the portion of the screen most used, the amount of reaching required to documents, etc. A high VDU position (top of the useable screen level with the eyes) and placement of the copy holder as high as possible under the VDU is generally to be recommended (Fig. 14.8).

Reading and writing tasks

The same principle of improving visual angles for a positive effect on posture applies to more traditional reading/writing-type tasks. However, for writing tasks there is a trade-off between improving visual angles and creating elevated and unsupported postures for the arm when writing. These can increase tension in the upper arm and scapular stabilizing musculature.

A look at furniture design in previous generations shows that clerical workstations were usually sloping. Good posture was considered a sign of good manners and furniture was designed to facilitate this. Current fashion has flat, horizontal surfaces for reading and writing tasks, capable of multipurpose use. The low, flat desk demands a poor flexed posture for the neck and spine for reading and writing tasks (Fig. 14.9). There is evidence that small amounts of slope can have a significant effect on posture.

Bendix & Hagberg (1984) compared sitting posture for three different desk slopes – 45, 22 and 0 degrees – for reading and writing tasks.

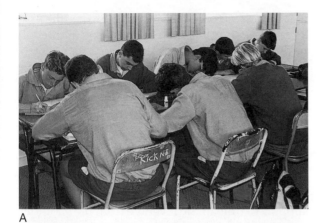

A

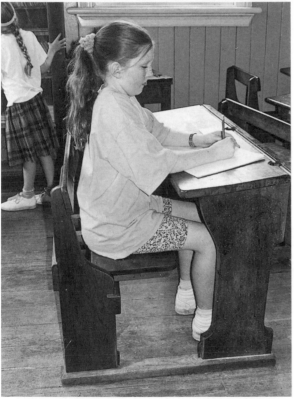

B

Figure 14.9 Low flat desks for reading/writing tasks lead to flexed spinal postures and excessive neck tension. Small changes in the slope can create relatively large improvements in posture. The modern school environment (A) is in contrast to an old fashioned school desk (B).

They found that posture improved with increasing desk slope, with a 14 and 6 degree change towards the vertical of the cervical spine and trunk, respectively, when the 45 degree surface was compared to the 0 degree surface. The rating for acceptability was in favour of the 45 degree slope for reading but against either tilted surface for writing. Bendix & Hagberg suggest that reading matter should be placed on a sloping surface while the writing surface should be horizontal. Other studies have found significant postural advantage for reading/writing tasks with a 10 degree slope. De Wall et al (1991) studied ten subjects sitting at 0 and 10 degree sloping surfaces. They found that the position of the head and trunk were 6 and 7 degrees, respectively, more erect with the 10 degree surface and calculated an average decrease in force of 15% for the neck and 22% for the trunk. They concluded that: 'A reduction in the number of neck complaints could be expected'. Freudenthal et al (1991) also compared slopes of 0 and 10 degrees and found the position of the neck 8 degrees more upright and the trunk 9 degrees more upright with the 10 degree tilt. They calculated that this corresponded in reducing the moment of force 29% at L5–S1 and 21% at C7–T1. They noted:

Desks with a small slope have a relatively large effect on the position of the trunk and head. A great advantage of a desk with a slope of only 10 degrees is that it is easy to use whilst reading and not an inconvenience when writing. Pencil and paper do not slide down.

Both studies noted that some individuals showed much more pronounced improvements in posture than the average findings.

In conclusion, there are positive benefits to recommend a slope of 10 degrees for writing and, if reading documents are required, a greater angle has more positive benefits (Fig. 14.10). The worksurface height can also make a difference to spinal posture with clerical tasks and a low desk will encourage flexed postures to reduce visual distances. Bendix & Bloch (1986) studied 108 subjects with adjustable tables and chairs to determine preferred desk and seat heights. They recommended a table height of 4–6 cm above sitting elbow height. They noted that children preferred greater desk heights and recommended that a slanting worksurface should be 'even more recommendable than for adults'.

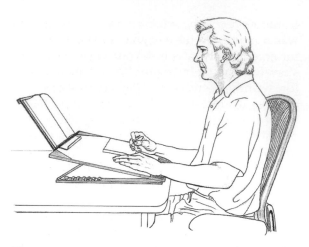

Figure 14.10 A well-designed workstation for reading/writing tasks involves a small slope for writing (10–15 degrees) with a greater slope for reading.

Mandal (1985), after extensive trials and postural analysis on preferred postures for schoolchildren, also recommended higher desks and chairs than usual, with tiltable worksurfaces. Ergonomists generally recommend worksurfaces 5–10 cm above elbow height for delicate or precision work such as sewing, craftwork or electronic assembly (Kroemar & Grandjean 1997, Pheasant 1997). At these heights it is important to have the arms supported on the worksurface rather than to use muscle tension to elevate the shoulders and arms.

It is difficult to recommend a general height for desks. The clinical ergonomics approach requires that people have a worksurface that suits them with regard to their personal anthropometry, their particular symptoms and the tasks involved. This means that educational institutions and employers should provide a range of workstation heights to ensure that everyone is catered for, not just those who cluster around the average. In conclusion, a worksurface 4–6 cm above sitting elbow height is recommended for reading and writing tasks, with additional heights considered for children and precision tasks.

Using the upper limb

The position of the arm has a significant effect on the amount of tension generated in the trapezius and levator scapula muscles. The further the arm is moved from the body – notably by abduction or flexion – the greater the muscle tension generated in these muscles. This muscle force can be magnified by manipulating tools or using a hand grip. The usual guidelines apply regarding muscle fatigue due to high loading or repetitive loading with insufficient breaks. Static loading can also be a risk factor for the scapular stabilizing muscles. Mouse or keyboard use has few EMG gaps, providing a prolonged static load (Hagberg & Sundelin 1986). Insufficient forearm support to unload the leverage from the shoulder muscles has been shown to elevate muscle tension levels, producing more rapid fatigue and loss of efficiency (Aaras et al 1997, Hermans et al 1998a).

Precision work and stressful work have been shown to increase activity levels of the shoulder and scapular muscles. Sporong et al (1998) monitored the EMG activity in five shoulder muscles in different arm positions and compared it with precision manual tasks in the same position. There was a 22% increase in average EMG readings in the precision tasks, with the levator scapula increasing to a high degree (20–40%) and the rhomboid major and trapezius to a lesser degree. The trapezius has been shown to be poor at utilizing rest periods after long periods of static contraction – it loses the ability to relax. This has been proposed as a risk factor in some subjects. Haag & Astrom (1997) compared trapezius EMG readings in medical secretaries with shoulder myalgia to those who had no symptoms. They found more frequent EMG gaps in the healthy medical secretaries. The lack of EMG gaps can be due to a combination of:

- static loading with little opportunity for relaxation
- increased stress levels
- personality factors
- muscle fatigue processes.

SUDDEN FORCE INJURIES

The neck is very prone to sudden force injuries, particularly from whiplash-type injury, where a sudden force is applied and the unstable head and neck hyperextend or hyperflex. A stumble or fall providing an unexpected peak force can provide a similar type of injury. A very common form of sudden force injury is a blow to the head, which can provide a sudden acceleration injury, or where the head comes into contact with something while already moving, which can provide a deceleration force injury. These injuries are all similar in nature and the degree of trauma is related to the forces of the head and neck relative to the body and the planes and range of movements involved. There is usually a combination of planes of movement and a combination of traumatized tissues, including ligamentous, neuromuscular, facet compression, neural traction and inflammatory processes.

This type of injury requires more specialized assessment and management, particularly when severe and serious tissue damage is suspected or when neurological symptoms develop. Clinically, they should be managed conservatively to begin with to allow the inflammatory processes to diminish and the soft tissue healing processes to proceed. Ice is very helpful in the acute inflammatory stage. Every effort should be made to maintain normal mobility within pain barriers to enhance fluid flow, reduce neuromuscular sensitivity and reduce disability. This will enhance effective recovery and minimize the risk of complication. As the inflammation settles, gentle mobilization up to the tissue pain barrier is helpful, but care should be taken to avoid stress on any traumatized tissues. Immobilization using collars should be avoided where possible. Exceptions can be made for short periods with acute situations but the use of collars should be minimized. Any such reduction in mobility will reduce healthy fluid exchange and proprioception and encourage sensitization of muscle spindles, producing increased stiffness and disability. As the soft tissue healing progresses, more active manual therapy and rehabilitation can be used. In a landmark study, Mealy et al (1986) compared 61 whiplash patients randomized into an early mobilization group with a group given 2 weeks in a soft collar with rest prior to mobilization. The two groups were assessed on a linear analogue

scale (where 0 was completely free of pain and 10 was maximum pain thought possible) prior to treatment, and at 4 and 8 weeks. The early mobilization group had scores of 5.7, 2.8 and 1.7, respectively, while the soft collar group scored 6.4, 5.1 and 4. Mobility was significantly improved in the active group at 4 and 8 weeks. Mealy et al (1986) concluded that: 'Initial immobility after whiplash injuries gives rise to prolonged symptoms whereas a more rapid improvement can be achieved by early active management without any consequent increase in discomfort'.

There is evidence that whiplash-type injuries can lead to widespread sensitization and the presence of trigger points. Buskila et al (1997) compared 102 patients with neck injury (74 were motor vehicle trauma, 28 were single event and work-related) with 59 patients with leg fractures. The neck-injury patients had a much higher presence of tender points in the upper body and 21.6% of the neck-injured patients fulfilled the diagnostic criteria for fibromyalgia syndrome, compared to 1.3% of the leg-injured patients. Quality of life and physical functioning were significantly more impaired in the patients with neck injury. This study suggests that neck injuries may produce an accelerated progression to a type of chronic pain syndrome.

There is a great deal of literature about the ramifications of whiplash syndrome and its behavioural and physical genesis. This literature will not be renewed here except to say that it has remarkable similarity to other chronic pain and chronic overuse syndromes. Significant trauma with multiple tissue damage to a highly innervated region close to the central nervous system has the capacity to accelerate the normal processes of chronicity. The whiplash syndrome should be recognized early on in the history and the full LOAD model applied with the manual therapy and clinical ergonomic management models.

DEGENERATIVE CHANGE

There is evidence that cervical degenerative change begins at a young age. Hole et al (1995) found that cervical mobility in all planes declines with age, and that the change is most noticeable in early adulthood, in the 20–29 and 30–39 age groups. They estimated the decline at 4 degrees in flexion and lateral flexion, 6–7 degrees in extension and 4–7 degrees in rotation, per decade over 20.

The pattern of degenerative change is similar to the lumbar spine, with fissuring, erosion and general thinning of the articular cartilage of the zygapophyseal joints and accompanying osteophytosis. Narrowing of the intervertebral disc is accompanied by osteophytosis at the vertebral end-plate margins. At radiological examination, 90% of males over 50 and 90% of females over 60 exhibit degenerative changes, most commonly at the C5–6–7 levels (Fig. 14.11).

MRI studies show greater sensitivity to degenerative changes at earlier age groups and have shown that 25% of asymptomatic subjects under the age of 40 demonstrate disc degenerative change, this increases to 60% in subjects over 40. Dai (1998) examined 260 patients with cervical spine disorders and compared their MRI changes to functional radiographs. He found a high incidence of degenerative change, which significantly increased with age, at all levels of the cervical spine. He also found an association between early degenerative change and segmental instability.

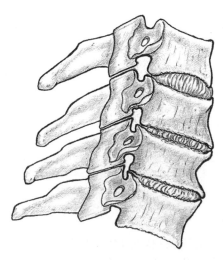

Figure 14.11 The typical pattern of cervical spine degenerative change. This affects 90% of people over 60, most commonly at C5–6–7 levels. The narrowed intervertebral foramen increases the risk of nerve root insult.

He proposed that loss of disc height produces a laxity in the facet joint capsule, resulting in segmental instability. Progressive degenerative change tends to restabilize the segment. There would seem to be a link between early degenerative change, combined with relatively youthful mobility, being likely to increase the degree of instability and aberrant segmental motion.

There is poor correlation between degenerative changes and symptoms, and many asymptomatic subjects demonstrate degenerative changes on MRI. However, the presence of degenerative change, particularly at a young age, will increase the sensitivity of the cervical spine to poor posture and biomechancial loading and increase the risk of developing symptoms. As in the lumbar spine, where a history of poor sitting posture has been linked with teenage Scheuermann's condition and early onset of intervertebral disc problems, head and neck postures in youth may predispose to early degenerative problems, instability and chronic neck problems in the cervical spine. Degenerative change in the lower cervical spine increases the possibility of compromise of the nerve root as it exits through the spinal canal. This may be from a bulging intervertebral disc, a fragment of disc material or from osteophytes at the uncinate processes or apophyseal joints. This most commonly occurs at the C5–6–7 levels affecting the C6–7–8 nerve roots.

SYMPTOMS ASSOCIATED WITH NECK INJURY

Headaches

Headaches are common in all age groups. They are often associated with neck or head injuries and frequently accompany neck pain and stiffness. However, there are many other causes of headaches, including vascular, meningeal, toxic and infectious, and sound differential diagnosis is important.

The so-called tension or cervical headache remains one of the most common causes. It is usually suboccipital, with pain radiating to the frontal, orbital or temporal regions. It can fluctuate in intensity and may be accompanied by light-headedness, fatigue and poor concentration. It tends to be aggravated by stress and poor posture and is eased by massage of the suboccipital pressure points. Frequent tension or cervical headaches can often be a primary presentation, often related to neck muscle tension and stiffness, although the subject may not necessarily be aware of any cervical dysfunction.

The pathophysiology of tension headache is poorly understood. Bogduk (1994) proposes that any afferent stimulation of tissues in the C1, C2 and C3 spinal nerves can produce referred pain to the head and suboccipital regions via the trigeminocervical nucleus. According to Bogduk (1994):

The receptive field of the upper three cervical nerves includes the joints and ligaments of the upper three cervical segments, their posterior and anterior muscles, the sternocleidomastoid and trapezius muscles, the dura mater of the posterior cranial fossa, and the vertebral artery. All of these therefore, become possible sources of cervical headache.

A number of researchers have been able to reproduce headaches in volunteers by applying stress to the upper cervical tissues, in particular the suboccipital extensor muscles and the occiput–C1 and C1–C2 joints. Other plausible explanations for cervical headache are suboccipital extensor muscle hypoxia and fatigue, and dural traction from the deep suboccipital extensors. Hack et al (1995), in a series of 11 cadaveric examinations, reported finding a connective tissue bridge between the rectus capitis posterior minor muscle and the spinal dura, and there has been speculation that the pain sensitive dura may be a source of headaches.

Hurwitz et al (1996) reviewed the literature for trials of manipulation and mobilization for headache. They concluded that 'Although some data indicate benefits of manipulation or mobilisation for patients with headaches, … the sparsity and quality of the data prevent a firm conclusion being reached'.

However, they found trials that did show some positive effects. The highest quality randomized, controlled trial demonstrated improved outcomes for chiropractic manipulation over amitriptyline 4 weeks after the conclusion of 6 weeks' treatment.

Manual therapy, including manipulation, showed short-term benefits (gone by 5 weeks) over cold packs for patients with post-traumatic headache of at least 1 year's duration. Physiotherapy (including mobilization) and acupuncture both showed statistically significant improvements for chronic muscle tension headaches at 4 weeks, with physiotherapy greater than acupuncture. Niere & Robinson (1997) analysed the treatment outcome of 112 headache patients presenting for manipulative physiotherapy. At the 2-month follow-up there were statistically significant improvements in frequency, duration and intensity. Of the 95 completed questionnaires, 62 indicated improvement of more than 50% and 29 of less than 50%. In eight series of case studies, 82% of 764 subjects self-reported at least temporary improvement, while 4% became worse and 7% reported no change (Hurwitz et al 1996).

Migraine typically affects about 15% of most populations. In recent years, the consensus has emerged that both neurological and vascular components are relevant and probably interrelated (Schoenen & Sandor 1999). Migraine sufferers often have frequent tension headaches. The frequency of migraine attacks can be influenced by the relative condition of the upper cervical musculoskeletal structure and thus treatment to this region can have an influence on the frequency of migraine attacks. Hurwitz et al (1996) cite a randomized, controlled study where migraine patients receiving chiropractic manipulation showed a reduction in frequency and intensity with statistically significant reduction in pain intensity. Toohey (1997) completed a retrospective study of migraine patients seeking osteopathic treatment. Of 52 questionnaires sent, 39 responded and 35 met the International Headache Society guidelines for the diagnosis of migraine. Thirty four reported benefit from treatment and the improvement in frequency, duration, severity and effect on activity levels were statistically significant.

Dizziness and vertigo

Dizziness is commonly associated with neck dysfunction. It can be positional – where it is associated with certain movements and follows a predictable pattern – or acute and episodic. The subject remains controversial and the differential diagnosis can be difficult. Many patients with dizziness report improvement with treatment to cervical structures and this parallels the improvement in neck symptoms (personal observation). However, because of the potentially serious effects of vertebrobasilar insufficiency, these cases must be managed carefully. Mechanisms that can create dizziness are: vertebrobasilar insufficiency and reflex vertigo.

Vertebrobasilar insufficiency

The vertebrobasilar system provides the circulation to the vestibular nuclei. Insufficiency of blood flow can be caused by intrinsic factors, such as atherosclerosis, or by extrinsic factors. Extrinsic factors can involve compression of the vertebral artery by muscles, osteophytes or excessive rotation at the atlantoaxial region. Symptoms are more likely to occur with cervical dysfunction if there is a pre-existing occlusion of vertebrobasilar blood flow due to other factors. Vertebrobasilar insufficiency is likely to be accompanied by other symptoms such as nausea and visual or sensory disturbances. Dizziness is likely to be the most common and predominant symptom. Age and degenerative change are likely to be significant factors. Manual therapists utilizing rotation should be extremely careful, particularly where there is a history of dizziness. Full neck rotation to the upper cervical spine should be minimized (see p. 191 for further discussion on this subject).

Reflex vertigo

The vestibular nuclei receive proprioceptive information from the muscles and joints of the upper cervical spine. A disturbance of this proprioceptive activity is widely thought to be capable of causing a disturbance in balance (for reviews see Bogduk (1994) and Bontoux (1998)). The key difference between ischaemic and reflex vertigo is that reflex vertigo is not accompanied by other features of brainstem ischaemia or cardiovascular disease (Bogduk 1994). Reflex vertigo is more likely to be acute, accompanied by muscle spasm and restricted mobility, and provoked by movements within the normal range.

ASSESSMENT OF NECK PAIN

Case history

An accurate and detailed case history is an important part of understanding the nature of the problem. The information collected should include:

- The duration of present problem.
- Whether it has happened before.
- Whether there is any history of trauma.
- The pattern of pain – When does it come on? What makes it better/worse? Can it be reproduced? Associations with any particular exposures such as work, or any particular postures.
- Description of the pain – location, type of symptoms (pain, stiffness, referred pain).
- Whether there are neurological symptoms – numbness, paraesthesia, nerve root pain, loss of strength or coordination.
- Whether there are frequent headaches or episodes of dizziness.
- The main daily exposures and how these affect the pain – driving, sleeping, work postures, sitting, relaxing, etc.

Postural assessment

The overall spinal posture should be assessed while standing. This should include:

- pelvic levels
- spinal postural alignment – presence of kyphosis or scoliosis
- position of scapulae, height of shoulders
- atrophy or hypertrophy of muscles of the shoulder and neck
- cervical spine posture, head position.

Mobility testing

This should include:

- full rotation

- upper cervical rotation (tested in neck flexion)
- flexion/extension
- sidebending
- oblique extension.

Active movements will give an idea of the region and the tissues involved. It is important to differentiate between restrictions in mobility due to stiffness or due to pain. Stiffness and tension suggest a neuromuscular phenomenon, while pain is suggestive of compression or stretching of a sensitized structure. In an acute, traumatic-type injury there may be sensitivity to ligament stretch; in a non-traumatic injury this is less likely. Sidebending will stress the uncovertebral joints. Oblique extension will cause a lower cervical facet joint compression and reveal sensitivity of these structures. Oblique extension will also narrow the intervertebral foramen and will accentuate any nerve root involvement. When assessing flexion/extension it is wise to try to avoid full excursion of these movements to prevent exacerbating an injury.

If there are any signs of pain, or if neurological symptoms extend into the upper limb, a neurological screen should be completed. This can include:

- Reflexes:
  - biceps – C5 nerve root
  - brachioradialis – C6 nerve root
  - triceps – C7 nerve root.
- Muscle strength:
  - deltoid – C5 nerve root
  - biceps, wrist extensors – C6 nerve root
  - triceps, wrist flexors – C7 nerve root
  - Pinch strength – C8 nerve root
  - Abductor digiti minimi – T1 nerve root.
- Dermatomes (Fig. 14.12).

The cervical spine is readily accessible for palpation and can provide valuable guidance to the source of the symptoms and the tissues involved. Palpation should be done in the prone position with the head and neck in neutral or slight flexion. It can be complicated by muscle spasm in the acute stage and degenerative change and widespread tenderness in the chronic phase. The cervical articular pillars can be readily identified

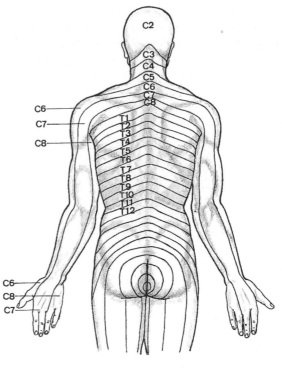

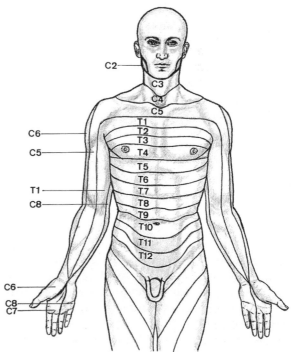

Figure 14.12 Dermatomes of the upper limb give a guide to the level of nerve root involvement.

and palpated for sensitivity or misalignment. The region of the intervertebral foramen can be gently palpated for sensitivity on the anterior aspect of the articular pillar. The cervical musculature can be readily accessed for palpation, with the exception of the cervical flexors. The muscles should be palpated for the degree of tension, sensitivity and presence of trigger points, with both sides compared. Careful note should be taken of the conscious ability of patients to relax their muscles.

Passive movements should be assessed with the patient in a supine position. With the compressive effects of gravity removed from the neck, and the postural muscles relaxed, there is usually more joint movement in passive testing. If there is a marked increase in mobility it suggests a muscular component to any joint restrictions previously noted. If there is still considerable stiffness this suggests a degenerative component. If there is still considerable pain or spasm this should be carefully assessed as to its origins. In the prone position the scalenes and sternocleidomastoid muscles can be readily palpated. At this point the practitioner has enough information to make a working diagnosis and can make a decision to proceed with treatment and whether further imaging is required. If there is a consistency between the presenting symptoms, the active and passive mobility and the palpatory findings, it is safe to proceed. Any inconsistencies should be further explored. Further imaging, such as X-ray, should be considered in cases of trauma, significant neurological involvement or history of chronicity. X-rays will generally help confirm a diagnosis and make it possible to assess the degree of degenerative change.

Most cervical problems represent a combination of pain sources and symptoms, with increased joint sensitivity, muscle spasm and facet compression. This may well be complicated by degenerative change and nerve root sensitivity. Once the primary joints and muscles have been identified, manual therapy is very successful for management of the acute stage, based on reducing muscle tension/spasm, and decompression and mobilization of the affected segments.

MANUAL THERAPY

A clear distinction needs to be made between injury due to trauma and injury due to fatigue and dysfunction. A recent traumatic injury that has some soft tissue damage will need a more conservative approach to avoid overstressing the damaged tissues while encouraging active rehabilitation with supportive therapy to optimize the healing process.

Trauma will frequently create a secondary neuromuscular reaction that is amenable to treatment in the early stages of injury. In fact, addressing the early neuromuscular dysfunction will assist active rehabilitation and may prevent some of the tendency towards chronicity that is common following cervical spine trauma (Buskila et al 1997). A non-traumatic injury where there is muscle tension and fatigue accompanied by joint dysfunction can be treated more positively to restore normal function. In all cases it is important to try to ascertain the key factors responsible for the symptoms in order to understand the nature of the injury. In acute or recurrent cases there is increasing emphasis on patient education and modification of risk factors. It is important not to provide simplistic explanations as to the cause of the injury, such as overemphasizing a previous or minor trauma. This reduces the incentive of the patient to become involved in management of current risk factors.

Although neck pain is as common as back pain, it rarely leads to the same incidence of work-related disability. An acute injury may sometimes necessitate a few days from work but it rarely threatens work status. Most people can continue to work with a neck injury, although there is often a need for pain avoidance techniques – such as limiting certain movements, or avoiding certain exposures. The upright neutral cervical posture is relatively stress free on the cervical spine and is usually one of the more comfortable postures with neck symptomatology. Being able to manage upright, neutral cervical postures in the sitting and standing positions means that an injured person can have a reasonably normal life with normal social interaction while avoiding painful movements.

Muscle release techniques

The accessibility of the muscles to palpation and to direct contact, combined with the additional mobility of the cervical spine, provide great advantages for using muscle release techniques.

Muscle spasm is an essential component in the pain–spasm–dysfunction cycle. Tight muscles restrict joint mobility and fluid dynamics, increase the biomechanical forces, increase the afferent/efferent output and contribute to neuromuscular fatigue processes. Muscle tension can lead to increased stress on facet joints and intervertebral discs, which can complicate or exacerbate the injury. An effective method of relieving tight muscles is an important part of the practitioner's armoury. This method can vary from deep massage or deep friction techniques, to trigger point therapies and postisometric releases such as muscle energy techniques. In mobile areas such as the cervical spine and scapulothoracic region it can be helpful to gradually stretch the tissue being treated during application of the technique, to assist the reduction in sensitivity of the muscle spindles.

Mobilization or articulation

When the muscles have been released and the limits to mobility can be reached without provoking pain, mobilization techniques can be used to enhance mobility and function. Mobilizations are usually performed at the functional limit to mobility. They are rhythmic, repetitive and provide a stretching to soft tissues. This improves mobility, encourages fluid exchange and reduces proprioceptive sensitivity. Mobilization is a very effective technique in the cervical spine. The additional mobility of the cervical spine, and the ability to use the head for providing extra leverage, gives a variety of planes for mobilization and a number of different methods of approaching a particular joint or tissue. The head can be used to provide traction to distract facet joint surfaces and mobilization can then be superimposed under traction while the facet joints, intervertebral discs and intervertebral foramina are separated.

Manipulation

The use of spinal manipulation was introduced in Chapters 8 and 13. The cervical spine is a rewarding area for the skilled manipulator. Its additional mobility and ready accessibility allow for precise use of leverages to achieve the release of the desired joints with a minimum of force required. It is also the most difficult area of the spine to develop manipulative competency. Supporting the weight of the patient's head while establishing physiological locking (combinations of flexion/extension plus rotation plus sidebending plus shear) while still maintaining physical and psychological relaxation of the patient (and practitioner!) in preparation for a thrusting manoeuvre is not always easy. Cervical manipulation should never be forceful. The additional mobility and the close presence of neurovascular structures makes forceful manipulation a dangerous proposition. If there is a good feel for physiological locking, manipulation should require only minimal additional force of very small dimensions. However, the additional force needs to be very quick to beat the reaction time of the muscle spindles and to avoid stimulating a protective reaction by the cervical musculature. This requires experience and sensitivity to the feel of physiological locking and confidence in the ability to balance the need for speed while using minimum additional force. The point of physiological locking is rich in soft tissue proprioception and this is not a position that should be held for more than a few seconds – it can cause a neuromuscular or inflammatory reaction.

Manipulation is not without risk. It is important to be aware of this, and to take steps to minimize it. While complications are very rare they can be very serious and patients have died following cervical manipulation. Hurwitz et al (1996) have completed a thorough literature review of the complications of cervical manipulation. They calculate the risks of complications at one in 1 million, with a rate of serious complications of six per 10 million and death of 3 per 10 million. It is important to keep these figures in context; Hurwitz et al list the complication rates from NSAIDs as one per 1000, from surgery as

15.6 per 1000 and death rates from cervical spine surgery as 6.9 per 1000.

The serious complications generally involve insults to the veretebral artery as it passes through the cervical spine. It is thought that manipulation can set up an inflammatory reaction in the artery that occludes circulation with consequences such as brainstem and/or cerebellar infarction, Wallenberg's syndrome (obstruction of the posterior/inferior cerebellar artery) and locked-in syndrome (occlusion of the basilar artery). For this to occur it is generally recognized that there has been some previous reduction in vertebrobasilar circulation due to anomalies, fibrous bands or artherosclerosis. A number of precautions can reduce the risk of vertebrobasilar insult:

- Always perform premanipulative testing of the vertebral artery.
- Avoid manipulation if there are signs of vertebrobasilar ischaemia. Cease immediately if these develop as a result of treatment.
- Avoid manipulation and mobilization in full rotation, and use other planes of movement to minimize the amount of rotation used.

Research into the efficacy of manual therapy

Aker et al (1996) completed a review of the literature relating to conservative management of mechanical neck pain. They identified nine randomized, controlled trials, using various types of manual treatment (mobilization, manipulation and massage) that met their eligibility criteria. Two trials compared manipulation with mobilization. One showed no significant difference between the groups and one showed significant improvement for the manipulation group. Aker and colleagues pooled five trials that compared manual treatment in combination with other treatment that used similar control groups. The pooled effect at 1–4 weeks following treatment was equivalent to 16.2 points on a 100-point scale, with similar effect sizes for acute, subacute or chronic patient groups. Aker et al (1996) conclude: 'There is early evidence to support the use

of manual treatments in combination with other treatments for short term pain relief, but in general, conservative interventions have not been studied in enough detail to assess efficacy or effectiveness adequately'.

Hurwitz et al (1996) completed a review of the literature of manipulation and mobilization of the cervical spine. They found that two of three randomized, controlled trials for acute neck pain showed short-term benefit for manipulation. The pooling of three randomized, controlled trials comparing cervical spine manipulation for subacute or chronic neck pain showed an improvement on the 100 mm visual analogue scale of pain at 3 weeks of 12.6 mm. Hurwitz et al (1996) concluded:

Manipulation, mobilization or physiotherapy probably are all more effective than muscle relaxants or usual medical care in producing short-term pain relief among some patients with acute or chronic neck pain and that manipulation is slightly more effective than mobilization or physical therapy.

The long-term results of manipulation cannot be determined.

A more recent randomized, controlled trial of 119 chronic neck pain patients, with pain lasting at least 3 months, compared the results of manipulative care with intensive training of the cervical musculature and with physiotherapy (Jordan et al 1998). All patients also received a home exercise programme and attended a group session neck school of approximately 1.5 h. Each category received treatment twice a week for 6 weeks. All groups reported significant improvements regarding self-reported pain (approximately 50%), and disability, following treatment, which were maintained at 4 and 12 months' follow-up. Medication levels decreased markedly through all groups through the follow-up period. There were no significant differences between groups at any assessment period. Pain levels appeared to decrease more quickly in the manipulative group and patients in the training group demonstrated greater endurance in the neck muscle extensors. It should be noted that the common exercise programme and neck school meant that the modalities examined had some homogenous elements that would tend to dilute differences in outcome, especially for the impressive long-term outcomes. Jordan et al (1998) stated: 'The authors of this study believe that one of the reasons why the current results were maintained was the effort put into self-reliance during neck school sessions as well as during individual therapy sessions'.

Skargren et al (1997) followed up 323 low back and neck pain patients in a randomized, controlled trial comparing chiropractic (mainly manipulation) to physiotherapy (mainly active rehabilitation). Treatment was at the discretion of the therapist. A highly significant improvement in pain, function and general healthcare related to back or neck problems could be measured in both groups, according to all variables, both immediately after the treatment and at the 6-month follow-up. No differences in outcomes or costs could be seen between the two study groups. A higher proportion of chiropractic patients felt their expectations were fulfilled. Both groups had an equal number of recurrences (nearly 50%) and also a higher proportion of chiropractic patients had additional treatments (52%) than in the physiotherapy group (25%). It should be noted that the chiropractic care was in private clinics, which might be seen as more attractive, compared with public primary care facilities for physiotherapy.

ADJUNCTIVE THERAPY

Two review papers have assessed the available research for different modalities. Gross et al (1999) conclude that: 'There is little information available from the trials to support the use of physical modalities for mechanical neck pain. There is some support for the use of electromagnetic therapy and against the use of laser therapy with respect to pain reduction'.

Aker et al (1996) reported positive results from studies using pulsed electromagnetic therapy, acupuncture, active exercise with stretching, heat and massage. They reported no significant improvements from studies using vapocoolant spray and stretch, exercise with drugs and education, laser therapy, infrared, traction, transcutaneous electrical nerve stimulation (TENS) and educational advice. They concluded that: 'There

is little information available from clinical trials to support many of the treatments for mechanical neck pain. In general conservative interventions have not been studied in enough detail to assess efficacy or effectiveness adequately'.

Exercises

Exercises can be a useful adjunctive treatment with neck injured patients. Neck symptoms are often associated with reduced range of motion and increased levels of muscle tension. Exercises can help control these features, reducing muscle sensitivity and creating an awareness of the degree of muscle tension. This assists in giving patients a feeling that they have some control over their symptoms. Rehabilitation exercises to improve muscle strength and coordination can improve muscle efficiency, reduce cumulative fatigue and improve recovery processes.

Exercises to improve mobility

Mobility will be better achieved in the standing than sitting positions because sitting increases the cervical curve and reduces lower cervical facet mobility. Each exercise should be performed approximately five times on each side, alternating sides. The exercises can be performed as part of a daily or twice-daily routine to enhance mobility and recovery. It is often worthwhile choosing a couple of key exercises and doing these regularly throughout the working day or during key exposures that have been identified as contributing to the problem:

- Cervical rotation. Gently rotate the neck to each side. Hold at the limit of mobility for 5 s (Fig. 14.13).
- Cervical sidebending. Gently sidebend the neck, approximating the ear to the shoulder while keeping the nose and chin in the midline. An effective method of increasing the muscle stretch is by holding down the shoulder opposite to the sidebending (Fig. 14.14). These exercises can also be used to unload an intervertebral foraminal nerve root compression by sidebending away from the site of nerve root entrapment.

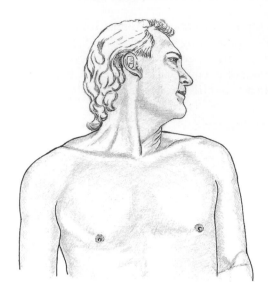

Figure 14.13 To improve rotation rotate the head from one side to the other, holding for 5 s each side.

- Cervical flexion/extension. In the sidebending position, roll the head forwards and backwards, holding for approximately 3 s at the limit of motion in each direction (Fig. 14.15). Repeat five times on each side. This stretch can also be enhanced using one hand to hold the opposite shoulder down.
- Neck rolling in flexion. With the head and neck gently flexed, rhythmically roll the head from side to side while keeping the chin in the midline (Fig. 14.16). Repeat five times each side.
- Upper cervical flexion. With head and neck erect, use finger pressure on the chin to tilt the head down and back (Fig. 14.17). Hold for 3 s, repeat three times.

Start with gentle stretches. The pressure can be increased gradually but should never be strong. Try to avoid holding stretches for too long as there is a significant amount of torsion and proprioception at the limits of joint mobility. In general, try to avoid holding full flexion and extension postures because of the excessive forces involved.

- A gentle and effective method of stretching the cervical extensors is to lay supine with the occiput supported on a platform about 5 cm

A

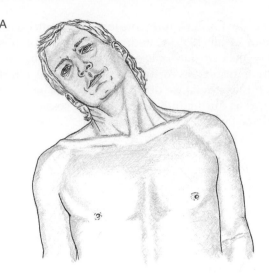

B

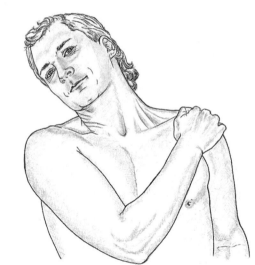

Figure 14.14 A: To improve sidebending sidebend the ear toward the shoulder, keeping the nose and chin in the midline. Hold for 5 s. Alternate sides five times each side. B: The stretching can be increased by holding the opposite shoulder down.

high. The effect of gravity on the midcervical spin gently stretches the upper cervical extensors (Fig. 14.18). This relaxing position can be assumed for 5–10 min after prolonged episodes of neck extensor activation. Breathing or relaxation techniques can be used to enhance this process.
- Shoulder circumduction. Rhythmically circumducting the shoulder and scapula region

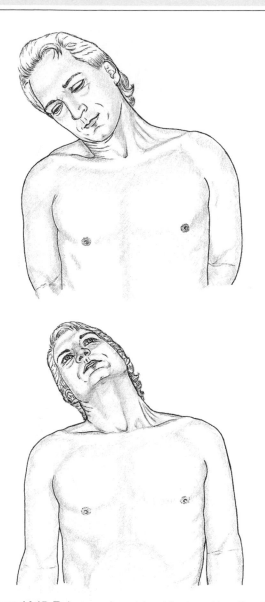

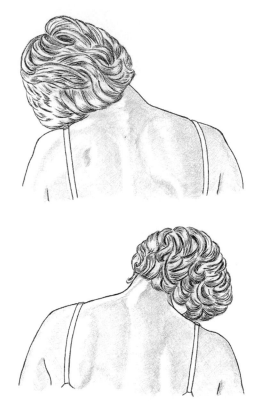

Figure 14.16 To stretch the cervical extensors with the head and neck gently flexed, the head should be rhythmically rolled from side to side while keeping the chin in the midline. Repeat about five times on each side.

Figure 14.15 To improve forward and backward bending, in the sidebent position the head and neck should be rolled forwards and backwards holding each position for 3 s. Repeat five times on each side.

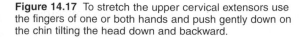

Figure 14.17 To stretch the upper cervical extensors use the fingers of one or both hands and push gently down on the chin tilting the head down and backward.

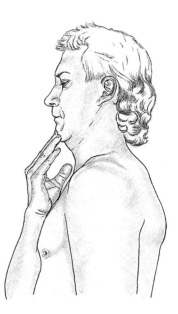

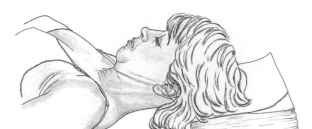

Figure 14.18 Lying with the occiput supported on a 5 cm platform can be an effective method of gently relaxing the cervical extensors.

is a method of stretching the scapula stabilizers and providing alterations of muscle length for muscles that have had long periods of static contraction (Fig. 14.19). Repeat five times clockwise and anticlockwise.

- Shoulder shrugging with an exaggerated shrugging action, then rapidly dropping the shoulders with expiration, is a method of teaching the trapezius and levator scapula muscles to relax after long periods of static tension (Fig. 14.20). It recreates a contraction/relaxation cycle. Repeat three or four times regularly throughout working day.

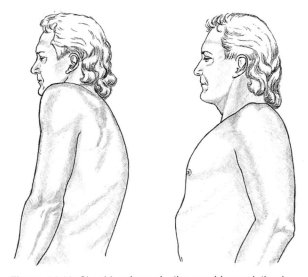

Figure 14.19 Shoulder circumduction provides variation in muscle length, muscle fibre recruitment and neuromuscular proprioception.

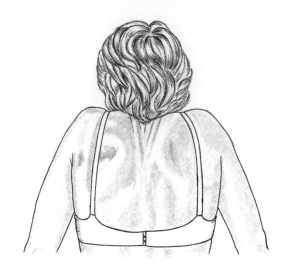

Figure 14.20 Shoulder shrugging recreates a contraction/relaxation cycle during long periods of static contraction.

Exercises for rehabilitation/stabilization

With the growing emphasis on stabilization exercises to prevent low back chronicity, and increasing evidence of their efficacy, there has been increasing interest in applying the same principles to the cervical spine. The research and practice is in its infancy but some of the early results have been encouraging. Although the incidence of neck/shoulder pain is similar to low back pain (LBP), the morbidity and costs associated with it are a lot lower. This has reflected in a lower priority for research and an emphasis on lower-cost interventions. Jull (1997) places emphasis on the deeper neck muscles, including the flexors (longus colli and longus capitis) and the extensors (semispinalis cervicus and multifidus) as providing a continued tonic activity concomitant with a postural stabilizing role, and notes that these lose their endurance capacity in patients with neck pain. Jull recommends an exercise programme involving sustained submaximal muscle contractions to be performed throughout the day and during functional daily activities. These stabilizing muscles are then incorporated as coactivators during functional daily activities. This is very similar in approach to the lumbar stabilization philosophy, of which Jull is one of the research team. Jull (1997) and Grant et al (1997) recommend two exercises in a programme to enhance the function of the cervical and scapula stabilizers:

1. The cervical spine flexors are not amenable to direct palpation. They can be tested by use of an inflatable air filled pressure sensor. The test is conducted with the patient supine, with the head and neck in a neutral posture. The air-filled bag is placed under the suboccipital region and inflated to 20 mmHg. The patient is instructed to slowly flex the upper cervical spine with a gentle nodding action and hold the position steady for 10 s (Fig. 14.21). The aim is to increase the pressure by 10 mmHg and to be able to hold this for ten times 10 s. Grant et al (1997) report that not only do these muscles lose their endurance capacity with neck pain patients, but that retraining of these muscles parallels a reduction in symptoms.

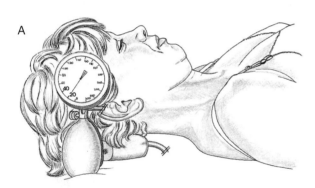

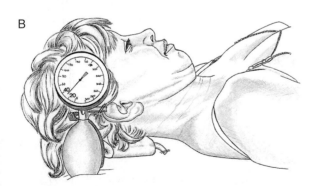

Figure 14.21 Retraining the holding capacity of the deep neck flexors. A: An air bag is placed under the suboccipital region and inflated to 20 mmHg. B: The patient gently flexes the head and aims to increase the pressure 8–10 mmHg and aims to hold this for ten periods of 10 s. Based on Jull (1997) and Grant et al (1997).

2. The patient is positioned prone with the arms abducted to 45 degrees and the elbows flexed to 90 degrees. The patient aims to retract the scapula using the lower trapezius while the arms remain on the plinth. The patient aims to hold this for ten periods of 10 s.

Grant et al (1997) describe a case report where a female subject with minor subclinical dysfunction demonstrated that an active stabilization programme, as described, paralleled a reduction in sensitivity of selected neural, muscular and articular structures (without any changes in measured postural parameters). However, the previously quoted ergonomic studies identify the muscles most subject to fatigue as the cervical extensors and the upper trapezius (whereas the Jull and Grant et al stabilization programme targets the flexors and the lower trapezius), and these are linked to postures used in the everyday working environment. This suggests that the Jull and Grant et al programme may be poorly targeted. Jull (1997) notes the importance of the cervical extensors but concedes there is not yet a method of testing these.

In the Jull and Grant et al programme the principles of lumbar stabilization exercises seem to be applied to the cervical region with little adaptation for the altered role of the cervical spine. The trunk flexors in the lumbar spine act via the thoracolumbar fascia to resist flexion forces and assist stabilization. There is no such demonstrated mechanism with the cervical flexors. While it is practical and advisable to limit intersegmental lumbar spinal mobility, it is more difficult to do this with the cervical spine where modern work environments often demand considerable segmental mobility and prolonged static loading in awkward postures. While a muscle can be trained to cope better with a demanding role, to do this without workplace modification and postural education is like putting the cart before the horse and there is little to recommend this specific approach as opposed to a more generalized exercise programme.

Jordan et al (1998) used a more generalized exercise programme for chronic neck pain and

compared the results to manipulation and physiotherapy (see p. 192) with impressive results
that were maintained at 4 and 12 months' follow-
up. The intensive training programme included:

- 5–6 min on a stationary bicycle.
- 10 min stretching programme for neck, shoulder, chest and scapular muscles.
- Intensive training of neck muscles on an
  apparatus using a built-in measuring device
  for isometric strength measurement. Flexion,
  extension and sidebending exercises were
  performed at 30% of EMG max, in series of 12
  repetitions. One series for flexion and three for
  sidebending and extension. The patients were
  re-evaluated every 14 days and the exercise
  levels adjusted.
- Strengthening of the shoulder, scapula and
  chest muscles using hand-held weights.
- Lateral pull-downs to strengthen latissimus
  dorsi.
- 5–6 min stationary cycling.

The programme was performed twice a week for
6 weeks, lasted 1–1.25 h and included a home
exercise component. Thirty four out of 40 (85%)
completed the programme and demonstrated
increased maximal extensor strength and isometric extensor duration, with an average 100%
increase.

Randlov et al (1998) compared the effectiveness of an intensive 3 month training programme
with a less intensive programme for females suffering from chronic neck/shoulder pain. The sessions were 1.5 h, three times a week for 6 weeks
(total 36 sessions) (Fig. 14.22):

- The light exercise group (A in Fig. 14.22) began
  with hot packs for 14 min, followed by 15 min
  stationary cycling and stretching exercises.
  The six exercises for the neck and shoulder
  region were carried out in one series of 20
  repetitions for each exercise.
- The intensive exercise group (B in Fig. 14.22)
  began with cycling and stretching for 10 min.
  The seven exercises were carried out with 20
  repetitions each series with five series per
  session. Shoulder exercises were carried out
  with increasing resistance.

Twenty five out of 41 (61%) and 27 out of 36
(75%) completed the light and intensive training
programmes, respectively. The 6 and 12 month
follow-up questionnaires were completed by
approximately 80% of the group. Both groups
showed improvements of MVC and isometric
endurance in flexion and extension. Activities of
daily living scores improved in both groups. Pain
levels also improved in both groups but tended
to relapse to baseline in the light exercise group
at 6 and 12 months, while the intensive group
continued to improve to 20% below baseline at 12
months. Pain-relieving medication was reduced
in the intensive group. The overall satisfaction
rate was 50% at conclusion and 60% at 12 month
follow-up. Randlov et al (1998) summarize as
follows:

The type of low-tech dynamic training used in either
of our two programmes resulted in both subjective
and objective improvements in patients suffering
from neck/shoulder pain, but there were no
statistically significant differences between the two
approaches. The subjective improvements were
maintained throughout the follow-up period.

The weakness of the study is the high drop-out
rate, only 41 of the original 77 completed the 12
month follow-up. Interestingly, the authors note
that the drop-outs were younger, stronger and
took less pain relief than the other participants,
and may have had less need to complete the programme (the opposite of LBP rehabilitation programme drop-outs). Only 5% of participants
were on sick leave (this figure is usually much
higher in LBP studies), which may have created
time management difficulties. The authors speculate that the lack of statistical difference
between the two studies may be because of the
lack of increased resistance in the neck muscle
exercises in the intensive group.

In summary, the evidence for exercise programmes for neck/shoulder pain is in its infancy.
There are suggestions that it provides good
medium- to long-term effects, with exercise programmes of increasing intensity providing additional long-term benefits. The trend from the
available evidence of treatments for manual
medicine, and manipulation in particular, is to
provide quicker, short-term improvements and

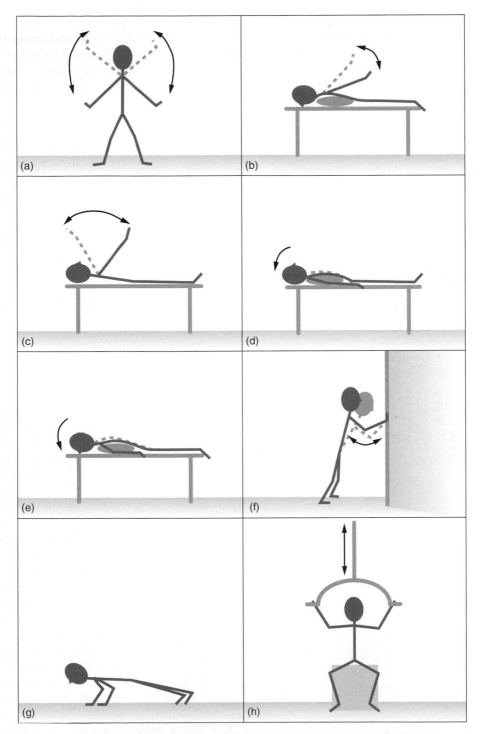

Figure 14.22 The exercise programme advocated by Randlov et al (1998) for chronic neck/shoulder pain in females. A = light group, B = intensive group. (a) Arm abduction: A + B (with increasing load); (b) shoulder retraction: A + B (with increasing load); (c) arm swing: A + B (with increasing load); (d) neck extension: A + B; (e) neck flexion: A + B; (f) push-away: A; (g) push-up: B; (h) lateral pull-down: B. Reproduced with permission from Randlov et al (1998).

treatment regimens incorporating exercise pro-grammes to assist long-term improvement.

Aerobic exercise

With the increased response of the trapezius to stress, and its reluctance to relax fully following long periods of static contraction, the neck/shoulder muscle groups would seem to be powerful benefactors from the physiological benefits of aerobic exercise (as outlined in Chapter 7). The principles of an aerobic exercise programme for neck/shoulder pain are:

- The head and neck should be in an upright, well-balanced posture, close to the centre of gravity.
- The arms and shoulders should not be elevated.
- The exercise should be rhythmic, emphasizing contraction/relaxation cycles rather than static contractions.
- The exercise should start easily, with grad-ually increasing dosage. Postexercise soreness is common and exercise should not be repeated until this is settled.
- As fitness increases and neuromuscular sen-sitivity decreases, postural alterations and higher arm actions can be better tolerated.

Brisk walking, jogging, dancing, aerobics and stepping could all be good forms of aerobic exer-cise. Cycling, and in particular road cycling, with the emphasis on forward-leaning postures, extended head position, significant body weight through the shoulders, and vibration, could create additional exposure to sensitized structures. Stationary cycling, which emphasizes upright postures and minimal forward lean, is acceptable.

Swimming should be done with caution. Freestyle with bilateral breathing and back-stroke are acceptable. Freestyle with unilateral breathing with its asymmetric movement pattern can create strain and dysfunction. Breast stroke should be minimized due to the neck hyper-extension it creates.

ERGONOMIC ADVICE

The primary ergonomic risk factors for neck pain were outlined on page 174, and the neuro-muscular exposures associated with different postures were described, and how these increase the risk of symptoms. Neck pain is so common and so often associated with very common ergonomic exposures that sound ergonomic advice and ergonomic assessment should never be overlooked. In chronic patients, or those with a history of recurrence, where there is an increas-ing likelihood that there is a mismatch between the neuromuscular demands of their environ-ment and their ability to adapt, there should be a systematic search for risk factors. These should be modified where possible to reduce the expo-sure, and the patient should be educated in the management of these risk factors to improve the match between exposure and recovery/adapta-tion. The primary ergonomic exposures are:

- head and neck postures
- arm positions
- forceful arm movements
- relaxing neck postures
- sleeping posture.

Head and neck postures

These should be as close to the centre of gravity as practical – the head and neck should be in balance with normal relaxed posture for the person without undue muscle tension required to hold the posture. Static postures where the head and neck are held in off-neutral postures should be avoided. These might include:

- rotation – an off-centre computer screen
- sidebending – telephone use
- flexion – a low flat work surface.

A certain amount of off-neutral postures is part of normal mobility and normal healthy usage, but where postures are required to be sustained for long periods head and neck posture must be optimized. The key points for optimizing pos-tures are:

- Visual angles are best 0–30 degrees below horizontal and centrally located.
- Where vision is required to manipulate imple-ments with the hand, such as writing or craft work, the optimum height is regarded as 5–10 cm above relaxed elbow height.

- For reading tasks, a slope in the region of 45 degrees assists the maintenance of neutral neck posture.
- For writing tasks, a slope of 10–15 degrees, 4–6 cm above elbow height assists posture.
- Overhead work is particularly stressful to cervical structures, particularly when combined with forceful arm movements. These postures should be minimized.
- Where suboptimal postures are required there should be increasing emphasis on task variety and breaks.
- Where there are exacting visual requirements below eye level, reclined (backward leaning) sitting postures should be avoided to avoid poking the neck forward (see Chapter 13 for good sitting postures).

Arm positions

The position of the arm is an important consideration for neck injury, as it can create tension through the scapular stabilizing muscles. The further the arm is positioned from the midline of the body, the greater the leverage on these scapular muscles and the greater the forces relayed through the cervical joints. The arm is in the most relaxed position hanging loosely by the body or being supported close to the body. The most common exposure to these muscles involves moving the arm forward into flexion – reaching to manipulate a keyboard or mouse – or laterally into abduction – working at a high work surface or reaching sideways to a poor mouse position. Straight arm postures create additional leverage.

The key points for optimizing arm and shoulder postures are:

- A worksurface at elbow height allows the most comfortable shoulder posture. Where visual requirements are needed at the worksurface, 5–10 cm above elbow height provides a trade-off between head and neck posture and shoulder posture.
- The worksurface should be close to the body to avoid forward reaching. The worksurface should be planned so the most commonly used tasks are closest to the body in the zone

of convenient reach and it should allow space to place the forearm during pauses to enable unloading the weight of the arm.
- If static arm positions are required these should aim to provide as little leverage and muscle tension as possible. There should be increasing emphasis on providing arm support to reduce the leverage. Variety and breaks should receive increased prominence.

Forceful arm movements

To generate force from the arm, the scapular muscles must be stabilized. The higher the force and the greater the distance, the greater the leverage developed and the more muscle tone is required for stabilizing. High force arm movements should be kept close to the body, where optimum body posture can utilize some of the stronger muscles, such as leg and trunk muscles, and reduce the leverages involved. The most common increases in exposure are:

- flexion – overreaching forward – being too far away from the object
- abduction – the object is off centre
- elevation – the object is too high.

Leverages can often be reduced by repositioning the object or repositioning the body, e.g. using steps to gain access to a high object.

Where these actions are repetitive, increased emphasis must be given to correct task design for work heights, tools and easy access. Where there is high force or repetition, or postures are suboptimal, increased emphasis must be given to work variety and breaks. For example, painting a ceiling should be interspersed with more convenient tasks.

Relaxing neck postures

During periods of relaxation we usually try to recline our trunk to reduce the constant demands of gravity. However, we often try to maintain concentrated vision for tasks such as reading and watching television. This can compromise neck and head positions, e.g. reading in bed or watching TV lying on the sofa. Key points to remember are:

- To minimize strain on the neck, the head should be rested on a surface to try and unload the weight, rather than using muscle tension to maintain a poor posture. High-backed chairs or sofas provide neck support.
- In reclined postures a visual angle slightly above horizontal reduces neck flexion – the more reclined the higher the visual angle (provided there is neck support).
- Frequent postural changes are often advisable.

Sleeping posture

Sleeping postures should maintain the head and neck in as close to neutral posture as possible, avoiding excessive torsion or flexed/extended postures. Most people prefer to sleep on their sides or in the recovery position. Sleeping on the front inevitably creates neck twisting and has been associated with increased neck pain. Most people change postures regularly throughout the night and using a malleable pillow that allows for changes of posture while still providing support for head and neck is very important.

Feather/down pillows provide the optimum balance between support and malleability without the 'bounce back' of rubber products. The pillow needs to be of the right density to provide neutral posture in the most favoured sleeping position. This can vary depending on the person's frame, width of shoulders, degree of kyphosis and softness of bed.

SUMMARY

- Neck pain is very common. It is associated with forceful upper limb movements, repetition, static contraction and poor posture.
- The highly mobile neck is particularly prone to muscle strain, lower cervical degeneration and sudden force injury. It can be complicated by headaches and vertigo.
- The trend from the available evidence of treatment is for manual medicine and manipulation to provide effective short-term improvement, and progressive exercise programmes to provide better long-term outcomes.
- Improvements in posture and ergonomics are important to reduce the incidence of and assist the rehabilitation of injury.

15

Shoulder pain

RISK FACTORS

In a comprehensive review of over 20 epidemiological studies that examined workplace factors and their relationships to shoulder tendonitis and non-specific shoulder pain (NIOSH 1997b) the researchers concluded:

- There is evidence for a positive association with highly repetitive work and shoulder musculoskeletal disorder (MSD). Of the six studies that included odds ratios, three were over 3 and three were 1–3.
- There is evidence for a relationship between repeated or sustained shoulder postures with greater than 60 degrees of flexion or abduction and shoulder MSDs. The evidence is strongest for highly repetitive or forceful work. The largest odds ratios (8.3–10.6) were associated with work above acromion height.
- There is insufficient evidence for a positive association between force or vibration based on currently available studies.
- Age, sporting activities and stress were found to be significant confounders.

Hagberg et al (1995), in their review on work-related musculoskeletal disorders, state: 'There is consistency across studies from a range of industries showing increased risk of shoulder tendonitis with repetitive and overhead work. Overhead work results in a high load on the rotator cuff tendons.'

ANATOMY

The shoulder complex is a highly mobile structure permitting a wide range of movement of the upper limb. The structure of the complex, with the acromioclavicular joint providing the only point of articulation to the trunk, is highly dependent on muscular stability.

The glenohumeral joint is a shallow ball and socket joint, allowing a significant degree of mobility – it is the most mobile joint in the body. The socket – the glenoid fossa – is relatively small compared to the articular surface of the head of the humerus. Its congruence with the articular surface of the humerus is increased by the glenoid labrum, a connective tissue attached to the periphery of the glenoid fossa. The ability of the scapula to move in coordination with the shoulder joint confers an additional degree of movement in all planes. The scapula is required to provide both mobility enhancement and a stable base for the glenohumeral joint. This requires careful neuromuscular coordination of the scapula. The movements of the scapula are elevation/depression, protraction/retraction and superior/inferior rotation. Disturbance of

the scapulothoracic rhythm places additional load on the glenohumeral joint. The clavicle acts as a stabilizing strut on the anterior aspect of the shoulder, keeping the arm free of the body wall and providing structural support and a brake to the mobility of the scapula and the head of the humerus. The clavicle articulates with the acromion process of the scapula forming the acromioclavicular joint. Efficient movement at the acromioclavicular and sternoclavicular joints is important for normal scapular and shoulder mobility. The coracoacromial arch is formed by the coracoacromial ligament spanning the gap between the acromion and the coracoid process. The coracoacromial arch protects the sensitive tendons below from irritation and prevents the humerus dislocating superiorly (Fig. 15.1).

The rotator cuff muscles

The supraspinatus, infraspinatus, teres minor and subscapularis muscles form the rotator cuff.

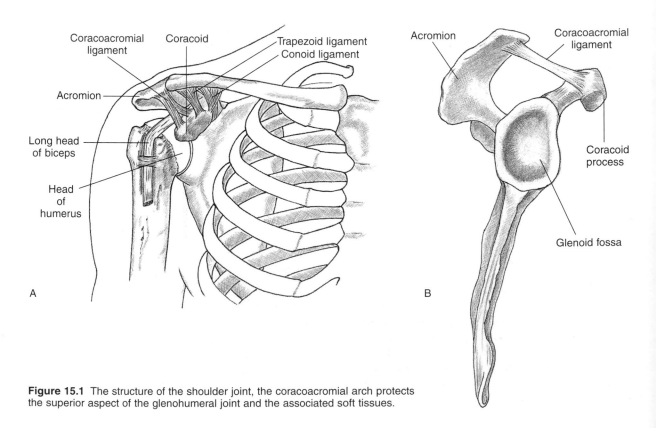

Figure 15.1 The structure of the shoulder joint, the coracoacromial arch protects the superior aspect of the glenohumeral joint and the associated soft tissues.

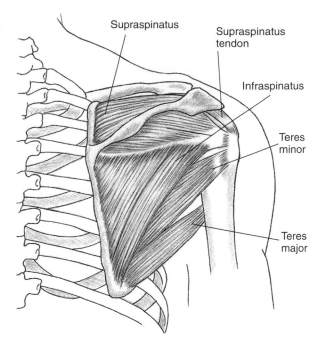

Supraspinatus

Supraspinatus tendon

Infraspinatus

Teres minor

Teres major

Figure 15.2 The posterior muscles of the rotator cuff are important stabilizers of the glenohumeral joint.

Their tendons reinforce the capsule of the glenohumeral joint and make a significant contribution to its dynamic stability (Fig. 15.2). They act to maintain optimum relationships of the articular surfaces of the glenohumeral joint when other more powerful muscles act on the joint.

Supraspinatus

The supraspinatus is deep to the upper fibres of trapezius. It arises in, and fills, the medial two-thirds of the supraspinous fossa, created by the scapula spine on the posterior aspect of the scapula. Its tendon passes under the coracoacromial arch and inserts onto the superior surface of the greater tubercle of the humerus. The supraspinatus abducts the arm and pulls the head of the humerus into the glenoid fossa. The supraspinatus is the principal muscle that resists carrying weights when the arm is hanging by the side. The supraspinatus is active during the mid-phase of the arm swing during walking but not at the limits of swing.

Infraspinatus

The infraspinatus arises from the medial two-thirds of, and fills, the infraspinous fossa. Its fibres converge on a tendon, which passes across the posterior aspect of the shoulder joint inserting into the middle facet of the greater tubercle of the humerus. The infraspinatus acts to externally rotate the arm. It is an important stabilizing muscle in abduction, flexion and throwing movements.

Teres minor

The teres minor is a relatively narrow muscle arising from the lateral border of the scapula and runs upward and laterally, inserting onto the lowest facet of the greater tubercle of the humerus. Its functions are closely related to the infraspinatus.

Subscapularis

The subscapularis arises from the anterior surface of the scapula filling the subscapular fossa. It crosses the front of the shoulder, joining the capsule inserting onto the lesser tubercle and the joint capsule on the front of the humerus. It acts to internally rotate and adduct the arm. It is active during the forward swing of walking and during early abduction.

Long head of biceps

The long head of the biceps is often regarded as part of the rotator cuff due to its intimate association with the joint capsule. It has some stabilizing function, assisting in maintaining humeral head position. It originates within the capsule of the shoulder joint as a long narrow tendon running from the supraglenoid tubercle and continuous with the glenoid labrum. It arches over the humeral head and descends in the intertubercular sulcus, where it is enveloped in a synovial sheath and retained by the transverse humeral ligament. Below this it joins the main belly of biceps muscle. The long head of biceps contributes to flexion of the shoulder and, if the

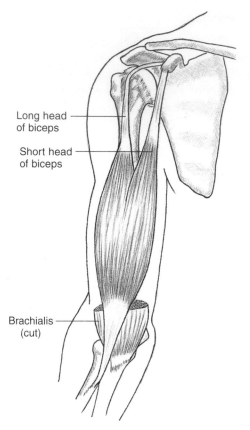

Figure 15.3 The long head of biceps tendon is a common cause of anterior shoulder pain.

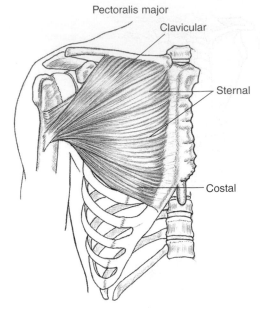

Figure 15.4 The pectoralis major is a powerful muscle that moves the raised arm down and across the chest, forward from extended positions and provides some internal rotation.

humerus is externally rotated, can also contribute to abduction. It is a common cause of anterior shoulder pain. Whether it is actively contracting or whether it is passively moving, the tendon must slide within the sulcus. This is a common region for increased friction, microtrauma and injury (Fig. 15.3). The long head of biceps is poorly vascularized and prone to degenerative change and rupture.

Global muscles

The global muscles of the glenohumeral joint are generally longer, bulkier and have more distal origins or insertions than the rotator cuff muscles, providing additional leverage. Their key role is that of strength production. They are important in manual handling tasks and sports where efficient and reliable production of strength is essential. The global muscles include the pectoral group (Fig. 15.4), latissimus dorsi (Fig. 15.5) and deltoid (Fig. 15.6).

NEUROMUSCULAR CONSIDERATIONS

The reduced muscle mass of the upper limbs compared to the lower limbs creates a higher physiological workload (blood lactate, peak VO_2). For the same workload the upper limb musculature will be more susceptible to fatigue and injury. The shoulder muscles are relatively small for the leverages that are required to stabilize or move the upper limb. The muscles do not have either the bulk or length required to produce large moments of force. When the shoulder is required to be stabilized in a non-neutral position the muscles often develop significant levels of tension. These levels of internal pressure are often increased by the bony surfaces that surround the infraspinatus, supraspinatus and subscapularis, limiting the ability of the muscle to expand and restricting the available surfaces for vascular supply. There has been considerable

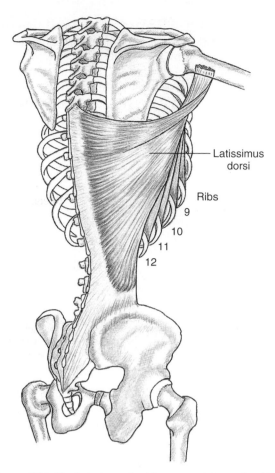

Latissimus dorsi

Ribs
9
10
11
12

Figure 15.5 The latissimus dorsi is a powerful muscle with strong leverages. It draws the raised arm down and backwards, providing some internal rotation.

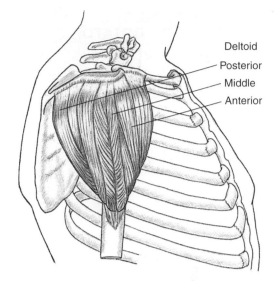

Deltoid
Posterior
Middle
Anterior

Figure 15.6 The deltoid muscle is very active in abduction, moving the arm away from the body, particularly in abduction over 90 degrees. In addition, the anterior fibres draw the arm forward and the posterior fibres extend the arm.

research interest in assessing the internal pressure of the shoulder stabilizers and determining at which joint positions the homeostasis becomes compromised (see Fig. 15.7). In the relaxed hanging position the rotator cuff muscles are electrically silent. The supraspinatus muscle resists any increase in load, such as carrying a weight or flexing the elbow to 45 degrees. During movements of the shoulder the rotator cuff muscles resist and control the translation of the humeral head, maintaining optimum relationship of the humeral head with the glenoid. This is particularly important in abduction movements where subscapularis, supraspinatus and teres minor counteract the strong upwards com-

ponent of the pull of the deltoid, and anterior and posterior deltoid control anterior and posterior translation. Any shortness or weakness in this group of muscles can lead to disturbed glenohumeral rhythm and subacromial impingement syndromes.

Sporrong et al (1995) reported that increasing grip strength is accompanied by increasing activation of the supraspinatus, infraspinatus and deltoid, particularly in elevated postures. The authors suggest this is a stabilizing mechanism. Sporrong et al (1998) showed that light manual precision work demonstrated increased EMG readings of the supraspinatus and infraspinatus, particularly in elevated postures, averaging 22%. Laurensen et al (1998) found that there was gradually increasing EMG of the 13 muscles tested when completing tasks that demanded both speed and precision with the arm hanging by the side. Supraspinatus showed the highest activity in all studied tasks. These studies illustrate that it is not just the posture of the upper arm that determines the rate of fatigue, but also that the tasks being performed must be taken into consideration.

PATHOPHYSIOLOGICAL MECHANISMS OF ROTATOR CUFF INJURY

The rotator cuff muscles have a considerable tonic activity in many arm postures. They can easily become fatigued and injured during prolonged, repetitive or static loading, particularly in non-neutral postures. They commonly refer pain to the anterior or lateral aspect of the shoulder. The duration of static postures is likely to be a significant factor. They can cause pain on a sudden increase in loading or on end-range movement or may exhibit a painful arc of movement, in abduction. They commonly ache at night in different sleeping positions. There are a number of plausible mechanisms of injury.

Ischaemia. Ischaemia of the muscle or its associated tendon due to persistent internal tension places a compromise on the vascular supply in rotator cuff injuries. Blood flow becomes compromised once the intramuscular pressure reaches 30 mmHg. The supraspinatus reaches this level at fairly low contraction levels due to the bony boundaries that prevent the muscle from expand-

ing. Jarvholm et al (1988) demonstrated that this threshold was reached by 30 degrees flexion at the shoulder joint (with flexed elbow). At 30 degrees of abduction (with straight arm) the intramuscular pressure of the supraspinatus reached over 80 mmHg, rising to 122 mmHg at 90 degrees abduction (Fig. 15.7). With a 2 kg hand load the intramuscular pressure reached 138 and 217 mmHg at 30 and 90 degrees of abduction, respectively. Jarvholm et al conclude:

Fatigue and shoulder pain related to elevated arm positions may be caused by muscle ischemia induced by the high muscular pressure. ... elevation abduction and hand load should be minimized to keep the load on the shoulder and the supraspinatus as low as possible.

Jarvholm et al (1991) compared the intramuscular pressure of four shoulder muscles at different loads of flexion and abduction. The highest pressures were in supraspinatus in abduction, followed by infraspinatus, with trapezius and deltoid showing much lower values. In flexion supraspinatus, infraspinatus and deltoid showed similar values with trapezius showing signifi-

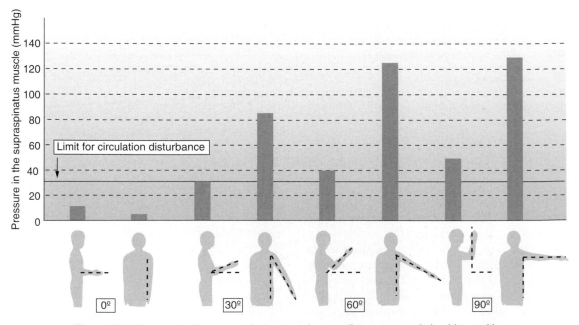

Figure 15.7 Pressure in the supraspinatus muscle according to arm and shoulder position.

cantly lower values. They concluded: 'Our findings may possibly explain the physiological stress on the rotator cuff muscles as compared with the deltoid and trapezius muscles in work with elevated arms'.

Delayed healing of microtrauma. This can be a significant factor, particularly in ischaemic zones due to static loading and the poorly vascularized zones identified in the supraspinatus and long head of biceps. Aged or degenerative tendons are more likely to be overloaded by repetitive or cumulative trauma. Accumulation of metabolites or debris can trigger a localized inflammatory response.

Impingement. Impingement on the underside of the acromion or coracoacromial ligament is considered to be a common cause of supraspinatus tendonitis. There is a critical angle of 80 degrees flexion or abduction where the greater tuberosity of the humerus approximates the coracoacromial arch. Above this the tuberosity is displaced downward increasing the subacromial space, leading to the painful arc of motion. The impingement can cause ischaemia, if the posture is static, and friction during repetitive movements, resulting in a reactive inflammatory process. Instability of the humeral head may increase the likelihood of impingement.

Degenerative change. This is part of the normal ageing process and can be accelerated in injury or overload situations. It is likely that injury occurs when a combined magnitude of cumulative loading and degenerative change occurs (Fig. 15.8). Degenerative change in the tendons leads to increased risk of microruptures, reactive inflammation, cell death and calcium deposition. There is a reduced tensile strength and an increased recovery period. The tendons of supraspinatus and long head of biceps have zones of avascularity where the tendon is particularly prone to degenerative change. Osteophytic spurring on the underside of the acromion process and on the greater tuberosity reduces the subacromial space and increases the likelihood of impingement. Frost (1995) compared MRI examinations of the rotator cuff from symptomatic and asymptomatic subjects. He found evidence for grade 1 and 2 degenerative change of 68.5% in symptomatic

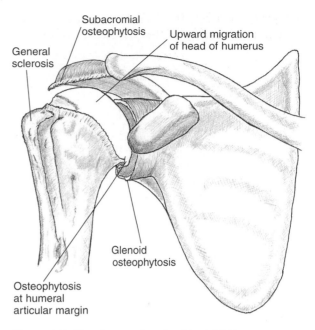

Figure 15.8 The degenerative shoulder joint. The combination of degenerative change and magnitude of load can lead to inflammatory change and injury in the tendons of the rotator cuff.

subjects compared to 66.7% in asymptomatic subjects (where grade 0 is normal and grade 3 is complete rupture). The results suggest that it is not the presence of degenerative change that is significant but the degree of exposure to poor postures.

Bursitis. This has long been described as a cause of shoulder pain and in particular an enlarged or degenerative subacromial bursa as a cause of impingement. Its use as a diagnosis seems to be falling from favour. It is likely that an enlarged bursa will coexist with a tendonitis or a degenerative problem.

EXAMINATION OF THE SHOULDER JOINT

As in all injuries, a thorough case history is important:

● Was there a recent trauma involved that would suggest a soft tissue injury. If so, what was the nature of it – a fall onto an outstretched hand forcing the head of the humerus superiorly? Landing on the tip of the shoulder (acromioclavicular joint)? A wrenching injury trying to control a heavy object (rotator cuff injury)?

- Is there a history of previous trauma that might suggest an accelerated degenerative process?
- Is it associated with a recent exposure to non-neutral postures, for example, overhead work?
- Are there any long-term exposures that may have contributed to a cumulative injury?
- Where is the pain? What is the pain pattern? What factors make the pain better or worse?
- Are there any other symptoms such as stiffness, weakness, numbness, paraesthesia or grating?

The pain from shoulder soft tissue injury is usually positional in nature, aggravated by movements that stress the injured tissues and relieved by positions that unload them. This can cause a dramatic increase in pain with certain movements or joint postures. In the acute stage patients may guard against movement and attempt to keep the shoulder supported and out of harm's way. In the subacute phase they will often have sharp pains when using the arm to reach something, having temporarily forgotten about the pain. Isolating those movements that aggravate the pain is very helpful with diagnosis. The absence of change of the nature of pain with position is suggestive of cervical spine or nerve root involvement. The shoulder region is a common site for referred nerve pain from the lower cervical nerve roots. Testing movements of the head and neck to see if they influence the pain can help with differential diagnosis. A patient with an acute nerve pain will often hold the shoulder elevated to relieve brachial plexus tension, which can create secondary tension in the shoulder elevators.

Any numbness or tingling should be thoroughly investigated. The most common causes are of cervical nerve root origin and these symptoms are suggestive of more than just a shoulder soft tissue or degenerative injury.

Muscle weakness is a common sign associated with shoulder injuries, particularly in abduction. Vollestad et al (1995) demonstrated that an injured shoulder had an EMG reading 50% higher than the non-injured shoulder during exhaustive submaximal contractions, suggesting an inefficiency in performance. He also demonstrated that this inefficiency was negated by pain blockade or manual therapy.

Observation

- Is the shoulder at the same level as the other one – trapezius height and bulk, acromion levels, acromioclavicular congruity?
- Are there any obvious signs of muscle wasting?
- Can the shoulder hang normally and swing normally when walking?
- Poor scapula position – flexed as in a kyphotic spine, or protracted – will create additional glenohumeral stress in non-neutral shoulder postures.

Active movements

- Flexion/extension.
- Abduction/adduction.
- Abduction/adduction in 90 degree flexion.
- Internal/external rotation in 90 degree abduction.
- Combined movements: collar sign – reaching behind the head to touch the collar – and scapula sign – reaching behind the back to touch the scapula.

Both sides should be compared. Careful note should be made of glenohumeral and scapulothoracic rhythm, to determine which components are restricted, particularly in abduction. Patients will often learn to compensate for poor glenohumeral abduction/flexion by exaggerating and elevating scapular movements and by swaying the trunk (Fig. 15.9).

To test for subacromial impingement, Neer's test is valuable. With the patient sitting, the practitioner stabilizes the scapula with one hand over the acromion and passively raises the arm into abduction with a hold under the forearm (Fig. 15.10) A modification of this involves moving the arm in an anterior/posterior plane. A positive test reproduces the patient's discomfort

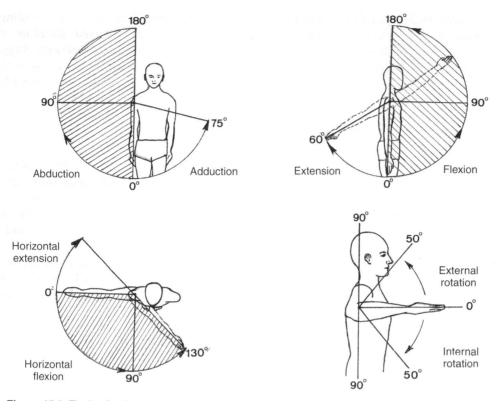

Figure 15.9 Testing for the range of active movements at the shoulder joint.

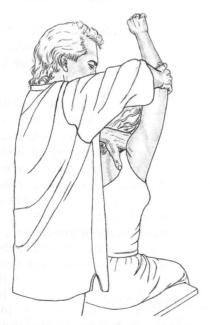

Figure 15.10 Neer's test will recreate the patient's symptoms if a subacromial impingement is present.

as the rotator cuff impinged under the stabilized coracoacromial arch.

Any dysfunction of scapular or glenohumeral mobility should prompt examination of the sternoclavicular and acromioclavicular joints. Good mobility of these joints is necessary for scapular elevation and rotation.

Any restrictions in motion will need to be compared with passive mobility to ascertain whether the restriction is functional – related to neuromuscular structures or more structural such as degenerative change or adhesive capsulitis. Passive mobility is best tested in reclined positions where the patient is more relaxed and finds it easier to 'unguard' the shoulder musculature. The degree of passive restriction and the end feel can be helpful in diagnosis. When the end point of the restriction has been established it should be investigated. A gritty end point suggests degenerative change; a bouncy end point suggests muscle tension. If it can be gradually increased by traction and repeated movement it suggests a neuromuscular cause causing some kind of impingement or compression of the joint. A stubbornly resistant restriction in more than one plane of movement, particularly noticeable in abduction and rotation, suggests adhesive capsulitis. This can be quite easy to identify in the postacute stage when the adhesions are well established, but can represent a diagnostic challenge in the acute case.

Resisted muscle tests

Resisted muscle tests can help isolate dysfunctional muscles. The key movements to test are:

- abduction at 45 degrees and 90 degrees (supraspinatus and middle deltoid)
- flexion at 90 degrees (anterior deltoid)
- flexion 90 degrees with external rotation (long head of biceps)
- arm abducted 90 degrees, elbow flexed 90 degrees, externally rotated – test internal rotation (subscapularis)
- arm abducted 90 degrees, elbow flexed 90 degrees, internally rotated – test external rotation (infraspinatus and teres minor).

Palpation

The shoulder joint is readily accessible to palpation. With its generous degree of mobility and its easy accessibility to palpation, the shoulder joint rewards the manual therapist. A careful review of the musculature for increased tension and trigger points, the rotator cuff for thickened areas with increased sensitivity and the degree of clearance in the subacromial space can be very helpful in reinforcing good diagnosis. A deep palpatory technique is required to assess the supraspinatus in the supraspinous fossa, deep to the upper fibres of the trapezius, and a firm grip is needed to palpate its tendon in the subacromial space deep to the deltoid. Palpation is best performed in the prone position with the arm hanging over the side of the couch. This provides a joint neutral position with the traction effect of the weight of the arm increasing the space around the rotator cuff. Anterior shoulder structures are best palpated in the supine position.

The most common dysfunctional muscle is the supraspinatus. It is frequently found to be tense, shortened, thickened and very sensitive in the muscle belly and tendon. The next most common dysfunctional muscles are the infraspinatus/teres minor and the long head of biceps.

In acute injuries the findings are likely to be confined to one or two muscles; in the chronic situation there is more likely to be widespread muscle sensitivity in the rotator cuff group. Supraspinatus injuries nearly always involve the upper fibres of trapezius as an accessory abductor/elevator and sometimes the deltoid as an accessory abductor. This is probably the most common shoulder syndrome, often caused by working with abducted or elevated arm. The next most frequent is the anterior deltoid and long head of biceps strain caused by overreaching in flexion. An increasingly common problem is overexposure of the infraspinatus/teres minor muscle due to externally rotated arm positions for using a computer mouse (Fig. 15.11).

Imaging

X-rays provide a good screening tool for the osseous structure of the shoulder complex. This is particularly valuable in cases of trauma, to assess the degree of degenerative change and evaluate the subacromial space. However, they give little information on the soft tissue structures.

Arthrography and CT arthrography are useful for the assessment of capsular tears, rotator cuff tears and labrum lesions but are rapidly being replaced by MRI as the preferred modality.

Ultrasound is a low cost, non-radiation form of investigation that is becoming the treatment of choice for shoulder soft tissue injuries. It can effectively evaluate partial thickness tears of the rotator cuff and associated muscle tissue, tendonitis, tendon dislocation and synovial effusions.

For a thorough discussion of shoulder imaging see Souza (1994).

MANUAL THERAPY

The management of shoulder problems is largely based on empirical evidence as there is little

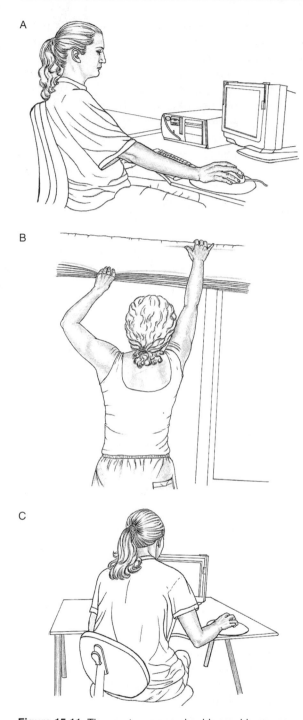

A

B

C

Figure 15.11 The most common shoulder problems are caused by: A: Abducted arm postures causing overstrain of the abductors – supraspinatus, upper fibres of trapezius and deltoid. B: Flexed arm postures involving the long head of biceps and anterior deltoid. C: Externally rotated arm postures exposing the infraspinatus and teres minor.

good quality evidence on which to base a treatment approach. Van der Heijden et al (1997) completed a literature review of the effectiveness of treatment for soft tissue shoulder injuries. The methodological quality of papers was generally poor, with only six papers including intervention groups of 25 or more. The authors concluded:

- Because of the small sample sizes and unsatisfactory methods of most trials, only a few randomised clinical trials of methods of physiotherapy in patients with soft tissue disorders allow firm conclusions on the effectiveness of treatment.
- When compared with placebo or another treatment ultrasound seems ineffective in patients with shoulder disorders.
- Evidence is insufficient to support the effectiveness of low level laser therapy, heat treatment, cold therapy, electrotherapy, exercise and mobilisation in such patients.
- Future trials should focus on the effectiveness of exercise and mobilisation in comparison to analgesics, non-steroidal drugs, steroid injections, and advice and a wait and see policy.

More recently, Green et al (1999), as part of the Cochrane collaboration, reviewed 31 trials on interventions for shoulder pain. They concluded:

- There is little evidence to support or refute the efficacy of common interventions for shoulder pain.
- Benefit of subacromial steroid injection over placebo for improving range of abduction was the only positive finding.

Nykanen (1995) found no difference in a study comparing pulsed ultrasound with placebo ultrasound and concluded: 'The results discourage the use of pulsed ultrasound therapy with the variables used for conservative treatment of the shoulder'.

Morrison et al (1997) completed a retrospective study of 616 patients suffering from subacromial impingement, based on a positive impingement sign at full elevation; 14% were classified as acute – less than 4 weeks, 37% subacute – 1–6 months and 40% chronic – more than 6 months. All the patients went through a rehabilitation programme that included a 3-week course of indomethacin, a physical therapy programme that included stretching exercises and a strengthening programme that emphasized the internal and external rotators. Sixty-seven per cent of patients had a good or excellent result, 28% went on to have surgical decompression and 5% declined surgery. Male/female results were similar, with improved results for acute cases and poorer outcomes for those aged over 60.

Ginn et al (1997) randomly allocated 66 patients with chronic shoulder pain to a control group (waiting list) or a 1 month individualized treatment programme based on stretching, strengthening and training dysfunctional muscle groups. The interventions were completed by ten physical therapists and the number of treatments varied between four and ten. Subjects in the treatment group showed improvement in pain-free abduction and flexion (22 and 16 degrees, respectively) and described a self-perceived improvement. There was no improvement in the control group. The authors conclude:

The results suggest that the physical therapy approach used in this study is effective in improving shoulder function in subjects experiencing pain of mechanical origin. The results provide little evidence of spontaneous recovery over a 1 month period.

Conroy & Hayes (1998) compared two randomly assigned groups (seven patients in each) receiving a comprehensive treatment programme for shoulder impingement (heat, active range of motion, stretching and muscle strengthening exercises, soft tissue treatment and patient education) with the intervention group receiving additional mid-range mobilization. The mobilizations involved anterior, posterior and inferior glides, and long axis traction. The programme involved nine sessions over 3 weeks and a home exercise component. Both groups improved equally on motion and function testing (abduction 27 degrees, elevation 24 degrees, internal and external rotation both 14 degrees). The mobilization group showed additional improvements, with statistically significant reduction in pain intensity over a 24-h period and reduced pain on subacromial compression testing, compared to the non-mobilization group. These studies (Conroy & Hayes 1998, Ginn et al 1997) indicate a positive short-term effect for a physical therapy and exercise programme, while Morrison et al (1997), with a large cohort and an average follow-up time of 27 months, demonstrated good long-term outcomes. Based on this limited number of studies, rehabilitation programmes would appear to be effective procedures for the management of shoulder problems.

Patients usually present for treatment with an acute manifestation of a shoulder problem. Like most acute injuries there is commonly a gradual recovery process and a successful resolution. Chronicity can develop if there is ongoing exposure to causative factors, particularly if combined with degenerative change. Thus treatment and exercise are helpful in the acute/subacute/recurrent phases, while management to keep exposures within the recovery threshold is critical in the recurrent and chronic phases.

In a rotator cuff strain the spasm reflex leads to a general shortening of the rotator cuff muscle group. This creates increased joint pressure, joint friction, increased afferent response and reduction of the subacromial space. A deep muscle release technique negates this spasm response, reverses these changes and provides a rapid improvement in function, mobility and strength. The muscle release technique will usually involve a direct pressure, such as the neuromuscular or myofascial release techniques, with the muscle in a lengthened position, using some type of lubricant. This will effectively lengthen the muscle, reduce the mechanoreceptor/nociceptor response and improve the fluid exchange. Clinical experience suggests that this is associated with an immediate improvement of mobility and an improvement in resisted muscle strength. This technique is particularly effective for the supraspinatus and infraspinatus. These muscles, having substantial osseous borders, are very sensitive to direct therapy. Cross-fibre, deep friction techniques are the method of choice for the rotator cuff tendons and encourage fluid exchange and cartilage repair in these tissues. This is best performed with the weight of the arm hanging over the side of the couch providing a joint distraction (Fig. 15.12).

Following muscle release techniques, the shoulder joint can be effectively mobilized to improve range of motion and stretch muscle tendons. Where mobility has been restricted

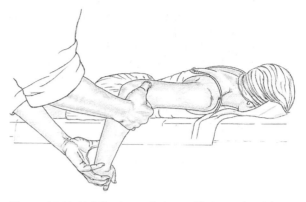

Figure 15.13 Mobilization technique with the patient lying prone, the upper arm being used as a lever and the practitioner's body weight providing the leverage.

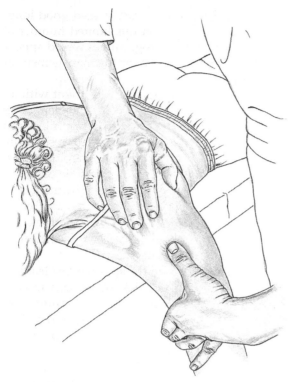

Figure 15.12 Deep friction techniques are best performed with the arm hanging over the side of the couch to provide joint distraction.

there is often shortening of the joint capsule and a reduced range of motion at the glenohumeral joint. Passive mobilization techniques can address this biomechanical inefficiency and improve the ability of the humeral head to clear the coracoacromial arch in elevated postures. This can be done in the prone, supine or side-lying positions using the arm as a very effective lever. Mobilization techniques should address the specific restriction in motion incorporating both traction and circumduction (Fig. 15.13).

Muscle energy techniques or thrusting techniques can provide additional impetus for mobilization of the shoulder joint if soft tissue barriers to mobility are identified. Exelby (1996) describes a technique for shoulder mobilization using an A/P glide at right angles to the plane of the gleno-humeral joint while the patient performs active movements in the plane that usually causes pain. The aim is to find a position where a previously painful movement becomes pain free. Exelby states: 'Pain free repetitions ensure sufficient corrective afferent input from the joint receptors and resulting reflex changes in muscle recruitment'.

A home exercise programme can be devised, incorporating the new movement pattern using taping to reposition the joint.

Mobility exercises for the shoulder

An injured shoulder joint will tend to develop increased muscle tension and subsequent muscular fatigue due to the increased afferent activity and the muscle tension reflex. If the shoulder is repetitively or statically used this can lead to shortening of the muscles and restrictions in joint mobility. Mobility exercises will effectively negate these processes and assist in maintaining normal joint mobility and function. They should be given to a patient as an adjunctive treatment to assist recovery and to provide postural variation during periods of exposure. As a general principle it is advisable to avoid exercises in positions above 90 degrees flexion or abduction (elbow above shoulder height) to avoid risk of impingement.

Stretching the anterior shoulder

1. With the arms behind the back, palms together and fingers interlaced, stretch backwards with the arms as far as possible (Fig. 15.14A). Hold for 3–5 s, repeat five times.

A

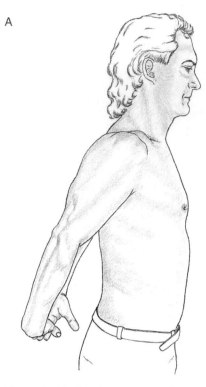

B

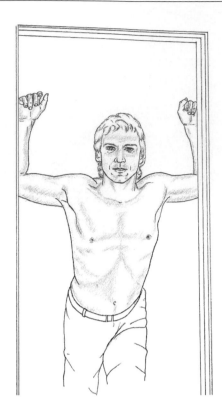

Figure 15.14 Exercises to stretch the anterior shoulder joint. A: The backward stretch with the shoulder internally rotated. B: The doorway stretch with the shoulder externally rotated.

2. With the forearms supported either side of a doorway and one leg in front of the other, gradually lean forward while bending the front knee (Fig. 15.14B). Hold for 5 s, repeat five times.

Stretching the posterior shoulder

1. Using the arm across the body and the forearm across the opposite shoulder, use the other hand to pull on the elbow (Fig. 15.15A). Hold for 5 s, repeat five times.
2. A variation of this places the shoulder in external rotation, by placing the wrist in the temple region (Fig. 15.15B).

Stretching into rotation

1. Improving external rotation. With the arm across the chest and the elbow flexed to 90 degrees the shoulder can be stretched into external rotation using the other arm as a lever. This stretches the joint capsule and the internal rotators.
2. Improving internal rotation. With the back of the hand in contact with the posterior aspect of the top of the pelvis, the other hand can be used to provide a leverage into internal rotation. This stretches the joint capsule and the external rotators.

Passively stretching into abduction and flexion

Active stretching into abduction and flexion causes large muscular forces which can exacerbate tendonitis and impingement syndromes. By hanging the hand over a horizontal surface the weight of the arm can be unloaded and the position of the body can determine the amount of elevation/stretch and the degree of traction (Fig. 15.16A). Side-on positioning creates an abduction stretch and front on positioning creates a flexion stretch (Fig. 15.16B).

A

B

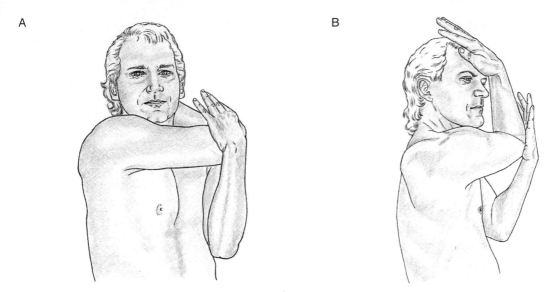

Figure 15.15 Exercises to stretch the posterior shoulder joint. A: The across-the-body stretch. B: A variation of this with the shoulder externally rotated.

A

B

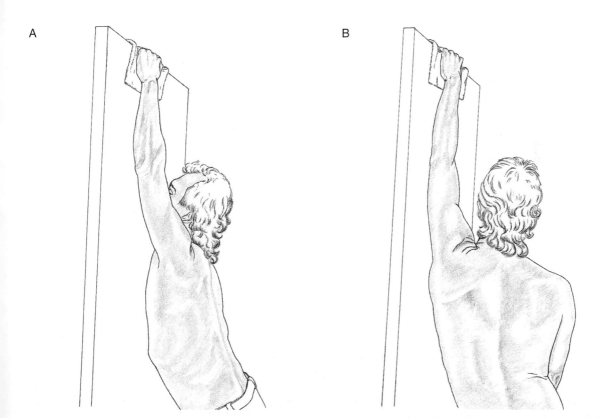

Figure 15.16 A strong passive abduction or flexion stretch can be created by hooking the hand over a horizontal rail to unload the weight of the arm while using the body weight and position to create a stretch. The orientation of the body determines whether the stretch is into flexion (A) or abduction (B).

Rehabilitation exercises

An exercise programme should be specific for the person concerned and the tasks that he or she is required to do. A sedentary desk worker will need to develop the ability to maintain static loads for long periods without fatiguing. A manual worker may need to develop the ability to repeatedly perform high demand loads, while a sportsperson may be required to develop peak power. However, all individuals will require an ability to maintain and coordinate the scapulohumeral stabilizers to maintain efficient biomechanics.

With the patient lying prone, the shoulder just off the surface and the arm just below the horizontal (Fig. 15.17A), the arm should be held in the following positions:

- abduction/elevation
- 30 degrees forward of this position
- 30 degrees backward of this position.

With the patient standing (Fig. 15.17B) the following postures are recommended:

- the arm straight, flexed to 60 degrees, palm facing down
- same arm position midway between abduction and flexion
- same arm position in abduction.

The patient should aim to hold each position for 10 s, followed by a rest period, with ten repetitions of this cycle. A weight can be incorporated to increase the muscle tension developed. Only small weights are required as there are substantial leverages involved with the weight at arm's length. The emphasis of the exercise is to improve muscle control and stamina rather than strength. The weight used, and the number of sets performed, can be increased as tolerance and adaptation to the exercise occurs. When the exercises have been mastered, subtle movements in one or more planes of movement can be incorporated in the different postures to create more dynamic stability.

To develop the glenohumeral rotators this is best performed in the standing posture with the shoulder relaxed and the elbow flexed at 90 degrees. An elasticated device can be used to

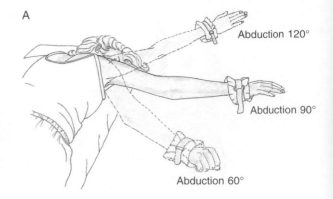

A

Abduction 120°

Abduction 90°

Abduction 60°

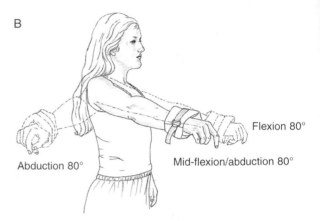

B

Flexion 80°

Abduction 80°

Mid-flexion/abduction 80°

Figure 15.17 Strengthening the shoulder stabilizers using various arm positions to develop sustained contraction strength. A: Lying prone. B: Standing.

resist rotational movements. From this position the shoulder can resist rotation internally and externally and hold in these positions against resistance. The patient should aim to produce approximately 30% of maximal voluntary contraction, and aim to hold this for ten repetitions of 10 s. Once adaptation has occurred the degree of tension and the number of repetitions can be adjusted. Morrison et al (1997) advocate strengthening the rotator muscles first in cases of impingement, and holding a magazine between the elbow and the trunk to create a forced deltoid relaxation (Fig. 15.18). The rotators form the lower cuff and strengthening these to the exclusion of deltoid and supraspinatus provides a net downward force on the humeral head, theoretically increasing the subcoracoacromial space.

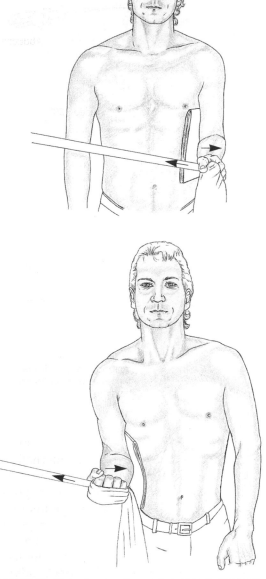

Figure 15.18 Strengthening the rotators is best done with the arm by the side, the elbow flexed, and pushing against elasticated resistance at approximately 30% of available strength.

With this exercise programme some key points to remember are:

- avoid holding the scapula elevated
- avoid holding end-range joint positions
- finish the exercise programme with 10 min of light aerobic exercise designed to re-establish contraction/relaxation cycles and restore blood supply
- to avoid fatigue, the exercises should not be performed prior to the working day.

For more dynamic, sports-orientated exercise programmes for shoulder rehabilitation, see Souza (1994).

ERGONOMIC ADVICE

It is often possible for the clinician to assess the tension pattern of the shoulder joint and link these with postures that may be responsible for building up muscle strain and advise the patient accordingly. For example, tense scapula elevators and glenohumeral abductors in a computer operator suggest the keyboard height is too high. Tense external rotators suggest a poor mouse position. It is often easy to give patients practical advice to remedy these factors. A painful arc of motion suggests overuse of elevated arm postures. A more detailed discussion of the ergonomics of computer use appears in Chapter 16.

Manual handling

- Overhead work should be minimized.
- 30 degrees abduction or flexion of the shoulder joint is a critical angle for efficient muscle physiology. Shoulder position should be maintained below these angles as much as possible.
- Leverages should be reduced where possible – distance, force, weight and grip strength.
- If suboptimal postures are necessary for sustained periods there should be an emphasis on providing support surfaces for unloading the weight of the arm.
- In a review paper Kilbom (1997) reports that the rate of repetition acceptable to different parts of the upper limb varies with repetition rates of greater than 2.5/min for the shoulder demonstrated as being at risk for injury.

Repetition is linked to the other ergonomic multipliers of force, posture, duration and static loads, and there is no guarantee that cycle times longer than this are risk-free.

● Work variety and breaks are important.

The shoulder joint generally works in conjunction with the rest of the upper limb. There is synchronous coordination of the muscles of the fingers, wrist, forearm, elbow, shoulder and scapula. It is not appropriate to examine one joint in isolation, either in the clinical or the workplace environment. A more detailed discussion on the ergonomics of the upper limb will appear in Chapter 16.

SUMMARY

● The highly mobile glenohumeral joint with its relatively small muscles and long leverages is very prone to developing muscle and tendon injuries. Degeneration of the joint and the tendons are common complications of injury.

● Injury is associated with sustained or repetitive postures with over 60 degrees of flexion or abduction.

● The shoulder joint is readily accessible to palpation and accurate biomechanical testing.

● Manual therapy and progressive exercise programmes have shown good outcomes.

● Management of postural and ergonomic exposures are important to prevent recurrence and chronicity.

16

Elbow, forearm and wrist pain

Many of the muscles in this region cross more than one joint and a regional view with a full examination of the upper limb is appropriate for any localized symptoms. While the symptoms will be most noticeable in one area there is likely to be more widespread dysfunction in the joint/muscle/tendon complex. For example, an extensor tendinitis (tennis elbow) is likely to have involved overuse of the extensor musculature and will be accompanied by muscular fatigue and trigger points, with some increased wrist compression or wrist tendonitis. In fact, the tennis elbow may very well have been preceded by a general myalgia as the complex approached its injury threshold. Injuries in this area are often not as anatomically precise as diagnostic labels would suggest. Ranney et al (1995) investigated 146 female workers in repetitive industries and the most common finding in the forearm region was myalgia, which frequently occurred in conjunction with epicondylitis (36% of 42 cases) but more frequently as a primary symptom without coexisting epicondylitis. Ranney expresses some surprise that forearm myalgia is not more commonly described in the literature[1].

As injuries become more chronic they very commonly affect neighbouring muscles and joints. This phenomenon is explained in Chapter 4. A sometimes confusing picture emerges where discomfort in different muscle groups or joints will become more apparent on different occasions.

---

[1] Don Ranney is a particularly skilled clinical examiner. His description of the examination of the forearm region is recommended (Ranney 1997).

Diagnosis in the forearm region is usually made by eliciting pain on resisted movement of the appropriate tissue. This is reinforced by positive findings on palpation. It may be accompanied by muscle weakness, particularly in chronic cases.

EPICONDYLITIS

Epidemiology

Lateral epicondylitis is far more common than medial epicondylitis. The dominant arm is most commonly affected; bilateral epicondylitis is uncommon. The extensor carpi radialis brevis (ECRB) is considered to be the most common portion of the common extensor tendon group involved. The ECRB, with a small insertion area on the lateral epicondyle, is considered to have a biomechanically poor position for withstanding high loads.

Lateral epicondylitis is most common in the 40–50 year age group, with incidence reducing after retirement. Male and female incidence is similar. It is common in occupations that have a high amount of manual work, particularly with forceful actions involving flexion/extension and pronation/supination of the wrist. The non-work-related incidence is also common – particularly related to sports such as tennis and golf, and activities such as painting and gardening.

Risk factors

In a review of six papers on lateral epicondylitis (Hagberg et al 1995), the authors conclude that: 'The epidemiologic literature does not make a convincing case for lateral epicondylitis being work related'.

The authors may have considered the high incidence of cases related to non-work situations in coming to this conclusion. A more recent, and very thorough, epidemiological review reached different conclusions (NIOSH 1997b). A review of over 20 studies relating to epicondylitis which assessed the evidence for different types of exposure concluded that:

- There is insufficient evidence for support of an association between repetitive work or postural factors and elbow musculoskeletal disorders.
- There is evidence for an association with force and epicondylitis. The majority of the 14 studies found a positive association.
- There is strong evidence for a relationship between exposure to a combination of risk factors (e.g. force and repetition, and force and posture) and epicondylitis. There are consistent data reporting the highest incidence of epicondylitis in jobs and tasks that are manually intensive and require high work demands in dynamic environments, for example mechanics, butchers, construction workers and boilermakers.
- This is consistent with evidence in the sports and biomechanical literature.

Two of the most important confounders are age and duration of employment. The incidence of epicondylitis has been found to peak during the fourth and fifth decades and to decrease after retirement.

Pathophysiology

There are three common causes of epicondylitis:

- a load, or period of loading, of flexion/extension and pronation/supination on the common extensor or common flexor tendon greater than the functional capacity of the tissues
- a long period of cumulative load, combined with age-related change
- local trauma to the common extensor tendon. This is postulated to disrupt the collagen fibre network and create an inflammatory response.

The precise pathological process is still keenly debated. The most common hypothesis relates to repetitive loading at the bone/tendon junction, which exceeds the strength of the collagen fibres causing ruptures, microruptures and inflammatory change. This leads to the secondary formation of fibrosis and granulation tissue. Other authors propose that repetitive loading leads to avascularization and subsequent inflammatory change. Some authors describe inflamed bursae and pinching of synovial fringe. The combination of sustained loading (as in gripping a tennis racquet) and the fatigue process that develops during isometric contraction may render the tendon more susceptible to peak loads (when hitting the ball).

Bauer & Murray (1999) showed that EMG readings of the ECRB while playing tennis were of earlier onset and longer duration, with higher levels of activation, in tennis elbow subjects than in controls. The authors propose that these EMG changes 'would contribute to increased strain on the injured soft tissue and promote muscle fatigue. Both the increased strain and the fatiguing aspects of the activation strategy would be counterproductive to the healing process'. This provides further evidence of the progressive inefficiency of injured muscle and the resulting increase in strain and fatigue to the injured tissues.

Anatomy

The muscles that move the wrist and fingers have their muscle bellies in the forearm and transmit their power to the wrist by long tendons that cross the wrist and insert into the carpal, metacarpal or phalangeal bones (Fig. 16.1). Most of the forearm muscles also traverse the elbow, and by means of a short tendon insert on, or just above, the humeral condyles. Overstrain of the wrist extensors at their origin is commonly known as tennis elbow while overstrain of the wrist flexors is known as golfer's elbow. The pain is usually located on the extensor or flexor surface of the upper one-third of the forearm. Diagnosis is made by tenderness on palpation over the epicondyle and reproduction of pain by resisted flexion or extension. Introducing finger movements, ulna or radial deviation and pronation or supination can help isolate the particular muscles involved. Extensor carpi radialis brevis and longus are strong wrist extensors and stabilizers, and also act to radially deviate the wrist. Extensor carpi ulnaris extends and ulna deviates. Extensor digitorum is a strong wrist extensor and also extends the metacarpophalangeal and interphalangeal joints.

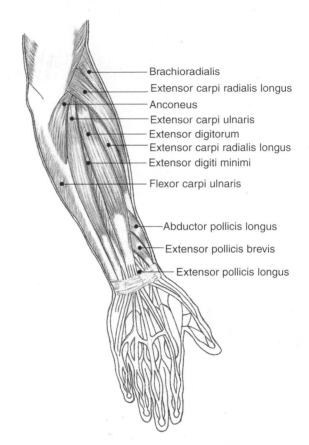

Brachioradialis
Extensor carpi radialis longus
Anconeus
Extensor carpi ulnaris
Extensor digitorum
Extensor carpi radialis longus
Extensor digiti minimi
Flexor carpi ulnaris
Abductor pollicis longus
Extensor pollicis brevis
Extensor pollicis longus

Figure 16.1 The wrist extensors of the forearm.

The superficial flexors of the forearm arise from a common tendon at the medial epicondyle of the humerus (Fig. 16.2). Flexor carpi radialis (FCR), flexor carpi ulnaris (FCU) and flexor digitorum superficialis (FDS) are regarded as the main wrist flexors; while FCU will also ulna deviate, FCR will radially deviate and FDS and flexor digitorum profundus can also flex metacarpophalangeal and interphalangeal joints.

Epicondylitis often occurs concurrently with strain and tension in the associated muscles and the tendons that cross the wrist. Careful palpation can isolate the muscles involved and the extent of the injury. It is important to try and link the injury to the causative postures. This will help the patient identify the problem and modify the exposure. Pronator teres and pronator quadratus are the muscles responsible for pronation (palm down) movements (Fig. 16.3) while supinator

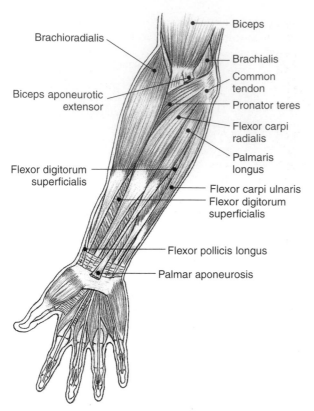

Figure 16.2 The superficial wrist flexors of the forearm.

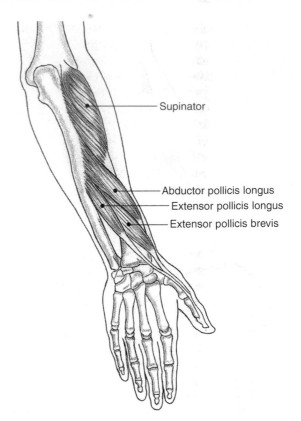

Figure 16.3 The pronator quadratus and pronator teres are the principal muscles acting to move the palm facing down.

and biceps are the principal muscles rotating the forearm to bring the palm up (Fig. 16.4).

TENDON INJURIES OF THE WRIST AND HAND

Epidemiology

There appears to be no particular predisposition to any particular age group or sex. Some reports describe increased incidence in females and in aged tendons, although these personal factors are of minimal significance compared to biomechanical factors. Tendon injuries seem to most often occur following prolonged or repetitive biomechanical loading, unaccustomed activity, an increase in normal activities or resuming activity after a prolonged absence. There are also reports of symptoms developing following relatively normal activities following trauma to the tendon.

Risk factors

Meta-analysis of eight epidemiological studies (NIOSH 1997b) concludes that:

- There is evidence of an association for any single factor (repetition, force or posture) and hand/wrist tendinitis.
  - The risk ratio for the seven studies examining repetition ranged from 1.4 to 6.2, with the reviewers concluding that the midgroup estimates of 2.5–4.1 are likely to most accurately reflect the true risk ratio.
  - There is strong evidence of an association between work that requires forceful exertions, with all five studies showing positive risk ratios.
  - There is strong evidence of an association between work that requires extreme postures, with all five studies showing positive risk ratios.

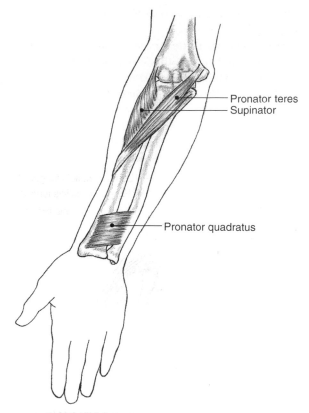

Figure 16.4 The supinator acts to bring the palm facing up.

- There is strong evidence that jobs that require a combination of risk factors, such as highly repetitive, forceful hand exertions, increase the risk for hand/wrist tendinitis.
- The prevalence of hand/wrist tendinitis ranged from 0 to 14% in unexposed groups to 4 to 56% in exposed groups. The wide range of prevalence rates reflects the variability in diagnostic criteria.
- There is no evidence that the associations reported can be explained by gender, age, or any other factors.

Anatomical features

Six muscles have tendons that cross the flexor surface of the wrist and are capable of creating a wrist flexion movement: the palmaris longus, the flexor carpi radialis, the flexor carpi ulnaris, the flexor digitorum superficialis, the flexor digito-

rum profundus and the flexor pollicis longus. The first three are primary wrist movers and the last three are flexors of the digits with secondary action at the wrist. The position of the FCR and FCU allow them to radially and ulnarly deviate the wrist respectively. The extensor surface of the wrist is crossed by nine muscles (Fig. 16.5). The extensor carpi radialis longus and brevis and the extensor carpi ulnaris (ECU) are primary wrist extensors. The other six are primarily finger extensors (extensor digitorum, extensor indicis and extensor digiti minimi) and thumb extensors (extensor pollicis longus and brevis (EPB), and abductor pollicis longus (APL)) that act secondarily on the wrist. The APL and EPB are both capable of radially deviating the wrist, although this is usually an unhelpful action and detracts from the prime action on the thumb. This unwanted action is opposed by synergistic contraction of ECU.

The hand and wrist complex is operated by a total of 42 muscles, most of which cross multiple joints. In order to perform precision movements

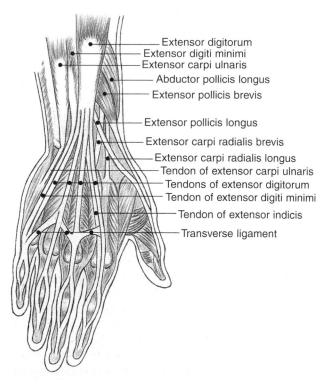

Figure 16.5 The extensor tendons at the wrist.

or to develop strength, there is a requirement to stabilize joints that are unwanted for mobility and to place these in optimum positions to provide power and precision for the muscles performing tasks. An apparently simple task, such as closing the hand to grasp an object, is of considerable mechanical complexity. The muscles involved in a particular task vary according to the particular demands of the task – the shape of the handle, the movement performed, the amount of force required, etc. The variety of permutations is almost infinite. Movements of the wrist are generally balanced by the wrist extensors. Finger flexion generally includes wrist extension and blocking of wrist flexion to create stability and limit flexion to the more distal joints. There are generally reciprocal motions between the wrist extensors and finger flexors to maintain optimum tendon length/tension, without which both precision and strength diminish considerably.

Motion of the thumb is generally balanced by abductor pollicis longus allowing flexor pollicis longus to act as a flexor of the metacarpophalangeal and interphalangeal joints. Different postures of the thumb can be produced by the interplay of flexor and extensor forces.

Pathophysiology

These injuries can be related to overload of the tendon causing a classic tendinitis, or a failure at the musculotendinous junction causing a peritendinitis. This typically involves a cumulative load greater than the recovery processes of the tissues. The pathological processes are thought to involve mechanical effects (such as viscous deformation, creep and microfailure), physiological processes (such as reduced vascularity, fatigue and inflammatory processes) and cartilagenous disorganization. Tenosynovitis is caused by inflammatory change produced by friction between the tendon and its sheath, or the tendon and neighbouring structures. Inflammatory change or trauma can increase the amount of friction. These different types of tendinitis frequently coexist and can sometimes be difficult to differentiate. They are usually associated with trigger points or areas of increased muscle tension in the related muscle

groups. Common tendon injuries at the wrist include:

Wrist extensor or flexor tendonitis. The tendons involved depend on the wrist position and the muscles activated during the involved tasks. For example, keyboard use commonly involves wrist and finger extension. Mouse usage commonly involves ulna deviation and first finger extension (clicking a mouse button). These movements can be exaggerated in workplaces where there are poor ergonomics or there is poor technique – such as an inability to touch-type (Fig. 16.6). The extensors are more commonly involved than the flexors. There is usually more than one tendon involved. The most common tendons involved are extensor carpi radialis longus and brevis and flexor carpi radialis and ulnaris. There is usually no pain on passive movement, symptoms are reproduced by resisted movement and grip strength is frequently diminished.

De Quervain's tenosynovitis. This involves overuse of the abductor pollicis longus and the extensor pollicis brevis. These muscles both originate on the distal third of the radius, while APL inserts on the base of the first metacarpal and EPB on the base of the first phalanx. Both muscles have a stabilizing role in position and orientation of the thumb in addition to providing muscular force, as in using the space bar while typing.

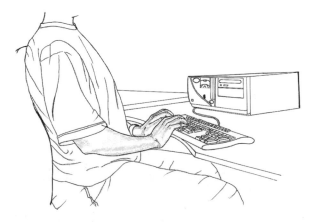

Figure 16.6 Keyboard use commonly involves wrist extension and repetitive finger flexion/extension, particularly where there is insufficient wrist support or poor typing technique.

Trigger finger. This occurs when there is an enlargement of the digital flexor tendons and these no longer have a smooth excursion through the tendon sheaths and the ligamentous pulleys that guide the tendon (Fig. 16.7). It is usually associated with increased friction and a history of high force grip or pinch grip, with high repeti-

tion, especially if there is a local pressure over the sheath of a finger or thumb flexor tendon. There will be a noticeable snapping or catching and sometimes an inability to extend the digit. There is usually a palpable nodule in the tendon.

ERGONOMIC FACTORS OF THE FOREARM

Grip

Grip strength is greatest when the wrist is in the neutral position. If the hand is placed palm up in the lap and allowed to relax, this constitutes the neutral position – with the wrist in about 20 degrees of extension and the metacarpal and interphalangeal joints semi-flexed with the fingers slightly separated. At this point the soft tissue tension is in equilibrium with no undue tension. Any deviation away from this position, particularly into wrist flexion, reduces grip strength by diminishing the capacity of the finger flexors to achieve optimum length. It is desirable for tool handles to be designed to allow postures approximating the neutral position to optimize grip strength and neuromuscular efficiency.

In the classic power grip (Fig. 16.8A) the fingers and thumb form a fist around a handle to achieve maximum contact and grasp to enable its manipulation. The optimum angle of the handle is 100–110 degrees to maintain a neutral wrist posture while allowing for the differing lengths of the digits. There are three variations of the power grip (Mital & Kilbom 1992):

1. force parallel to the forearm as in a saw
2. force at an angle to the forearm as in a hammer
3. torque about the forearm as in a corkscrew.

The size of the handle is an important determinant of grip strength. Pheasant (1991) recommends:

● 40 mm diameter handle for exerting a force along the long axis of a handle (e.g. rake)
● 50–65 mm for exerting a rotational torque about the axis of the handle (e.g. screwdriver)
● 65–75 mm for exerting a rotational torque on a spherical handle (e.g. doorhandle)
● 90–130 mm for exerting a rotational torque on a disc-shaped handle (e.g. screwtop lid).

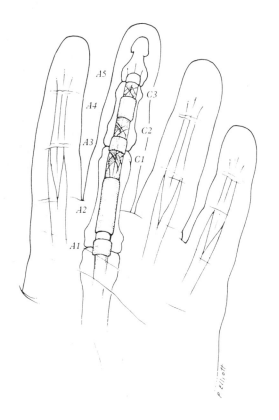

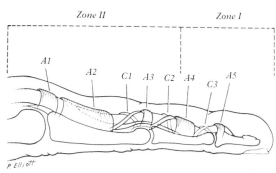

Figure 16.7 The arrangement of the annular and cruciate pulleys of the flexor tendon sheath. Tendonitis of the digital flexors can prevent smooth excursion of the tendon within the sheath. Reproduced with permission from Williams et al (1995).

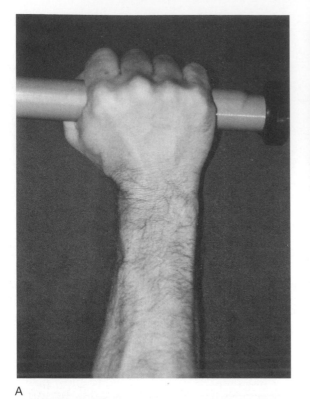

A

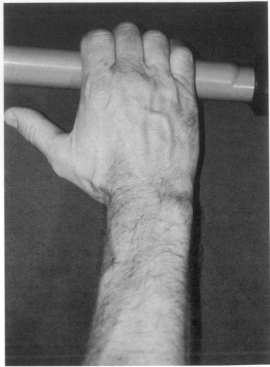

B

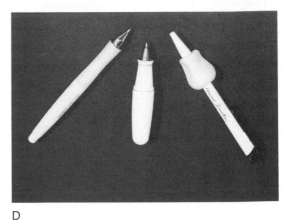

D

C

Figure 16.8 Different hand grips provide optimal efficiency for the appropriate task. A: The power grip provides maximum strength and control but sacrifices precision. B: The hook grip provides moderate strength with reduced effort and control. C: The pinch grip provides maximum precision and control but has little power. D: Examples of ergonomic pen designs that help reduce the fatigue in the wrist and finger musculature.

Pheasant (1997) makes the following recommendations for handle design and the efficient transmission of force from the user to the object:

1. It is more effective to impart a force perpendicular to a handle rather than along its axis (compression rather than shear). If shear is required a knob on the end will give better grip.
2. Grip surface area should be maximized to ensure pressure distribution over as large an area as possible. All sharp edges or other surface features that cause pressure hotspots should be removed.
3. Handles of circular cross-section and appropriate diameter will be most comfortable, with no hotspots. Greater purchase will be provided by rectangular or polyhedral sections but will be less comfortable. In general, where two planes meet the edges should be rounded.
4. The surface should be neither too smooth nor too slippery. Heavily varnished or rubber handles seem to be better than metal or plastic.
5. Grip length should be 100–125 mm.
6. If the palm of the hand is required to pass through a handle, as in the handle of a suitcase, a rectangle of 115 mm × 50 mm is required. For a finger or thumb, 35 mm will allow insertion, rotation and extraction.
7. Bend the tool to fit the task rather than bend the wrist.

The hook grip (Fig. 16.8B) can be used to suspend or to pull objects where manipulation is not required. This reduces wrist extension and reduces the activity of the wrist extensors. As the need for precision increases the object tends to be gripped more between the fingertips of the digits

where proprioception is most sensitive and fine motor adjustments are more easily achieved.

There are a number of variations of the precision grip: holding a thread in a pinch grip between finger and thumb, holding a dart in a pinch grip with two fingers, the lateral pinch grip as in holding a key and the classic pen-holding position (Fig. 16.8C), which uses elements of both the pinch and lateral pinch grip. These precision grips, where the additional flexion of the fingers and thumb are accompanied by additional extension of the wrist, combined with careful concentration and precision manipulation, can be quite demanding, particularly when associated with high force, long duration or repetition. Use a power grip for power and a precision grip only if precision is required, as the precision grip has on average only 20% of the power developed by the power grip.

Gloves can be an important protective factor for injury prevention. However, they can reduce proprioceptive sensitivity and usually require an increased grip strength to maintain a firm grasp. The thicker and stiffer the material (e.g. leather) used the greater the effect.

Vibrating hand tools create a multiplier effect for injury risk and often lead to increased muscle tension in an attempt to create stability. In addition, vibration has a fatiguing effect on neurovascular processes. (For further discussion on the design and selection of work tools see Pheasant (1991, 1997), Mital (1991) Mital & Kilbom (1992).)

The pen grip is one of the most commonly used precision grips and is a common source of discomfort in the hand and forearm. Most people will have experienced writer's cramp at some time, and the evocative description by Ramazzini in Chapter 4 places it in a historical context. Fernstrom & Ericson (1997) found significantly higher EMG readings for the hand and wrist when a pencil was used compared to keyboard or mouse usage. The slim, hard, round ballpoint pen is a particularly poor ergonomic design and can easily be improved upon by adding a rubber sleeve. The grip should be slightly wider than conventional – in the 15–30 mm range. The surface should be slightly scalloped, or of a compressible structure, to allow an increased contact

---

Case history

The author recently took up sea kayaking and, after an initial burst of enthusiasm, developed right wrist extensor tendinitis. This has been successfully ameliorated by changing the pull phase of the right-hand stroke from a power grip to a hook grip, and ensuring a full relaxation of the right grip during the left-hand stroke. This both reduced the load on the right wrist extensors tendons and ensured a full contraction/relaxation cycle to improve neurovascular physiology.

area and reduce point pressure (Fig. 16.8D). A good quality rollerball or fountain pen with low rolling resistance is helpful. Grooves or serrations on the contact surface are unhelpful.

Repetition

There is epidemiological evidence of frequency and duration of repetitive work being a risk factor in disorders of tendons and adjacent tissues, with work cycles shorter than 30 s, or occupying more than 50% of work duration, being of particular concern. In a review paper, Kilbom (1997) reports that the rate of repetition acceptable to different parts of the upper limb varies, with repetition rates of greater than the following demonstrated as being at risk for injury:

- 2.5/min for the shoulder
- 10/min for the elbow and wrist
- 100–200/min for the fingers

Repetition is linked to the other ergonomic multipliers of force, posture, duration and static loads, and there is no guarantee that cycle times longer than this are risk-free.

Computer keyboard

Use of the computer keyboard has been associated with forearm overuse injuries. There is increasing evidence of a dose-related response (Hochanadel 1995, Johnson et al 1997), with over 4 h a day regarded as a critical threshold (Veierstad 1998). In a cross-sectional study of 260 computer operators, Berqvist et al (1995) found an association between musculoskeletal disorders and VDU workers where there were suboptimal ergonomics. These included: static postures, lack of opportunity to take breaks, lack of forearm support and high keyboard position.

Serina et al (1999) measured mean joint angles of 25 subjects at standard, individually adjusted workstations. They found a significant usage of non-neutral postures:

… a majority of subjects typing with a mean wrist extension greater than 15 degrees and more than one quarter of subjects with a wrist angle greater than 30 degrees. 41% of subjects typed with an ulna deviation

greater than 20 degrees. Wrist angular velocities and accelerations were rapid during typing and flexion/extension velocities were comparable to wrist motions of industrial workers with high injury risk.

Tittiranonda & Burastero (1995) questioned 78 computer operators working over 4 h per day; 62% reported wrist or hand pain. When joint postures were compared between symptomatic and non-symptomatic users, the symptomatic users showed greater wrist extension (right: 21.5 and 17.7 degrees, left: 14.3 and 11.8 degrees) and increased right ulnar deviation (12.3 and 7.1 degrees). The researchers concluded that ulnar deviation and wrist extension were related to hand discomfort.

Martin et al (1998) measured the forearm muscle load of 20 young healthy touch-typists. They found extensor muscles were continuously active with a mean tonic load of 10% MVC and peak loads of 25–30% MVC, with about half this load for forearm flexors. The prime movers were extensor carpi ulnaris and flexor carpi ulnaris, while high tonic loads were demonstrated in extensor carpi ulnaris, extensor digitorum communis and extensor indicis proprius and flexor digitorum superficialis. They found that muscle load increased linearly with typing speed. The authors concluded that extensor muscle load is high considering the duration and repetitiveness of typing tasks.

There are a number of alternative-design keyboards that try to improve wrist angles and reduce the rate of fatigue and discomfort. These keyboards usually have either a fixed or variable split design, so the two halves can be angled to reduce wrist ulna deviation (Fig. 16.9). They often have a fixed or adjustable 'tent' so the keyboards can be raised toward the centre, reducing the degree of pronation. Other variables that are often manipulated are the tilt of the keyboard and the shape of the keypad. These are sometimes dished to reflect the different lengths of the digits. With so many different designs it is difficult to make generalized conclusions about the efficacy of these keyboards in preventing injury. It is clear that they are not going to be a major factor in preventing overuse injuries, although there are many people who are enthusiastic converts. In general:

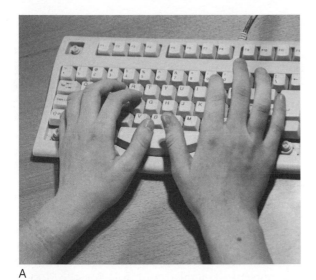

A

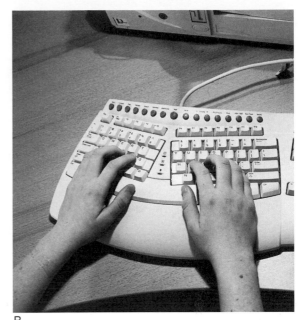

B

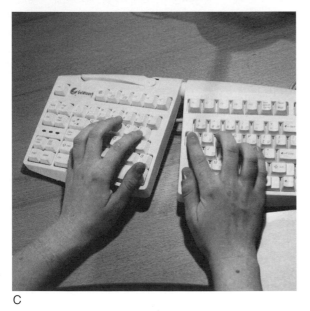

C

Figure 16.9 Keyboard design can affect upper arm posture. A: The traditional keyboard design creates an ulna deviation. B: The split keyboard reduces the ulna deviation, but the extra width can create a problem. C: The adjustable split keyboard with removable numeric pad and resited function keys reduces ulna deviation and provides for better mouse position.

- A new-style keyboard does have some initial effect on productivity. Studies have shown that productivity and error rates return to normal within 12 h of use (Swanson et al 1997).
- The alternative keyboards generally do lead to wrist angles that are closer to neutral, particularly with regard to ulna deviation and extension.
- Short-term studies of up to 2 weeks' duration have not shown improvements in levels of musculoskeletal pain or discomfort (Swanson

et al 1997), with both groups reporting increased pain in the back, neck, shoulders and wrists from the beginning to the end of the experimental period (Smith et al 1998).
- In a longer-term study of 6 months' duration, comparing a standard keyboard with three alternative keyboards (Titteranonda et al 1997), one alternative keyboard rated significantly higher than the others, including the standard keyboard, for comfort, ease of use and overall design. However, a different alternative

keyboard rated significantly higher for effort required and significantly lower for hand/wrist comfort.

In summary, it would seem that the type of keyboard is not likely to be as significant a factor to the injury risk as the amount of time spent keying, job variety, frequency of breaks, typing technique and other organizational or personal factors. However, it does seem that the best of the alternative keyboards confers some advantages in posture and rate of fatigue. The split keyboard design to reduce pronation and extension seems to have a higher acceptability than the tented design (Zecevic et al 2000). An adjustable split would have some obvious advantages over a fixed split in adjusting to individual anthropometric characteristics.

Alternative keyboards should only be recommended on a trial basis, as some users dislike them. However, a symptomatic user is likely to benefit from a good alternative keyboard and more likely to be motivated to make the transition. Keyboards should be as flat as possible to reduce wrist extension. Built-in wrist support has obvious advantages and it is better to have a specialized, good-quality product than a poor quality support attached to the keyboard.

Hedge et al (1999) tested the effects of a downward-tilting keyboard tray, complete with a broad, flat, smooth palm rest at the same angle as the keyboard (Fig. 16.10). Twenty-three subjects and 15 controls were pretested and then retested later after the subjects had used the configuration for 3 weeks. The results showed significant improvements in wrist posture, seated posture and musculoskeletal discomfort for the downward tilt group. There were no significant changes in the control group. Over 80% of move-

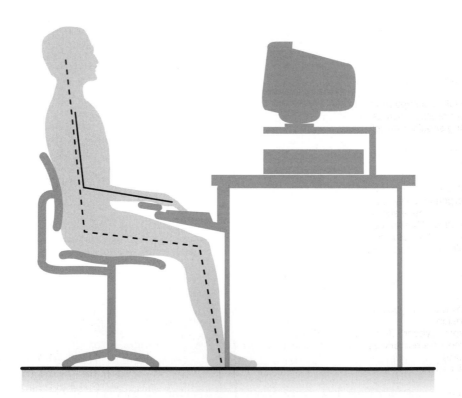

Figure 16.10 The downward tilt keyboard tray as tested by Hedge et al (1999) showed improved postures, comfort ratings and user acceptability. Reproduced with permission from Hedge et al (1999).

ments were in the wrist neutral zone compared to 50% with the control group. The downward tilt group showed a strong preference for the downward configuration compared with their previous arrangements, with no loss of performance. There was no training or instruction given to the subjects and the reported improvements were allied to the improved postures.

Typing technique has been proposed as a risk factor. The evidence is conflicting. Touch-typing would seem to be important to enable good posture and to avoid exaggerated hand movements. Zecevic at al (2000) found that subjects who had extended wrists on a standard keyboard tended to retain this (with reduced angles) on alternative keyboards.

Box 16.1 Keyboard use

- The keyboard should be at elbow height (olecranon process) when sitting in the working posture with the upper arms relaxed by the trunk and palms resting on the lap.
- The keyboard should not be tilted toward the user.
- There should always be desk space of 10–12 cm in front of the keyboard to enable unloading of the weight of the arms in opportunities available for rest.
- Additional wrist support at the level of the keyboard enables increased opportunity for unloading shoulder muscles and improving wrist angles.
- A wrist rest that supports the forearm and moves in the horizontal plane can effectively unload the weight of the arm in all keyboard postures and is an excellent aid in chronic cases.
- Some ergonomic keyboards that create neutral wrist postures have shown some advantage in some studies. They can be helpful in reducing symptoms but should be subject to trial.
- The optimal configuration based on current research suggests that the following configuration would promote the most joint neutral postures and would be most likely to minimize fatigue and discomfort:
  - downward-tilt keyboard tray (to reduce extension)
  - the split keyboard (to reduce ulna deviation)
  - a removable numeric pad (to improve mouse posture)
  - a wrist support at the same height and angle of the keyboard (to optimize the opportunity for EMG gaps) with some possible advantage to a mobile support.
- Work variety and breaks should be emphasized.

Computer mouse

Pointing devices are becoming an increasingly important part of computer work and their use has been shown to increase productivity for word processing. Continued software development has placed increasing emphasis on their use and some software applications make primary or even exclusive use of these devices. The mouse is the most commonly used device and is usually placed alongside the keyboard on the side of the dominant arm. The additional reach, beyond the keyboard to the mouse, has been shown by many studies to elevate, abduct, flex and externally rotate the shoulder, extend the elbow and ulnar deviate the wrist. This leads to significantly higher EMG readings in the associated muscle groups, which remain higher for the entire period of mouse use without any evidence of microbreaks (Harvey & Peper 1997). Karlqvist et al (1994) compared the postures of 12 mouse users to 12 keyboard-only users at their own workstations during text editing tasks. They found that the mouse users had greater angles of shoulder flexion, abduction and external rotation. The mean figures for mouse users were (with keyboard users in brackets) 6.2 (–7.5), 11.7 (8.6), 12.1 (–9.3), respectively. They found a mean ulnar deviation of 17.6 degrees for mouse users, with 30% of the time spent with greater than 30 degrees deviation. The non-mouse users had a mean ulnar deviation of 1.8 degrees with no time spent with greater than 30 degrees. The researchers concluded that: 'our observations showed long periods of strenuous working postures for mouse operators compared to non-mouse operators'.

The mouse usually takes second priority to the keyboard for position and the poor postures related to mouse use are more related to the demands of the keyboard placement than the requirements of mouse usage. Karlqvist et al (1998) showed lower EMG readings and higher comfort ratings with shoulders in neutral posture compared to the usual abducted or flexed postures (keyboards were conveniently removed to provide neutral postures). Karlqvist concludes: 'The VDU operators in the study preferred a table position for the mouse that was close to the relaxed neutral posture of the arm combined with arm support'.

Harvey & Peper (1997) showed reduced EMG readings for right upper trapezius, right lower trapezius/rhomboids and right posterior deltoid using a centrally located trackball compared to a mouse right of keyboard.

Improved mouse position and therefore shoulder and wrist posture can be gained by:

Reducing the width of keyboard. Most keyboard designs have a numeric pad and a block of function keys on the right. The function keys can be relocated to alternative sites or the numeric pad can be an optional extra on a separate removal pad (some keyboards now offer these features). Cook & Kothiyal (1998) found significantly less middle and anterior deltoid EMG readings when the mouse was situated adjacent to a keyboard without a numeric pad than when compared to a standard keyboard. They noted improved postures in the upper and lower arm, but noted that wrist posture remained poor in all positions with use of a standard mouse.

Using the mouse on the left side of the keyboard. Studies suggest that most computer users, following an adjustment period, can become accustomed to left-hand mouse usage for word processing tasks without loss of productivity. Hoffmann et al (1997) found no difference in performance between preferred and non-preferred hands during simple mouse tasks.

Placing increased emphasis on keyboard commands as a substitute for mouse usage. There is little evidence to show that any other pointing devices have any significant ergonomic advantage over the mouse once the overreaching to the mouse has been negated. These alternative methods (trackballs, touch screens, trackpoints, etc.) often have reduced sensitivity of pointer function and require increased use of wrist and finger flexors. Fernstrom & Ericson (1997) compared four different types of human–computer interaction for use with word processing tasks. The keyboard-mounted trackpoint reduced strain on the shoulder muscles but increased the loading on the muscles in the hand and forearm. The mouse with mobile arm support reduced load on the shoulder but also increased load on the forearm, although to a lesser degree than the trackball. Use of the keyboard shortcuts reduced loading on the shoulder but increased loading on the wrist. The extra reach required for mouse usage produced the highest shoulder EMG readings, which could be reduced when using a mobile arm support, though at the expense of increased wrist movements. There were no clear winners from this study. Karlqvist et al (1999) showed reduced shoulder elevation and reduced muscular activity, but greater wrist extension and use of the finger flexors, when using a trackball. Twelve of the 20 subjects showed preference for the computer mouse. Burgess-Limerick et al (1999) reached similar conclusions. 'Exposure to extreme ulnar deviation and wrist extension was observed in the use of computer mouse and trackball. The trackball involved decreased ulna deviation and increased wrist extension'. Karlqvist et al (1999) advised that:

- An input device offering natural shoulder joint positions with supported arm and few arm movements causes a low shoulder muscle activity.
- An input device offering natural hand/wrist joint positions with supported forearm/wrist and a balanced pointer, designed for the size of the hand gives a low forearm muscle activity.

Alternatives to the mouse should be offered on a trial basis and the degree of acceptance will vary according to the person, the design of the workplace, the computer hardware and software and the type of task being performed.

The traditional mouse design requires use of the forearm in pronated (palm facing down) posture while the most relaxed position of the forearm is in a neutral position midway between pronation and supination – note the position of the arm when hanging relaxed by the side. Some recent mouse designs reduce the amount of pronation required by providing an angled surface to the top of the mouse (Fig. 16.11). This both reduces the degree of pronation and the tendency for ulnar deviation during mouse excursion. Another recent mouse design is more along the lines of a joystick, which completely eliminates wrist pronation and allows a natural hand position. Aaras & Ro (unpublished data)

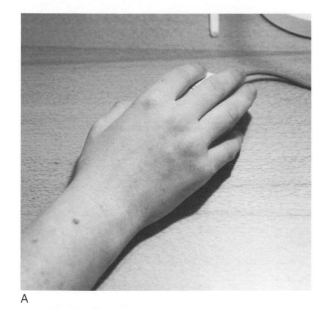

A

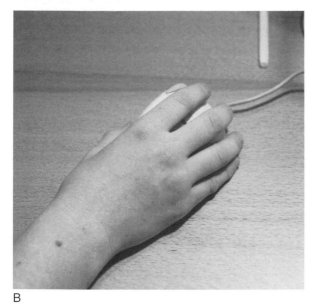

B

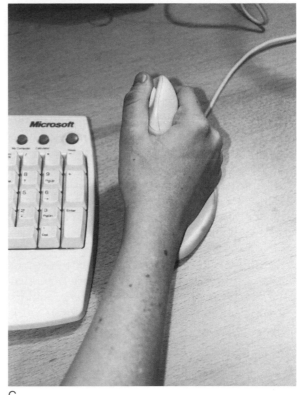

C

Figure 16.11 Mouse designs can make a difference to wrist posture and loading on forearm musculature. A: Traditional mouse design creates wrist extension, pronation and ulna deviation. B: An improved mouse design reduces non-neutral wrist postures. C: The joystick mouse design has shown improved posture, lower EMG readings and reduced discomfort.

compared a joystick mouse with a conventional mouse in 67 users with a history of shoulder and forearm pain. At 6 month follow-up the joystick group had a significant reduction in neck, shoulder, forearm, wrist/hand pain and headaches. The traditional mouse group remained largely unchanged. In another study, Aaras & Ro (2000) documented significantly reduced EMG readings of trapezius, extensor carpi ulnaris and extensor

digitorum using the joystick mouse with reduced static load, reduced medium load and increased periods under 1% MVC, both with and without forearm support.

The continuous and prolonged nature of muscle loading during mouse usage represents a risk factor even when the shoulder is relatively neutral. Jensen et al (1998) studied 149 subjects using computer-aided design (CAD) for at least

5 h a day and using predominantly puck and digitizer and/or mouse. The researchers made the point that the digitizer is usually placed in front of the operator and the shoulder posture is more neutral than for exclusively mouse usage. Despite this, the prevalence of symptoms in these operators was extraordinarily high. Based on 149 returned questionnaires (62% response rate) the 12 month prevalence of symptoms was hands/wrists 52%, elbows 41%, shoulders 54%, neck 70%, upper back 38% and lower back 54%; with 7 day prevalence between 25% and 50% of these figures. The symptoms were much more prevalent in the arm operating the mouse; hand/wrist and elbow problems were significantly higher in women while neck, shoulder, upper and lower back affected both sexes in similar proportions. The researchers note that EMG levels were similar to keyboard operators but not as high as other types of repetitive work using hand tools:

Thus for the CAD operators the actual level of muscular activity does not seem to explain the high prevalence of musculoskeletal symptoms. More likely, repetitive movements without postural variation may require prolonged activation of shoulder and forearm muscles and thereby present a risk for developing musculoskeletal symptoms.

Thus intervention aimed at improving the exposure should limit the length of time CAD work is performed with a mouse by introducing other tasks.

Yet again, the evidence reveals that providing neutral postures and minimizing EMG readings is not enough to prevent injury. Increasing emphasis must be placed on providing more dynamic work environments, with increased job variety, to create healthy neuromuscular homeostasis.

Wrist and forearm support

Holding the arms in a position for keyboard and mouse usage requires a static load on the shoulder muscles. Long periods of static loading have been linked with overuse injuries and this has been proposed as responsible for a dose-related response for injury risk with computer work (see Chapter 4). Any opportunity to unload the weight of the arms is likely to reduce the rate of

---

Box 16.2 Mouse use

- The mouse position should be at the same height and as close to the keyboard as possible, minimizing external rotation and abduction/flexion of the shoulder.
- Some 'ergonomic' keyboards have additional width, which encourage is abducted shoulder postures.
- Most people can adapt to a left-hand mouse position for word processing tasks and this usually provides better shoulder postures. Keyboards with removable numeric pads allow a better mouse position for right-hand mouse usage.
- Ergonomic mice or other pointing devices that encourage neutral postures of the shoulder, forearm, wrist and fingers are preferable to the conventional flat mouse.
- There should be a support surface available for resting the arm while using the mouse.
- Work variety and breaks should be emphasized.

---

muscular fatigue and reduce the risk of symptoms. The research literature largely supports the proposition that availability of forearm and wrist support is beneficial for computer users.

Aaras & Ro (1998) and Aaras et al (1998) completed a study comparing computer users who had the opportunity to support the forearms on the desk surface compared to users who were unable to. The group that had forearm support showed a reduction in the mean static load of the trapezius from 1.5% MVC to 0.2% MVC, and a significant reduction in the intensity of shoulder pain.

The minimum wrist support provided should be 10–12 cm of desk surface in front of the keyboard. There is persuasive evidence that provision of additional wrist support at the same height as the keyboard both reduces wrist extension angle and allows increased opportunity for resting the arms while maintaining neutral wrist posture. Albin (1997) studied subjects with and without use of a gel wrist rest and found that using the wrist rests facilitated more neutral wrist postures, with average wrist extension reducing from 11.93 degrees to 3.46 degrees. Subjects also reported improved subjective comfort ratings for the hands and wrist.

The supports should have a large surface area to avoid pressure points; they should be compliant to spread the surface load and should be low friction. This type of support is designed for use during pauses and breaks – not for use during typing.

Mobile forearm supports allow lateral movements of the forearms while unloading the weight of the shoulders during active working periods as well as during breaks (Fig. 16.12). Feng et al (1997) found 'the horizontal moveable arm support was more effective in reducing the EMG levels of the shoulder muscles than other supports'. Karlqvist

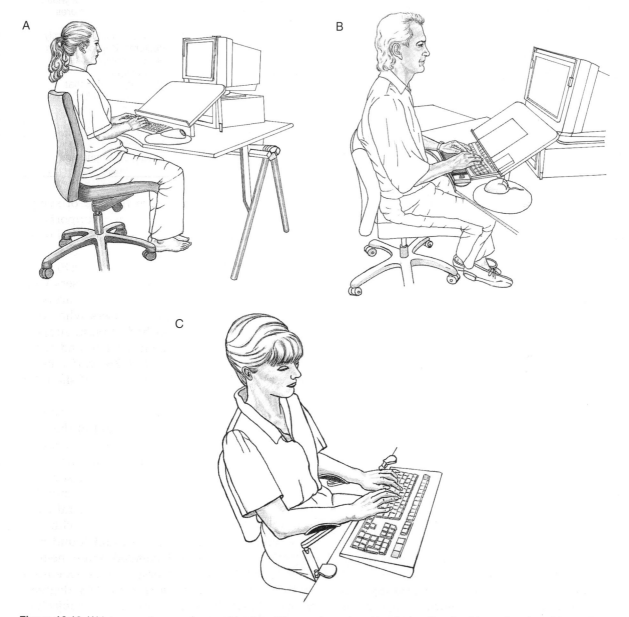

Figure 16.12 Wrist support can make considerable difference for reduced loading on the shoulder and neck and improving wrist angles. A: Using the table top as support during keyboard pauses and during mouse usage is essential to create rest periods in neck, shoulder and arm musculature. B: Providing added wrist support reduces wrist extension and can increase availability for rest periods. C: A mobile forearm support reduces loading to neck, shoulder and forearm during all keyboard and mouse usage.

et al (1998) found 'arm support markedly reduced muscle load in the neck/shoulder region'. These mobile arm supports have saved the careers of people with chronic symptoms, allowing them to continue work when otherwise they would be unable to. However, they should not substitute for a full ergonomic appraisal of the working environment.

Laptop computers

The increasing popularity of laptop computers is a major concern. They have significant compromises in design that affect posture to a degree that represents a significantly increased risk for computer users. The screen and the keyboard are attached to form a single unit, so inevitably there are compromises in head and neck posture to allow for a low visual angle, and elevation of shoulders and scapula to allow for an elevated keyboard position. Straker et al (1997) compared 16 subjects in a cross-over design and found a significantly greater neck angle and head tilt when using a laptop compared to a desk-top computer. The 6 degree change in neck angle was estimated to increase the torque at C7 by 9%. After 20 min use there was a clear trend for increased discomfort and visual fatigue among laptop users. These compromises will be exaggerated for tall users. The keyboard and pointing systems are miniaturized and these will create exaggerated ulna deviation for keyboard usage and finger/wrist flexion for mouse usage. Male or large dimension users are particularly at risk of having to adapt to the constrained postures.

It is a relatively simple intervention to plug in an external keyboard and mouse and elevate the screen to a good visual angle when using the laptop in a desk-type situation. These are relatively cost-effective procedures that make a dramatic difference to working postures (Fig. 16.13).

EXAMINATION OF THE FOREARM

As with all musculoskeletal injuries it is important to gain a thorough understanding of the nature of the injury, its history, any related traumas, current or predisposing exposures, any barriers to normal

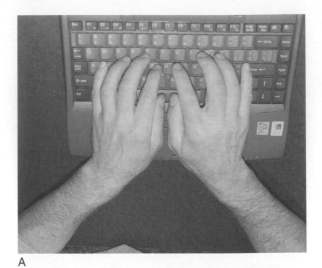

A

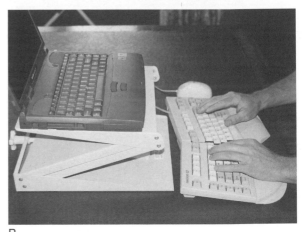

B

Figure 16.13 Laptops are a significant injury risk due to the compromises in posture they create. Note the exaggerated ulnar deviation (A). It is a relatively cost-effective intervention to attach an external keyboard and mouse and to raise the screen to improve visual angles (B).

recovery and to ascertain the pattern of pain and any aggravating or relieving factors.

A good clinical examination is an important component in establishing a working diagnosis. This should encompass the active and passive movements of the elbow, wrist and hand, and resisted movements of the muscle groups.

The elbow should be tested for full flexion, full extension and a degree of hyperextension. With the elbow in full extension, pronation of the forearm and flexion of the wrist provides maximum stretch of the wrist extensor complex and will usually reveal any tenderness or restriction. Pronation and supination can be tested with the elbow flexed to 90 degrees, loosely holding a pencil in the thumb-up position. There should be 70–80 degrees of supination and marginally less pronation. These movements can also be resisted in these positions.

Wrist flexion and extension can be compared in the prayer and reverse prayer postures (Fig. 16.14), which provide a symmetrical comparison. Resisted flexion/extension is best tested with the fist lightly clenched using a resisting force against the metacarpals (extension) and the middle phalanges (flexion). Resisted extension over the middle finger differentiates between the primary wrist extensors or the finger extensors. A general circumduction movement of the wrist will assess general wrist flexibility and radial and ulna deviation. Overall grip strength is a valuable test, comparing both sides and to the age-/sex-matched norm. Grip strength weakness is often a feature of the more chronic cases. Re-evaluating grip strength provides some marker of recovery.

Full finger and thumb flexion/extension should be tested and resisted, thumb circumduction is a useful mobility test. Pinch grip between thumb and each finger is a valuable test for overall strength and presence of pain. Finkelstein's test is the classic test for de Quervain's tenosynovitis (Fig. 16.15). The patient should make a fist with the thumb clenched inside the fingers, and while stabilizing the wrist with one hand and the thumb with the other, the practitioner should move the wrist into ulna deviation. A positive test will cause pain at the extensor pollicis longus or extensor pollicis brevis over the styloid process.

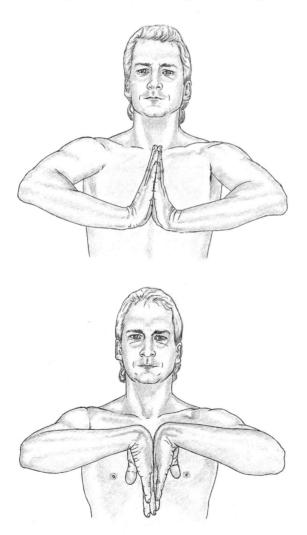

Figure 16.14 The prayer and reverse prayer positions for testing wrist mobility.

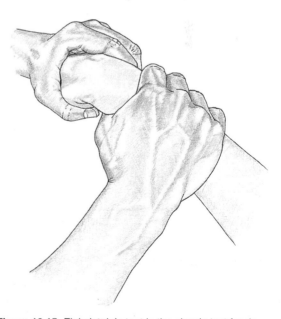

Figure 16.15 Finkelstein's test is the classic test for de Quervain's tenosynovitis.

The case history and physical examination will provide a working diagnosis. This can then be confirmed by palpating the suspected site of injury for tenderness, and to reproduce the typical pain pattern. Palpating while challenging the tissue with a demanding task (such as the appropriate resisted muscle test) will further reinforce the diagnosis. A careful examination should be made at neighbouring muscles and joints, as pain from more than one source is very common, particularly in chronic cases. Neuralgic pain in the forearm can mimic pain of soft tissue origin. A careful examination should be made of the cervical spine to test for dysfunction, particularly in the lower cervical and thoracic outlet regions. It is not unusual to find a patient who appears to have a classic epicondylitis that has not responded to the usual local treatments make a prompt recovery when the cervical or thoracic spine is treated.

Diagnosis in the forearm region is relatively straightforward because the tissues are readily accessible to palpation and because of the very specific nature of the contractile mechanisms. Diagnosis is not complete until the exposure that is responsible for the symptoms has been identified.

MANAGEMENT

The very acute injury may require some short-term rest and ice to reduce the inflammation or swelling and to prevent further injury. However, early mobility is recommended, within pain levels, while limiting the exposure of awkward postures and high force muscle contractions. Relative rather than absolute rest is recommended, by reducing hours or reducing exposures to hazardous tasks. The degree of activity can gradually be increased and supported with soft tissue treatment, mobilization, hydrotherapy and exercise.

Orthotic devices

The use of orthoses remains controversial. Jansen et al (1998) measured maximum grip strength and EMG readings in uninjured subjects while performing a variety of tasks using three types of wrist orthoses and compared these to no orthosis. There was a significant reduction in wrist extensor EMG readings during lifting tasks, while measured grip strength decreased significantly despite higher EMG readings. The authors concluded that none of the orthotic designs can be recommended as protection for patients with lateral epicondylitis during heavy gripping tasks. Based on a background of increasing evidence of immobilization tending to delay recovery and inhibit normal neurovascular homeostasis, orthotic devices should be used with caution. The use of a counterforce strap or tennis elbow band around the upper forearm for the management of epicondylitis is a popular intervention. Some studies showed an increase in pain-free grip strength and reduction in EMG readings of wrist extensors. Snyder-Mackler & Epler (1989) found reduced EMG readings of extensor digitorum communis (EDC) and extensor carpi radialis brevis, using indwelling electrodes at 80% MVC in healthy subjects, with the use of elbow braces compared to control values. This was non-significant with a standard tennis elbow band and significant with an aircast band. The effect was greater for EDC than ECRB. It is postulated that the use of these straps limits the tensile force on the epicondyle by redistribution of the muscle tension to fibres distal to the band. There may also be a counterirritant effect from reflex stimulation of the skin. This device does not have the disadvantage of limiting joint motion and the detrimental neurovascular effects. There is a case to be made for using these devices for early rehabilitation in heavy manual workers and sportspeople, where it is difficult to modify the peak exposures. However, the redistribution of forces may create a different type of injury. They should be used judiciously and not as a substitute for careful analysis and reduction of exposures.

Manual therapy

The use of deep friction techniques to tendon insertions and muscle release technique to muscle tissue is a valuable part of the management process. The soft tissues in this region are easily accessible to manual therapy. These tech-niques provide a neurovascular response that increases fluid flow throughout the affected soft tissues and reduces the muscular tension associ-ated with injury. It also provides a valuable aid to diagnosis and assessment of recovery. A tendon injury should always have the muscles that attach to the tendon released to reduce the resting tensile forces of the muscle/tendon complex and allow an improved therapeutic response. The neighbouring muscle groups and the muscle antagonists may also have developed an increased tonus.

The general increase in tissue tension around these injuries will often create a restriction in mobility of the wrist and elbow. In an analysis of 123 patients, Solveborn & Olerud (1996) found:

Practically all measured ROMs [range of motions] of the elbow and wrist were found to be limited in patients with unilateral radial epicondylalgia. The restriction of the ROM in the patients with right arm symptoms was most evident for active and passive wrist flexion, active and passive wrist extension, and passive pronation. Patients with left arm symptoms had significant restriction of the ROM for active and passive wrist flexion and pronation and for elbow extension.

Mobilization techniques to restore joint mobility will reduce tensile and friction forces around the joint. Particular attention should be paid to elbow flexion/extension, forearm pronation/supination, the superior radioulnar joint and the intercarpal joints. Muscle energy release techniques can be used effectively to improve joint mobility. Mill's manipulation provides a mobilization of the head of the radius and a powerful thrusting stretch of the extensor muscle tendon complex (Fig. 16.16).

Vicenzino & Wright (1995) describe a lateral glide technique to the elbow, used successfully in a single case study of epicondylitis, which allows pain-free gripping exercise to be performed while the technique is being applied and subsequently in a home exercise programme (Fig. 16.17).

The intercarpal joints are frequently com-pressed with restriction of motion and crepitus following a forearm overuse injury. Mobilization of these joints is assisted by providing a degree of traction and using local pressure to the affected carpals with a circumduction movement of the hand and wrist.

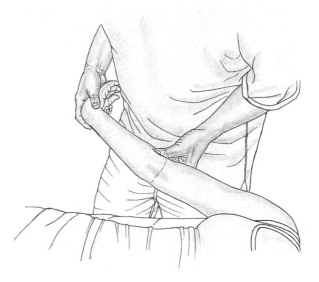

Figure 16.16 Mill's manipulation creates a powerful stretch on the extensor musculature and mobilizes the elbow, superior radioulnar joint and the wrist.

Exercises

Stretching exercises are valuable to regain mobil-ity following injury, to try and prevent develop-ment of increased muscle tension and to provide variation of neurological input during prolonged episodes of exposure.

Stretching the flexors is best performed with the elbow and wrist extended using the other hand grasping the palm to increase the leverage. It can be done in a predominantly wrist extended position and pronation and supination can be incorporated as a variation (Fig. 16.18).

Extensor stretching is performed with the elbow extended, the wrist flexed, and the other hand grasping the knuckles to provide addi-tional leverage (Fig. 16.19). This can also be done in a pronated or supinated position to provide variation.

These exercises should be done regularly throughout the day, moving through the differ-ent variations for about 30 s. Ideally, they should be done every hour during the working day in patients who have continual exposure to pro-longed loading, to encourage some neuromus-cular variation. Using the same elbow and wrist postures, primary contact can be made with the

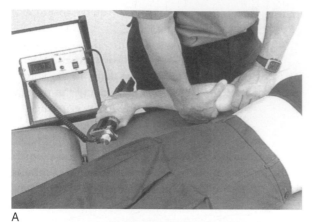

A

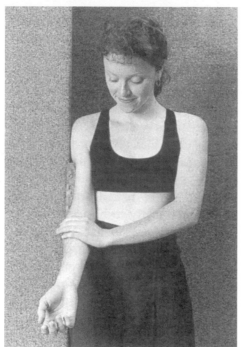

B

Figure 16.17 A lateral glide mobilization technique of the elbow. A: Performed by the practitioner. B: In a home exercise programme. Reproduced with permission from Vicenzino & Wright (1995).

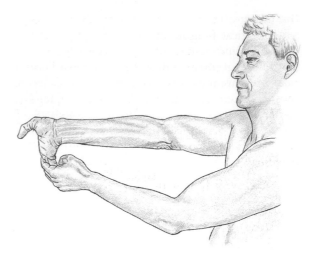

Figure 16.18 Exercises to stretch the wrist flexors should be performed with the elbow and wrist extended grasping the fingers with the other hand to provide additional leverage. Pronation and supination can be incorporated to provide variation. Flexor stretching in a supinated position.

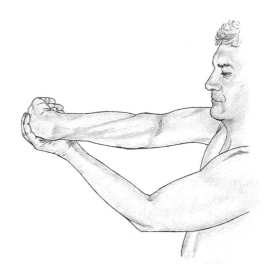

Figure 16.19 Exercises to stretch the wrist extensors are best performed with the elbow extended, the wrist flexed and the arm internally rotated, with the forearm fully pronated and the other hand grasping the knuckles to increase the leverage.

thumb to provide stretch of the associated muscle groups.

Wrist shaking and wrist circumduction are additional dynamic exercises that provide some muscle stretching with neuromuscular and proprioceptive variation. These will encourage relaxation of muscle groups during and after prolonged usage.

Rehabilitation exercises

Most chronic overuse injuries involve a mismatch between the demands upon the user and the capacity of the worker to meet those demands. Once the injury process has developed the changes of physiological fatigue and inefficiency associated with the injury usually compound this mismatch. Chronicity of forearm problems is often accompanied by a weakening of the grip strength of the most affected limb and a higher percentage of available muscle capacity will be required to continue normal tasks. Exercises to improve the available strength of the associated musculature are beneficial for the rehabilitation process. It is important to provide the appropriate level of exercise based on the symptom picture. Early prescription of physically demanding exercises will compound the muscle fatigue and injury cycle. To begin an exercise programme, the demands of the task upon injured tissue must be below the injury threshold.

In the early phase of the injury the key component of exercise is to re-establish normal muscle physiology – to develop a contraction/relaxation cycle that will improve fluid dynamics, encourage a postexercise relaxation and encourage normal neuromuscular homeostasis. A good example of this is the gripping of a soft rubber ball about the size of a tennis ball. This should be gripped for about 1 s at about 30% MVC, followed by 5 s relaxation. During the relaxation phase the arm should be supported and the hand maintained in its relaxed position. This can be repeated 10–20 times. As tolerance increases the length of time the grip is held can be gradually increased to 10 s and some wrist movements incorporated during that period, initially within an easy radius of the neutral wrist posture gradually incorporating a greater radius as symptoms allow. This can be done regularly throughout the day.

The second phase of exercise involves exercising specific muscle groups against resistance. Using a hand-held weight or an elasticated band for resistance works very well. This should aim to produce about 30% MVC with not more than 20–30 degrees of wrist movement. The 30% figure is based on the need to develop both strength and stamina without incurring a fatigue process. The patient will usually readily understand the concept of 30% but may find it hard to judge the required tension level. Some training with a dynamometer will help. In practice, if the

exercise creates postexercise fatigue or pain in the muscles being used, they are doing too much.

Resisted extension and resisted pronation can be performed in the palm down position; flexion and supination in the palm up position (Fig. 16.20). The exercise should start holding for 5 s, with 5 s relaxation and aiming for ten repetitions. This can be increased to 10 s and ten repetitions, aiming to do three sets. Initially, the exercise should be done once a day after any significant exposures, but the patient should aim to progress to three times per day. A more advanced stage involves performing radial and ulna deviation during the flexion and extension cycles. It should be made clear that the 30% MVC is not a constant

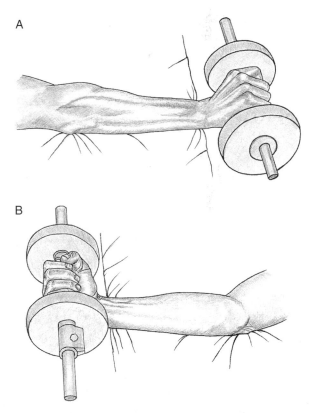

Figure 16.20 Resisted wrist movements using an elasticated band or a hand-held weight are helpful for forearm conditioning. Initially, sets of flexion and extension movements holding at 30% MVC should be used and pronation/supination and ulna or radial deviation can be incorporated. The length of time held and the number of sets can be gradually increased. A: Resisted wrist extension and supination. B: Resisted flexion and pronation.

force but will gradually increase with improving strength. These should be retested regularly with a dynamometer.

Pienimaki et al (1996) followed up 39 chronic tennis elbow patients, mean age 42.3, comparing a progressive exercise programme with local pulsed ultrasound. The patients were randomized into two groups, both groups were similar in pain scores, sick leave and duration of treatment. The patients underwent an 8-week intervention. The exercise group was trained in a four-step home exercise programme and visited the physiotherapist every other week for examination and to receive a more intensive programme. The patients performed the exercise programme four to six times per day. The ultrasound (US) group received pulsed ultrasound two to three times per week. At the 8 week follow-up, the exercise group had significantly better subjective and objective outcomes than the US group, with decreased pain at rest and under strain. The isokinetic torque of wrist flexion increased 45% (reduced 4% in US group) and maximal grip strength increased 12% (unchanged in US group). Of the eight subjects unable to work in the exercise group, six were able to return to work, while only three of nine returned to work in the US group. Long-term evaluation of the subjects was completed at 36 months (Pienimaki et al 1998), with 23 of the 30 (76.6%) completing the questionnaire. The exercise group had less physiotherapy, fewer medical visits and less sick leave than prior to the intervention, while the US group had more of each parameter following the intervention. Two patients in the US group (and none in the exercise group) were absent from work due to the tennis elbow condition. Patients in the exercise group had significantly reduced pain scores. Five patients in the US group subsequently had an operation, compared to one in the exercise group. The researchers concluded:

The progressive exercises evaluated in this study showed beneficial long-term effects compared to ultrasound treatment in terms of pain alleviation and working ability, and the functional overall condition of the exercise patients was also better. Exercise may be able to prevent chronicity and should hence be tried and recommended.

The progressive exercise programme (described in detail in Pienimaki et al 1996) consisted of:

- Step 1: slow fist clenching, resisted wrist movements (flexion and extension) and isometric wrist rotations with both hands on a stick.
- Step 2: resisted movements against an elastic band – flexion, extension, ulna deviation and radial deviation.
- Step 3: wrist rotatory movements using the table top as a support and pressing hands against a wall.
- Step 4: soft ball compression exercises, transferring buttons from one cup to another, twisting a towel into a roll plus wrist rotatory movements from Step 3.

The exercises were held for 8 s and were repeated for 10 × 3 series several times a day. They always finished with at least 30 s stretching in wrist flexion and wrist extension.

This programme showed impressive results, with demonstrable improvements in muscle power and efficiency. Caution must be taken when advising some of the more advanced exercises. The combination of force and extreme posture represents a hazard for both epicondylitis and hand/wrist tendinitis. Any exercise incorporating both these components must be done with great care, under supervision, and carefully graduated.

Home treatment routine

A home treatment routine can provide a helpful initiative towards recovery. It will have an important component of accelerating the rehabilitation process and provide powerful psychosocial benefits. If performed after the working day it can optimize the postwork recovery period. A suggested regimen might include:

- stretching exercises
- rehabilitation exercises
- 5 min ice
- 5 min massage
- stretching exercises.

SUMMARY

- Epicondylitis is a common finding in manual workers or active sports participants over the age of 40.
- It is associated with high grip force, and strongly associated with high grip force in combination with frequent repetition or deviated wrist postures.
- Wrist tendonitis is associated with repetition, force and deviated wrist postures, and strongly associated with combinations of these exposures. It is a common finding in exposed working populations.

- Forearm and wrist problems are more common in computer users who work with deviated wrist posture, notably wrist extension, ulna deviation and pronation.
- Good results have been reported with relative rest from exposures, combined with manual therapy, followed by progressive strengthening exercises.
- Management of ergonomic and postural exposures is critical in reducing incidence and preventing chronicity.

17

Nerve entrapments

NEUROLOGICAL SYMPTOMS

Normally, pain is felt following activation of nociceptor afferents and relayed to the spinal cord via nerve axons. Injuries generally cause a reduction in the threshold of nociceptor endings, rendering them more sensitive to further stimuli, this is known as peripheral sensitization. This tenderness created by the sensitization is termed allodynia. Further noxious stimuli will evoke an exaggerated pain response termed hyperalgesia. Persistent nociceptive input into the spinal cord can create a central sensitization. The peripheral and central sensitization usually fade quickly but, when there is persistent nociceptive stimulation, the central sensitization can be maintained indefinitely. During a state of central sensitization, non-nociceptive nerve endings, such as touch, and mechanoreceptors stimulated by movement can create a pain response known as secondary hyperalgesia. These pain responses are still primarily stimulated by peripheral stimulation of nerve endings.

Pain may also arise from injuries to the nerve tracts, this is known as neuropathic pain. These ectopic sites of neuropathic stimulus may also create a central sensitization, which can then stimulate a response of allodynia and hyperalgesia following peripheral stimulation of nerve endings. The nerve injury will create similar symptoms to the peripheral injury.

Thus persistent soft tissue injury can create nerve-type symptoms and a nerve injury can create soft tissue sensitivity in the related myotome and dermatome. Differential diagnosis can be very difficult in these cases and it becomes important to recognize that, in chronic cases, injury is rarely confined to neatly prescribed boundaries. This process seems to be particularly true of static posture-type injuries where the prolonged and unceasing afferent stimulation is more likely to create peripheral and central sensitization and secondary spread of symptoms.

A peripheral and central sensitization due to persistent peripheral nociceptor activity is more likely to trigger sites of ectopic neuropathic nerve impulses. Thus, what may at first appearance seem to be a cervical spine nerve root neuropathy may be being maintained by persistent peripheral nociception, and what seems to be a classic epicondylitis may well involve a cervical nerve root neuropathy. Chronic upper limb injuries are rarely simply demarcated to one region or one tissue and it pays dividends to explore the upper quadrant and explore the possibility of multiple cause and multiple effect.

NERVE ENTRAPMENT

Nerve entrapments refer to an incompatibility between the volume of a peripheral nerve and the anatomical space available to the nerve. This can be caused by acute injury, where the nerve is peripheral and subject to trauma, or it may be due to cumulative trauma. In the early stages the trauma will impair blood flow, oxygenation and the axonal transport system. If the nerve pressure is high, mechanical blocking of the depolarization process can occur. If a nerve is entrapped at one point there is increased susceptibility to mechanical pressure both distal and proximal to the impairment due to the diminished axonal flow.

CERVICAL RADICULOPATHY

Cervical radiculopathy is the compression of a nerve root as it exits the spinal column. This is most commonly due to a herniated disc or a narrowed intervertebral foramen and is often associated with degenerative changes in the lower cervical spine. The symptoms are usually acute pain radiating to the appropriate dermatome.

Tingling, numbness and loss of reflexes and muscle strength may be present. The symptoms will be aggravated by further closure of the intervertebral foramen by extension and sidebending of the cervical spine to the injured side. Imaging can be a useful aid in diagnosis. A review of cross-sectional studies of the incidence found an incidence of 1–5% with no evidence of any exposure–response relationship (Hagberg et al 1995). However, the studies reviewed were not designed to specifically assess the incidence of cervical radiculopathy, although this was one of many diagnostic categories investigated. The lower cervical spine is particularly stressed by flexion/extension movements and it is likely that these would be most at risk of producing radiculopathies, particularly in people with pre-existing degenerative change or instability. The flexion/extension may have a traumatic sudden onset, such as a whiplash injury or falling from a horse, or it may be associated with flexion/extension postures – tree pruning, fruit picking, window cleaning, etc.

These cases can be extremely painful and sometimes there is little respite from the neuralgia. Therapy should emphasize cervical movement away from the affected nerve root, to open the foramen and relieve the nerve pressure. The outcome is usually very good depending on the degree of degenerative change or trauma and the patient's capacity to avoid the cause.

THORACIC OUTLET SYNDROME

Thoracic outlet syndrome (TOS) is a neurovascular impingement syndrome at various anatomical sites where the brachial plexus and subclavian artery can be impinged as they pass from the cervical spine to the arm. The anatomical site of compression provides the labels commonly used: cervical rib or fibrous band compression, scalene syndrome, costoclavicular syndrome and pectoralis minor syndrome. Clarys et al (1996) recently described an axillary arch formed by variations of the latissimus dorsi or pectoralis major that is capable of causing neurovascular compression in abduction and external rotation of the shoulder. In an echographic study of 1321 subjects they found the axillary arch to be present in 8.5%, usually bilateral.

There is no clear consensus on diagnostic criteria for TOS and the diagnostic tests are unreliable. The result is that research in this area is poorly developed. TOS is often used as a dustbin diagnosis for upper limb neurological symptoms that have no obvious cause. A commonly recognized type is caused by the presence of a cervical rib or fibromuscular bands associated with the scalene muscles, which can impinge the lower branch of the brachial plexus resulting in ulna nerve symptoms. The more severe manifestations of this syndrome are well recognized, with pain and unilateral severe atrophy of the hypothenar muscles. There are characteristic changes in the electrical conductivity of the C8–T1 nerve roots and it is nearly always associated with cervical rib anomalies (Le Forestier et al 2000). The symptoms in these severe cases of identified malformations were progressive and insidious and represent one end of a spectrum of TOS. Many cases of cervical ribs do not develop TOS symptoms. The early diagnosis of TOS is extremely difficult (Ranney 1996). The symptoms include: arm–hand weakness, intermittent pain, burning, limb stiffness, paraesthesia and other neurovascular symptoms. There are a number tests used that increase the index of suspicion. These should not be regarded as positive unless they reproduce the patient's neurological symptoms. Adson's test involves deep inspiration, neck extension and turning the head away from the examiner (a modification involves turning the head toward the examiner). The examiner holds the patient's arm in abduction and external rotation (Fig. 17.1). This position is held for 10–20 s. A variation combines this with practitioner-induced costoclavicular compression. Classically, this test has involved palpating for obliteration of the radial artery but this gives no indication of neurological change and can lead to a high incidence of false negatives and false positives.

The candlestick test (Fig. 17.2) involves abducting the upper arms to 90 degrees with the arms in external rotation and the elbows flexed. This position should be held for 30 s. A reproduction of paraesthesia is regarded as a positive test. Grip

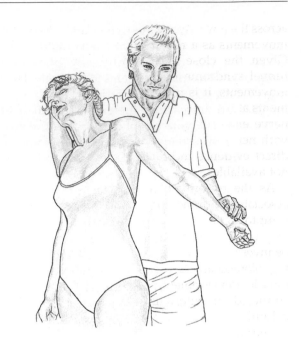

Figure 17.1 Adson's test.

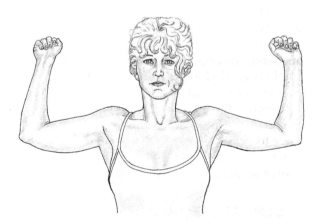

Figure 17.2 The candlestick test should be held for 30 s test for reproduction of neurological symptoms. Paraesthesia or reduction of grip strength suggest TOS.

strength can be tested in this position at the end of the period.

Hagberg et al (1995) reviewed six epidemiological studies that included TOS. They found rates of between 0.3% and 44%. When occupational groups were pooled, the odds ratio for exposure to repetitive arm movements was 4. They concluded that there was consistency across the few studies that showed repetitive arm movements as a risk factor for neurogenic TOS. Given the close relationship between carpal tunnel syndrome (CTS) and repetitive forearm movements, it is plausible that repetitive movements at the thoracic outlet could cause a similar nerve entrapment syndrome. This is consistent with nerve physiology as we know it, although direct evidence indicating exposure–response is not available.

As the majority of congenital malformations associated with the presence of TOS do not cause symptoms, and when they do cause symptoms they come later in life, other reasons should also be investigated. A multifactorial approach including biomechanical – posture, obesity, excessive muscle development, etc. – and ergonomic – abducted or externally rotated postures – is helpful.

Therapy should be directed at restoring optimum biomechanics to the cervicothoracic spine, mobilizing the first rib, establishing correct breathing patterns, scalene stretch and release and treating shoulder instability with particular reference to the shoulder elevators. Surgery is frequently disappointing and a recent study by Franklin et al (2000) following-up 158 cases of surgery found that at an average of 4.8 years follow-up 'those receiving surgery had 50% greater medical costs and were 3–4 times more likely to be work disabled' compared to a sample of workers with a TOS diagnosis who did not receive surgery.

ELBOW AND FOREARM

There are a number of sites around the elbow and forearm where nerve entrapments can take place. The most commonly affected nerve is the ulna nerve as it crosses the elbow. Compression occurs most commonly at two sites – the epicondylar groove and the point where the nerve passes between the two heads of the flexor carpi ulnaris – the cubital tunnel. Flexion movements stretch the ulna nerve and reduce the diameter of, and increase the pressure in, the cubital tunnel. These effects are enhanced by the contraction of the flexor carpi ulnaris. The results of these phenom-

ena are to reduce the circulation to the nerve and restrict the axonal flow of proteins. If the process is prolonged, the nerve can be damaged. The patient will complain of numbness and tingling in the little finger and the ulna border of the forearm. In severe cases, the ulna-mediated muscles may be weak – the patient may be unable to adduct the little finger or cross the middle finger over the index finger. The elbow flexion test, where the elbow is fully flexed and the wrist is fully extended for 1 min, is considered positive if paraesthesia or numbness occurs in ulna nerve distribution. The nerve is often tender to palpation in the epicondylar groove. It is quite common for compression of the ulna nerve at the elbow to be associated with additional compression in the cervical spine, thoracic outlet or more distally in the canal of Guyon. Treatment should involve mobilization of the neck, shoulder, elbow and wrist, neural stretching, avoidance of flexed elbow postures, during the day, and in sleeping postures.

The median nerve can be compressed at the elbow where it passes through a hypertrophied or swollen pronator teres muscle, or deep to a tense flexor digitorum superficialis muscle. Characteristically, contraction of the elbow, wrist and finger muscles causes tingling or pain in the thumb.

The radial nerve can be compressed where it enters or passes through the supinator muscle. The pain along the extensor aspect of the forearm can be reproduced by resisted supination. This condition can easily resemble or be associated with radial epicondylitis or wrist extensor muscle strain.

CARPAL TUNNEL SYNDROME

Carpal tunnel syndrome (CTS) involves the compression of the medium nerve at the wrist. It is characterized by pain, numbness and tingling in the median nerve distribution in the hand and fingers. Nocturnal pain is a common feature. The classic tests for CTS are Phalen's wrist flexion test – full wrist flexion held for 60 s – and Tinel's sign – tapping over the course of the median nerve at the carpal tunnel. If numbness, paraesthesia or tingling are produced, these tests are regarded as positive. Kuhlman & Hennessy (1997) found the most accurate test for diagnosis of CTS to be testing for abductor pollicis brevis weakness. This is performed by asking the patient to touch the pads of the thumb and small finger together. The examiner applies pressure over the thumb inter-phalangeal joint in the direction of the index finger while the patient attempts to resist. They found a positive result correlated with a positive nerve conduction test 66% of the time, while the figures for Phalen's and Tinel's were 51% and 23%, respectively. Electrodiagnostic nerve conduction tests are regarded as more sensitive indicators of nerve function, with about 90% sensitivity, but do not always correlate with symptoms.

There are a number of personal factors that can contribute to the incidence of CTS. Werner et al (1997) studied 527 workers in industrial and clerical settings:

- Obese workers were four times more likely to present with a median neuropathy than workers who were normal or slender.
- Industrial workers had twice the risk of clerical workers.
- Increasing age was related to an increasing risk.
- When only women were included in the model, the findings were similar but there was a more pronounced effect for BMI and industrial setting.

Diabetes mellitus, rheumatoid arthritis, Colles' fracture, narrow wrist, acromegaly, thyroid disorders, pregnancy and dysmenorrhea have also been linked to increased incidence of CTS. These conditions can contribute to reduced carpal tunnel volume and increased likelihood of elevated pressures. There are strong associations with jobs that have high repetition (odds ratio 2–5.5) and high force and high repetition (odds ratio 4–15). Cold and vibration have been identified as factors that amplify the risk. Hagberg et al (1995) in a review of the literature consider that: 'There is strong evidence supporting the contribution of work related factors to the development of CTS'.

In a review of 30 epidemiological studies relating to CTS, NIOSH (1997b) concluded:

- There is **evidence** of an association between highly repetitive work alone or in combination with other factors and CTS.

- There is **evidence** of forceful work and CTS.
- There is **insufficient evidence** of an association between CTS and extreme postures. Laboratory-based studies of extreme postural factors support a positive association.
- There is **evidence** of a positive association between work involving hand/wrist vibration and CTS.
- There is **strong evidence** of a positive association between exposure to a combination of risk factors (e.g. force and repetition, force and posture, and CTS).
- Epidemiologic surveillance data have consistently indicated that the highest rates of CTS occur in occupations and job tasks with high work demands for intensive manual exertion – for example in meat packers, poultry processors and automobile assembly workers.

There is a high reported incidence of CTS in computer operators, with incidence reports varying from 8 to 38%, compared with 5.6% for industrial manufacturing workers. Mathias et al (1998) examined 45 cases of CTS among computer operators and compared them with controls. They found the most significant factors in order of significance were:

- percentage of workday with computer
- working posture – increased trunk incline, wrist extension or ulna deviation
- anthropometry – small arms/wrists/hands.

The researchers found that, as the wrist deviates from neutral, the tolerance to exposure decreases.

Rempel (1996) reports that a carpal tunnel pressure of under 30 mmHg is required for healthy homeostasis of the median nerve. Normal resting pressure is 5–10 mmHg. Rempel et al (1997) reported that patients with CTS had an average lowest pressure of 19 mmHg – more than twice the pressure of control subjects. At 30 mmHg there is reduced venule blood flow, increased permeability and slow axonal transport; at 50 mmHg, reduced blood flow and epineural oedema. If the pressure is prolonged, the endoneural and synovial oedema may trigger a fibrosis. The pressures are primarily determined by wrist and hand function, with typing and mouse usage typically showing 40–50 and 60–80 mmHg, respectively. Non-neutral wrist postures elevate carpal tunnel pressures significantly, with the increase occurring on a parabolic scale towards extremes of wrist flexion/extension and with dramatic increases above 40 degrees of flexion/extension and 20 degrees of radial/ulna deviation (Rempel et al 1998). Rempel et al (1997) found that fingertip loading elevates carpal tunnel pressure and relatively small loads have a large effect, with the effect being greater than and independent of wrist angle. Prolonged elevated carpal tunnel pressures have been proposed to impair fluid exchange, cause vascular leakage oedema and, eventually, epineural fibrosis. Animal studies have found that 4 h of elevated pressure can cause 24 h of oedema and raised endoneural pressure. The increase in carpal tunnel pressure is thought to be due to migration of muscles and tendons, and changes in the volume of the tunnel.

In the early stages the symptoms can be episodic and related to the exposures. In the more advanced stages there can be scarring and adhesion of the nerve and the dysfunction of the nerve is continuous. In the initial stages the condition responds to manual therapy and modification of exposure, in latter stages surgery is usually successful.

Recent research has demonstrated the postures that result in the least carpal tunnel pressures (Rempel et al 1998, Weiss et al 1995). These involve essentially neutral positions of flexion/extension and radial/ulna deviation, 45 degrees pronation and 45 degrees metacarpophalangeal flexion. This is very similar to the neutral position previously described under wrist ergonomics and has implications for tool and brace design.

The ulna nerve can become irritated as it passes through the canal of Guyon, where the nerve is superficial to the transverse carpal ligament. It is often affected by direct pressure, as in cyclists, or a combination of pressure and vibration using hand tools, as in hypothenar hammer syndrome.

CTS is the most researched of the neuropathies and it is interesting to note that the risk factors are largely the same as for the overuse injuries of the muscle and tendon structures in the hand and wrist. Interventions to reduce the incidence of these overuse injuries are likely to be equally effective in reducing the incidence of CTS. Furthermore, these risk factors are similar for a broad range of soft tissue injuries and it is reasonable to suggest that they may be similar for other regional nerve complaints. While nerves have a quite different physiology compared with muscle and tendon complexes it would suggest that the same physiological principles regarding healthy homeostasis apply. The LOAD injury model developed in Section 1 may be similarly applicable to injuries and chronic pain syndromes involving the peripheral nerves.

HAND ARM VIBRATION SYNDROME

Hand arm vibration syndrome (HAV) is recognized as causing a characteristic symptom picture, including episodic numbness, tingling and blanching of the fingers, reduction in grip strength and finger dexterity and exaggerated pain response to cold exposure. Vibration appears to have independent effects on neurological, vascular and musculoskeletal tissues. In a substantial review, based on 20 studies (NIOSH 1997b), the authors conclude there is strong evidence of a positive association between high level exposure to HAV and vascular symptoms. There is substantial evidence that, as intensity and duration of exposure increase the risk and severity of symptoms also increase. NIOSH quote a number of studies that show that as the weight of the vibrating tool, and the intensity and frequency of vibration, reduce, the prevalence and severity of symptoms decrease.

There is evidence that prolonged exposure to vibration can cause progressive demyelination and fibrosis of the nerves around the wrist. Stromberg et al (1997) compared biopsies from the dorsal interosseous nerves of ten men exposed to vibration for between 17 and 30 years and compared them to 12 aged-matched controls. They concluded:

Demyelination may be the primary lesion in neuropathy induced by vibration followed by fibrosis associated with incomplete regeneration or with organization of oedema. Such changes may constitute a structural component in carpal tunnel syndrome among people exposed to vibration. This may help to explain the poor results achieved by carpal tunnel release in these patients.

18

Multiple tissue disorders

Some authors and researchers have chosen to include a separate category of injury for multiple tissue disorders. This is often described as occupational overuse syndrome (OOS), repetitive strain injury (RSI) or cumulative trauma disorder (CTD). These terms are often used when there is a collection of symptoms with no easily identifiable anatomical injury and where static or highly repetitive postures with multiple anatomical exposures are involved. Spread of symptoms is a natural consequence of chronicity, as neighbouring muscles and joints become affected, particularly when the cause of the early symptoms has often not been addressed. These terms often lead to confusion.

It is perhaps more helpful to think of the RSI, OOS and CTD acronyms as describing the gradual or cumulative process of injury, rather than a syndrome created by chronicity. The introduction of a new syndrome – divorced from anatomical location – allows these labels to become politicized and their very existence questioned. It also tends to create problems of definition. When does extensor muscle strain become OOS? And, in the case of mouse-user's syndrome – when neck, shoulder and forearm pain develop in close parallel – when does it become RSI? This confusion encourages scepticism of the whole concept and spawns increasingly new interpretations of newly defined syndromes. It is more important to understand the location of the injury, its characteristics and link these to the cause than to attach a label that has no clarity or insight.

There is general agreement that these multiple tissue injuries have increased dramatically in most countries since the late 1980s (Hagberg et al 1995).

There are many reasons for this trend, which have been discussed in Section 1. The types of exposure that cause these multiple tissue syndromes – prolonged static or highly repetitive tasks and their physiological and psychosocial consequences – have also increased in recent years.

Thus, if OOS, RSI, CTD or LOAD define the type of injury, the term should always be qualified to provide an anatomical description of the location of the injury be it single or multiple, unilateral or bilateral.

Management strategies for chronic injuries

Low back pain has traditionally been the dominating concern of musculoskeletal injury. In the last decade or so, there has been a dramatic escalation of neck, shoulder and arm problems, which now have similar incidence and morbidity to low back pain (LBP). It is becoming increasingly important to develop effective prevention and treatment strategies for these injuries.

In a significant and award-winning paper, Westgaard & Winkel (1997) reviewed the literature for intervention strategies for improved musculoskeletal health. In a thorough search, using strict inclusion criteria, they found 89 relevant research papers. Among their conclusions were:

- A reduction in mechanical exposure level may be beneficial for musculoskeletal health where mechanical exposure level is high. The situation is less clear where the mechanical exposure is low.
- There is little evidence to suggest that improved health can be achieved through redesign of the production system. Nevertheless, this intervention approach has validity and should be pursued. Organizational culture interventions tend to be more successful when there is management commitment and ownership of the process.
- All the accepted studies report no improvement associated with health education or training.
- Exercise interventions, possibly above a certain intensity level, can improve musculoskeletal health.

- Two studies using electromyographic biofeed-back reported positive outcomes in terms of shoulder and neck complaints.
- The studies involving multiple modifier interventions including early medical contact, physiotherapy, exercise, education, behaviour therapy/relaxation techniques, and modification of work duties all showed positive results.

They concluded by pointing out:

... it appears that the modifier interventions that actively involve the worker ... often achieve positive results. In contrast more passive measures do not appear equally successful. The following intervention strategies have the best chance of success:

- Organisational culture interventions with high commitment of stakeholders, using multiple interventions to reduce identified risk factors.
- Modifier interventions, especially those that focus on workers at risk, using measures that actively involve the worker.

Westgaard & Winkel (1997)

Ekberg & Wildhagen (1996) studied 93 patients who had been off work for at least 4 weeks with neck, shoulder or arm pain and followed them up 1 year after rehabilitation to identify what factors were associated with recovery and chronicity. The group who remained on sick leave for longest after rehabilitation contained more immigrants and slightly more women than the short duration group. The long-sick-leave group perceived their work as uncomfortable with monotonous sitting positions, high precision demands, higher job constraints, and less opportunity for stimulation and development.

Multiple regression analysis indicated that long term sickness absence was largely related to work conditions rather than individual characteristics. The results underscore the importance not only of treating the individual with musculoskeletal disorders but in particular of improving his or her work conditions.

Ekberg & Wildhagen (1996)

Feuerstein et al (1993) assessed 34 chronic work-related musculoskeletal disorders of the upper extremity with a minimum of 3 months' work disability. They were divided into two groups: one group of 19 receiving a comprehensive work rehabilitation programme including physical conditioning, work conditioning, home exercise programme, pain and stress management, ergonomic consultation and vocational counselling/placement. The other group of 15 (those considered ineligible for the programme) received normal care from their physician and other common modalities, such as physical therapy, chiropractic input and a rehabilitation nurse. Both groups were similar on pretreatment measures. Return to work status was assessed at 17–18 months, with 40% of the control group and 74% of the treatment group returning to work. Ninety one per cent of the treatment group were in full-time work, compared with 50% of the control group. This study demonstrated that a comprehensive rehabilitation programme showed superior outcomes to usual care. The study had a limited cohort and the groups were not randomly assigned. The authors noted that the return to work results were not as impressive as similar approaches to work-related LBP (80–88% return to work rates) and recommended greater emphasis on ergonomic modifications at the workplace to reduce the risks of repetition, force, awkward posture, work/rest cycles and workstyle.

While comprehensive rehabilitation strategies show validity for chronic problems, there is evidence that they may be unhelpful in acute injuries. Ekberg et al (1994) studied a cohort of 107 neck- and shoulder-injured patients with no more than 4 weeks' sick leave. One group had active, multidisciplinary rehabilitation for 8 weeks, while the other had traditional treatment – physiotherapy, medication, etc. The rehabilitation programme involved substantial time away from work and this 'sick role' may be the explanation for the significantly increased days of sick leave for the first year found in the rehabilitation group. At 90 days after completion of rehabilitation, 21% of the rehabilitation group and 63% in the traditional group were back at work, at 12 and 24 months the differences had disappeared. This study suggests that over-managing acute injuries that are more likely to resolve with traditional methods may be counterproductive.

The rehabilitation strategies for chronic neck, shoulder and arm injuries appear to be very similar to those involving LBP. The important components include:

- A graduated, individualized exercise programme designed to restore mobility and improve the duration and strength of muscle contraction.
- Reversal of deconditioning and a work hardening programme.
- An educational component to give ergonomic advice, education and control over symptoms.
- A psychosocial component to improve confidence and remove any negative beliefs or psychosocial factors that may be barriers to recovery.
- Employer support with modification of work tasks.

A successful outcome is less likely when there is prolonged time off work, advanced physical and psychosocial deconditioning, no job to return to, a physically demanding job, a poor psychosocial environment or compensation issues.

For further details, see the discussion on rehabilitation programmes in Section 2.

References

Aaras A, Ro O (1998) Supporting the arms at the table top during VDU work. In: Kumar S (ed) Advances in occupational ergonomics and safety. IOS Press, Amsterdam, pp 549–552.

Aaras A, Ro O (2000) Position of the forearm and VDU work. Proceedings of the IEA 2000/HFES 2000 Congress, **1**: 649.

Aaras A, Fostervold KI, Ro O, Thoresen M, Larsen S (1997) Postural load during VDU work: a comparison between various work postures. *Ergonomics*, **40**(11): 1255–1268.

Aaras A, Horgen G, Bjorset H, Ro O, Thoresen M (1998) Musculoskeletal, visual and psychosocial stress in VDU operators before and after multidisciplinary ergonomic interventions. *Applied Ergonomics*, **29**(5): 335–354.

Adams M, Dolan P (1995) Recent advances in lumbar spinal mechanics and their clinical significance. *Clinical Biomechanics*, **10**: 13–19.

Adams M, Hutton W (1985) Gradual disc prolapse. *Spine* **10**(6): 524–531.

Adams MA, McNally DS, Chinn H, Dolan P (1994) Posture and the compressive strength of the lumbar spine. *Clinical Biomechanics*, **9**: 5–14.

Adams M, McMillan D, Green T, Dolan P (1996) Sustained loading generates concentrations in lumbar intervertebral discs. *Spine*, **21**(4): 434–438.

Adams MA, Kerin AJ, Bhatia LS, Chakrabarty G, Dolan P (1999) Experimental determination of stress distributions in articular cartilage before and after sustained loading. *Clinical Biomechanics*, **14**: 88–96.

AHCPR (1994) Management guidelines for acute low back pain. Agency for Health Care Policy and Research, US Department of Health and Human Services.

Aker PD, Gross AR, Goldsmith CH, Peloso P (1996) Conservative management of mechanical neck pain: systematic overview and meta-analysis. *British Medical Journal*, **313**: 1291–1296.

Albin T (1997) Effect of wrist rest use and keyboard tilt on wrist angle while keying. IEA 97 Conference proceedings, **4**: 16–18.

Andersson GBJ (1985) Loads on the spine during sitting. In: Corlett NJ et al (eds) The proceedings of the first international occupational ergonomics symposium: ergonomics of working posture: Taylor and Francis, London, pp 309–318.

Andersson GBJ, Ortegren R (1974) Lumbar disc pressure and myoelectric back muscle activity during sitting. *Scandinavian Journal of Rehabilitation Medicine*, **3**: 115–121.

Andersson HI, Ejlertsson G, Leden I (1998) Widespread musculoskeletal pain associated with smoking. *Scandinavian Journal of Rehabilitation Medicine*, **30**: 185–191.

Armstrong TJ, Fine LJ, Goldstein SA, Yair R, Lifshitz YR, Silverstein BA (1987) Ergonomic considerations in hand and wrist tendinitis. *The Journal of Hand Surgery*, **12A**(5): part 2, 830–837.

Armstrong TJ, Buckle P, Fine LJ et al (1993) A conceptual model for work-related neck and upper-limb musculoskeletal disorders. *Scandinavian Journal of Work Environment and Health*, **19**(2): 73–84.

Axler CT, McGill SM (1997) Low back loads over a variety of abdominal exercises: searching for the safest abdominal challenge. *Medicine and Science in Sports and Exercise*, **29**(6): 804–810.

Balague F, Dutoit G, Waldburger B (1988) Low back pain in school children. A preliminary study. *Scandinavian Journal of Rehabilitation and Medicine*, **20**: 175–179.

Bartholomew JB, Lewis BP, Linder DE, Cooke DB (1996) Post-exercise analgesia: replication and extension. *Journal of Sports Sciences*, **14**: 329–334.

Bauer JA, Murray RD (1999) Electromyography patterns of individuals suffering from lateral tennis elbow. *Journal of Electromyography and Kinesiology*, **9**: 245–252.

Bendix T (1984) Seated trunk posture at various seat inclinations, seat heights, and table heights. *Human Factors*, **26**(6): 695–703.

Bendix T, Biering-Sorensen F (1983) Posture of the trunk when sitting on forward inclined seats. *Scandinavian Journal of Rehabilitation Medicine* **15**: 197–203.

Bendix T, Bloch I (1986) How should a seated workplace with a tiltable chair be adjusted? *Applied Ergonomics*, **17**(2): 127–135.

Bendix T, Hagberg M (1984) Trunk posture and load on the trapezius muscle while sitting on sloping desks. *Ergonomics*, **27**(8): 873–882.

Bendix A, Jensen CV, Bendix T (1988) Posture, acceptability and energy consumption on a tiltable and knee-support chair. *Clinical Biomechanics*, **3**: 66–73.

Bendix AF, Bendix T, Labriola M, Boekgaard P (1998a) Functional restoration for chronic low back pain. *Spine*, **23**(6): 717–725.

Bendix AF, Bendix T, Haestrup T (1998b) Can it be predicted which patients with chronic low back pain should be offered tertiary rehabilitation in a functional restoration programme? *Spine*, **23**(16): 1775–1784.

Bengtsson A, Henrikson KG (1989) The muscle in fibromyalgia – a review of Swedish studies. *Journal of Rheumatology*, **19**(16): 144–149.

Berqvist U, Wolfgastt E, Nilsson B, Voss M (1995) Musculoskeletal disorders among visual display workers: individual, ergonomic and work organizational factors. *Ergonomics*, **38**(4): 763–776.

Bigos SJ, Battie MC, Spengler DM et al (1991) A prospective study of work perceptions and psychosocial factors affecting the report of back injury. *Spine*, **16**(1): 1–6.

Bogduk N (1994) Cervical causes of headache and dizziness. In: Boyling J, Palastanga N (eds) Grieve's modern manual therapy, 2nd edn. Churchill Livingston, Edinburgh, **22**: 317–331.

Bogduk N (1997) Clinical anatomy of the lumbar spine and sacrum, 3rd edn. Churchill Livingstone, New York.

Bongers PM, de Winter CR, Kompier MA, Hildebrandt CH (1993) Psychosocial factors at work and musculoskeletal disease. *Scandinavian Journal of Work Environment and Health*, **19**(5): 297–312.

Bonney R (1995) Human responses to vibration: principles and methods. In: Wilson J, Corlett E (eds) Evaluation of human work. Taylor and Francis, London, pp 541–556.

Bontoux D (1998) Dysphagia, headache, and dizziness as symptoms of cervical spine disorder. *Revue of Rhumatisme* (English edition), **65**(5): 346–351.

Broom ND (1985) The collagenous architecture of articular cartilage – a synthesis of ultrastructure and mechanical function. *The Journal of Rheumatology*, **13**(1): 142–152.

Bureau of Labor Statistics (1999) Number of occupational injuries and illnesses involving time away from work for selected occupations 1993–1997, 1–10. United States Department of Labor, Washington.

Burgess-Limerick R, Shemmell J, Scadden R, Plooy A (1999) Wrist posture during computer pointing device. *Clinical Biomechanics*, **14**: 280–286.

Burton A, Clarke R, McClune T, Tillotson K (1996) The natural history of low back pain in adolescents. *Spine*, **21**(20): 2323–2328.

Buskilla D, Neumann L, Vaisberg G, Alkalay D, Wolfe F (1997) Increased rates of fibromyalgia following cervical spine injury. *Arthritis and Rheumatism*, **40**(3): 446–452.

Caffier G, Heinecke D, Hinterthan R (1993) Surface EMG and load level during long-lasting static contractions of low intensity. *International Journal of Industrial Ergonomics*, **12**: 77–83.

Carayon P (1995) Work pressure as a determinant of job stress and cumulative trauma disorders in automated offices. Premus 95 book of abstracts, 172–174.

Chaitow L (1996) Modern neuromuscular techniques. Churchill Livingstone, Edinburgh.

Charman RA (1994) Pain and nociception: mechanisms and modulation in sensory context. In: Boyling J, Palastanga N (eds) Grieve's modern manual therapy, 2nd edn. Churchill Livingstone, Edinburgh, pp 253–270.

Choi PYL, Mutrie N (1996) The psychological benefits of increasing exercise for women: improving employee quality of life. In: Kerr J, Griffiths A, Cox T (eds) Workplace health: employee fitness and exercise. Taylor and Francis, London, pp 83–100.

Cholewicki J, McGill SM (1996) Mechanical stability of the in vivo lumbar spine: implications for injury and chronic low back pain. *Clinical Biomechanics*, **11**(1): 1–15.

Clarys JP, Barbaix E, Van Rompaey JP, Caboor D, Van Roy P (1996) The muscular arch of the axilla revisited: its possible role in the thoracic outlet and shoulder instability syndromes. *Manual Therapy*, **1**(3): 133–139.

Clifford J (1993) Successful management of chronic pain syndromes. *Canadian Family Physician*, **39**: 549–559.

Cohen ML, Arroyo JF, Champion GD, Browne CD (1992) In search of the pathogenesis of refractory cervicobrachial pain syndrome. *The Medical Journal of Australia*, **156**: 432–436.

Conroy DE, Hayes KW (1998) The effect of joint mobilisation as a component of comprehensive treatment for primary shoulder impingement. *Journal of Orthopaedic and Sports Physical Therapy*, **28**(1): 3–14.

Cook CJ, Kothiyal K (1998) Influence of mouse position on muscular activity in neck, shoulder and arm in computer users. *Applied Ergonomics*, **29**(6): 439–443.

Croft P, Macfarlane G, Papageorgio A, Thomas E, Silman A (1998) Outcome of low back pain in general practice: a prospective study. *British Medical Journal*, **316**: 1356–1359.

CSAG (1994) Report on back pain. Clinical standards advisory group. HMSO, Norwich.

Dai L (1998) Disc degenerative change and cervical instability. *Spine*, **23**(16): 1734–1738.

Dennett X, Fry HJF (1988) Overuse syndrome: a muscle biopsy study. *The Lancet*, April 23: 905–908.

De Wall M, van Reil MPJM, Snijders CJ, van Wingerden JP (1991) The effect of sitting posture of a desk with a 10 degree inclination for reading and writing. *Ergonomics* **4**(5): 575–584.

DiGiovanna EI, Schiowitz S 1991 An osteopathic approach to diagnosis and treatment. Lippincott, Philadelphia.

Djupsjobacka M 1997 On motor learning, motor patterns and sensory feedback. Proceedings of the 13th triennial Congress of the International Ergonomics Association. IEA 97, **4**: 263–264.

Donceel P, Du Bois M, Lahaye D (1999) Return to work after surgery for lumbar disc herniation. *Spine*, **24**(9): 872–876.

Drury CG, Francher M (1985) Evaluation of a forward sloping chair. *Applied Ergonomics*, **16**(1): 41–47.

Edwards RHT (1988) Hypotheses of peripheral and central control mechanisms underlying occupational muscle pain and injury. *European Journal of Applied Physiology*, **57**: 275–281.

Ekberg K, Wildhagen I (1996) Long-term sickness absence due to musculoskeletal health: the necessary intervention of work conditions. *Scandinavian Journal of Rehabilitation Medicine*, **28**: 39–47.

Ekberg K, Bjorkvist B, Malm P, Bjerre-Kiely B, Axelsen O (1994) Controlled two year follow up of rehabilitation for disorders in the neck and shoulders. *Occupational and Environmental Medicine*, **51**: 833–838.

Exelby L (1996) Peripheral mobilisations with movement. *Manual Therapy*, **1**(3): 118–126.

Faas A (1996) Exercises: which ones are worth trying, for which patients, and when? *Spine*, **21**(24): 2874–2879.

Fallentin N, Jurgensen K, Simonsen EB (1993) Motor unit recruitment during prolonged isometric contractions. *European Journal of Applied Physiology*, **67**: 335–341.

Feng Y, Grooten W, Wretenberg P, Arborelius UP (1997) Effects of arm supports on shoulder and arm muscle activity during sedentary work. *Ergonomics*, **40**(8): 834–848.

Fernstrom E, Ericson MO (1997) Computer mouse or trackpoint – effects on muscular load or operator experience. *Applied Ergonomics*, **28**(5/6): 347–354.

Feuerstein M (1996) Workstyle: definition, empirical support and implications for prevention, evaluation and rehabilitation of occupational upper-extremity disorders. In: Moon SD, Sauter SL (eds) Beyond biomechanics. Psychosocial aspects of musculoskeletal disorders in office work. Taylor and Francis, London, pp 177–206.

Feuerstein M, Sult S, Houle M (1985) Environmental stressors and chronic LBP: life events, family and work environment. *Pain*, **22**: 295–307.

Feuerstein M, Callan-Harris S, Hickey P, Dyer D, Armbruster W, Carosella AM (1993) Multidisciplinary rehabilitation of chronic work-related upper extremity disorders. *Journal of Occupational Medicine*, **35**(4): 396–403.

Fisk J, Baigent M, Hill P (1984) Scheuermann's disease: a clinical and radiological survey of 17 and 18 year olds. *American Journal of Physical Medicine*, **63**: 18–30.

Franklin GM, Fulton-Kehoe d, Bradley C, Smith-Weller T (2000) Outcome of surgery for thoracic outlet syndrome in Washington State Worker's Compensation. *Neurology* **54**: 1252–1257.

Freudenthal A, van Reil MPJM, Molenbroek JFM, Snijders CJ (1991) The effect of sitting posture on a desk with a 10 degree inclination using an adjustable chair and table. *Applied Ergonomics*, **22**(5): 329–336.

Friedrich M, Gittler G, Halberstadt Y, Cermak T, Heiller I (1998) Combined exercise and motivation programme: effect of the compliance and level of disability of patients with chronic low back pain: a randomized controlled trial. *Archives of Physical Medicine and Rehabilitation*, **79**: 475–487.

Frost P (1995) Subacromial pain syndrome (SAPS). A comparison of findings by NMRI of the rotator cuff in slaughterhouse workers with and without SAPS. Premus 95 book of abstracts, 226–228.

Frost H, Lamb SE, Klaber Moffett JA, Fairbank JCT, Moser JS (1998) A fitness programme for patients with chronic low back pain. *Pain*, **75**: 273–279.

Ginn KA, Herbert RD, Khouw W, Lee R (1997) A randomized, controlled clinical trial of a treatment for shoulder pain. *Physical Therapy*, **77**(8): 802–809.

Grandjean E (1988) Fitting the task to the man. A textbook of occupational ergonomics, 4th edn. Taylor and Francis, London, pp 57–73.

Grandjean E, Hunting W (1977) Ergonomics of posture – a review of various problems of standing and sitting posture. *Applied Ergonomics*, **8**(3): 135–140.

Grandjean E, Hunting W, Nishiyama K (1984) Preferred VDT workstation settings, body posture and physical impairments. *Applied Ergonomics*, **15**(2): 99–104.

Grant R, Jull G, Spencer T (1997) Active stabilisation training for screen based keyboard operators – a single case studyz. *Australian Physiotherapy*, **43**(4): 235–242.

Graver V, Ljunggren AE, Loeb M, Haaland AK, Lie H, Magnaes B (1998) Background variables in relation to the outcome of lumbar disc surgery. *Scandinavian Journal of Rehabilitation Medicine*, **30**: 221–225.

Green S, Buchbinder R, Glaxier R, Forbes A (1999) Interventions for shoulder pain. The Cochrane Library. Update Software, issue 4.

Grieve G (1994) Bony and soft-tissue anomalies of the vertebral column. In: Boyling J, Palastanga N (eds) Grieve's modern manual therapy, 2nd edn. Churchill Livingstone, Edinburgh, pp 227–250.

Griffiths A (1996) Employee exercise programmes: organisational and individual perspectives. In: Kerr J, Griffiths A, Cox T (eds) Workplace health: employee fitness and exercise. Taylor and Francis, London, pp 1–28.

Gross AR, Aker PD, Goldsmith CH, Peloso P (1999) Physical medicine modalities for mechanical neck disorders (Cochrane review). In the Cochrane Library, issue 4.

Guest GH, Drummond PD (1992) Effect of compensation on emotional state and disability in chronic back pain. *Pain*, **48**: 125–130.

Hack GD, Koritzer RT, Robinson WL, Hallgren RC, Greenman PE (1995) Anatomic relationship between the rectus capitis posterior minor muscle and the dura mater. *Spine*, **20**(23): 2484–2486.

Hagberg M (1995) Work-related musculoskeletal disorders – illnesses or diseases. Second international scientific conference on prevention of work related musculoskeletal disorders. Premus 95 book of abstracts, 6–11.

Hagberg M, Sundelin G (1986) Discomfort and load on the upper trapezius muscle when operating a word processor. *Ergonomics*, **29**(12): 1637–1645.

Hagberg M, Silverstein B, Wells R et al (1995) In: Kuorinka I, Forcier L (eds) Work related musculoskeletal disorders (WMSDs): A reference book for prevention. Taylor and Francis, London.

Hagg GM (1997) Gap training – a new approach and device for prevention of shoulder/neck myalgia by EMG feedback. Proceedings of the 13th triennial congress of the International Ergonomics Association. IEA 97, **4**: 283–285.

Hagg GM, Astrom A (1997) Load pattern and pressure pain threshold in the upper trapezius muscle and psychosocial factors in medical secretaries with and without shoulder/neck disorders. *International Archives of Occupation and Environmental Health*, **69**: 423–432.

Haldorsen EMH, Indahl A, Ursin H (1998) Patients with low back pain not returning to work. *Spine*, **23**(11): 1202–1208.

Hamilton N (1996) Source–document position as it affects head position and neck muscle tension. *Ergonomics*, **39** 593–610.

Harreby M, Neergaard K, Hesselsoe G, Kjer J (1995) Are radiological changes in the thoracic and lumbar spine of adolescents risk factors for low back pain in adults? *Spine* **20**(21): 2298–2302.

Harvey R, Peper E (1997) Surface electromyography and mouse use position. *Ergonomics*, **40**(8): 781–789.

Hazard RG, Fenwick JW, Kalisch SM et al (1989) Functional restoration with behavioural support. *Spine*, **14**(2): 157–161.

Health and Safety Executive (1992) Health and Safety (display screen equipment) Regulations (1992). HMSO, Norwich.

Hedge A, Morimoto S, McRobie D (1999) Effects of keyboard tray geometry on upper body posture and comfort. *Ergonomics*, **42**(10): 1333–1349.

Hedman TP, Fernie GR (1997) Mechanical response of the lumbar spine to seated loads. *Spine*, **22**(7): 734–743.

Helme RD, Le Vasseur SA, Gibson SJ (1992) RSI revisited: evidence for psychological and physiological differences from an age, sex and occupation matched control group. *Australia and New Zealand Journal of Medicine*, **22**: 23–29.

Hermans V, Hautekiet M, Spaepen AJ (1998a) Relationship between posture and neck shoulder muscular effort. In: Kumar S (ed) Advances in occupational ergonomics and safety. IOS Press, Amsterdam, pp 202–205.

Hermans V, Spaepen AJ, Wouters M (1998b) Recovery of muscular effort after a sustained submaximal task. In: Kumar S (ed) Advances in occupational ergonomics and safety. IOS Press, Amsterdam, pp 230–233.

Hides JA, Richardson CA, Jull GA (1996) Multifidus recovery is not automatic after resolution of acute first-episode low back pain. *Spine*, 21(23): 2763–2769.

Hochanadel CD (1995) Computer workstation adjustment: a novel process and a large sample study. *Applied Ergonomics*, 26(5): 315–326.

Hocking B (1997) Some social and cultural anthropologic aspects of musculoskeletal disorders as exemplified by the Telecom Australia RSI epidemic. In: Moon SD, Sauter SL (eds) Beyond biomechanics: psychosocial aspects of musculoskeletal disorders in office work. Taylor and Francis, London, pp 145–158.

Hoffmann ER, Chang WY, Yim KY (1997) Computer mouse operation: is the left-handed mouse user disadvantaged? *Applied Ergonomics*, 28(4): 245–248.

Hofmann F, Schumacher M, Siegel A, Michaelis M, Stobel U (1995) Occupational epidemiology of low back disorders. Premus 1995 book of abstracts, 114–116.

Hole DE, Cook JM, Bolton JE (1995) Reliability and concurrent validity of two instruments for measuring cervical range of motion: effects of age and gender. *Manual Therapy*, 36(1): 36–42.

Hurwitz EL, Aker PD, Adams AH, Meeker WC, Shekelle PG (1996) Manipulation and mobilization of the cervical spine. A systematic review of the literature. *Spine*, 21(15): 1746–1760.

Jarvholm U, Palmerud G, Styf J, Herberts P, Kaderfors R (1988) Intramuscular pressure in the supraspinatus muscle. *Journal of Orthopaedic Research*, 6(2): 230–238.

Jarvholm U, Palmerud G, Karlsson D, Herberts P, Kaderfors R (1991) Intramuscular pressure and electromyography in four shoulder muscles. *Journal of Orthopaedic Research*, 9(4): 609–619.

Jaschinski W, Heuer H, Kylian H (1999) A procedure to determine the individually comfortable position of visual displays relative to the eyes. *Ergonomics*, 42(4): 535–549.

Jensen C, Borg V, Finsen L, Hansen K, Juul-Kristensen B, Christensen H (1998) Job demands, muscle activity and musculoskeletal symptoms in relation to work with the computer mouse. *Scandinavian Journal of Work, Environment and Health*, 24(5): 418–424.

Johannson H (1996) Pathophysiological mechanisms behind work related myalgia. Risk Assessment for Musculoskeletal Disorders conference proceedings ICOH 96, Copenhagen, 43–46.

Johannson H, Solka P (1991) Pathophysiological mechanisms involved in genesis and spread of muscular tension in occupational muscle and chronic musculoskeletal pain syndromes. A hypothesis. *Medical Hypotheses*, 35: 196–203.

Johnson PW, Rempel D (1995) A new technique for measuring fatigue in the finger flexor muscles resulting from low force work. Premus 95 book of abstracts, 298–300.

Johnson P, Lehman S, Rempel D (1996) Does muscle fatigue result from computer keyboard use? Risk Assessment for Musculoskeletal Disorders conference proceedings ICOH 96. 47–48.

Johnson P, Lehman S, Rempel D (1997) Does muscle fatigue result from computer keyboard use? Proceedings of the 13th triennial congress of the International Ergonomics Association. IEA 97, 4: 58–60.

Jonsson B, Stromqvist B (1996) Clinical appearance of contained and non-contained lumbar disc herniation. *Journal of Spinal Disorders*, 9(1): 32–38.

Jordan A, Bendix T, Nielsen H, Hansen FR, Hoste D, Wimkel A (1998) Intensive training, physiotherapy or manipulation for patients with chronic neck pain. *Spine*, 23(3): 311–319.

Jull G (1997) Management of cervical headache. *Manual Therapy*, 2(4): 182–190.

Kaderfors R, Forsman M, Quixia Z (1998) Motor unit recruitment in VDU tasks: a methodological analysis. In: Kumar S (ed) Advances in occupational ergonomics and safety, 2nd edn. IOS Press, Amsterdam, pp 206–209.

Kaderfors R, Forsman M, Zoega B, Herberts P (1999) Recruitment of low threshold motor-units in the trapezius muscle in static arm positions. *Ergonomics*, 42(2): 359–375.

Kadi F, Waling K, Ahlgren C, Sundelin G et al (1998) Pathological mechanisms implicated in localized female trapezius myalgia. *Pain*, 78: 191–196.

Kankaanpaa M, Taimela S, Airaksinen O, Hanninen O (1999) The efficacy of active rehabilitation in chronic low back pain. *Spine*, 24(10): 1034–1042.

Karasek RA, Theorell T (1990) Healthy work. Basic Books, New York.

Karlqvist L, Hagberg M, Selin K (1994) Variation in upper limb posture and movement during word processing with and without mouse usage. *Ergonomics*, 37(7): 1261–1267.

Karlqvist L, Bernmark E, Ekenvall L, Hagberg M, Isaksson A, Rosto T (1998) Computer mouse as a determinant of posture, muscular load, and perceived exertion. *Scandinavian Journal of Work, Environment and Health*, 24(1): 62–73.

Karlqvist L, Bernmark E, Ekenvall L, Hagberg M, Isaksson A, Rosto T (1999) Computer mouse and trackball operation: similarities and differences in posture, muscular load and perceived exertion. *Industrial Ergonomics*, 23: 157–169.

Katavich L (1998) Differential effects of spinal manipulative therapy on acute and chronic muscle spasm: a proposal for mechanisms and efficacy. *Manual Therapy*, 3(3): 132–139.

Keable D (1997) The management of anxiety: a guide for therapists, 2nd edn. Churchill Livingstone, Edinburgh, 16: 162.

Keegan JJ (1953) Alteration of the lumbar curve related to posture and seating. *Journal of Bone and Joint Surgery*, 35A(3): 589–603.

Keel PJ, Wittig R, Deutschmann R, Diethelm U et al (1998) Effectiveness of in-patient rehabilitation for sub-chronic and chronic low back pain by an integrative study treatment programme (Swiss multicentre study). *Scandinavian Journal of Rehabilitation Medicine*, 30: 211–219.

Kelsey JL (1975) An epidemiological study of the relationships between occupations and acute herniated intervertebral lumbar disks. *International Journal of Epidemiology*, 4: 197–205.

Kendall NAS, Linton SJ, Main CJ (1997) Guide to assessing psychosocial yellow flags in acute low back pain: risk factors for long term disability and work loss. Accident Rehabilitation & Compensation Insurance Corporation of New Zealand and the National Health Committee, Wellington, NZ.

Kilbom A (1997) Repetitive work of the upper extremity: guidelines for practitioners. Proceedings of the 13th triennial Congress of the International Ergonomics Association. IEA 97, **4**: 66–68.

Ko H, Park BK (1997) Facet tropism in lumbar motion segments and its significance in disc herniation. *Archives of Physical Medicine and Rehabilitation*, **78**: 1211–1214.

Koes BW, Bouter LM, Beckerman H, van der Heijden GJMG, Knipschild PG (1991) Physiotherapy exercises and back pain, a blinded review. *British Medical Journal*, **302**: 1572–1576.

Koes BW, Bouter LM, van Mameren H et al (1992) The effectiveness of manual therapy, physiotherapy, and treatment by the general practitioner for nonspecific neck and back complaints. *Spine*, **17**(1): 28–35.

Koes BW, Scholten RJPM, Mens JMA, Bouter LM (1995) Efficacy of epidural steroid injections for low-back pain and sciatica: a systematic review of clinical trials. *Pain*, **63**: 279–288.

Koes BW, Assendelft WJJ, van der Heijden GJMG, Bouter LM (1996) Spinal manipulation for low back pain. *Spine*, **21**: 2860–2873.

Konz S (1998a) Work/rest: Part 1 – Guidelines for the practitioner. *International Journal of Industrial Ergonomics*, **22**: 67–71.

Konz S (1998b) Work/rest: Part 2 – The scientific basis (knowledge base) for the guide. *International Journal of Industrial Ergonomics*, **22**: 73–99.

Korr I (1955a) The concept of facilitation and its origin. In: Peterson B (ed) The collected papers of Irwin M Korr. American Academy of Osteopathy, Colorado Springs, pp 148–151.

Korr I (1955b) Clinical significance of the facilitated state. In: Peterson B (ed) The collected papers of Irwin M Korr. American Academy of Osteopathy, Colorado Springs, pp 152–157.

Korr I (1973) The facilitated segment: a factor in injury to the body framework. In: Peterson B (ed) The collected papers of Irwin M Korr. American Academy of Osteopathy, Colorado Springs, pp 188–190.

Korr I (1975) Proprioceptors and somatic dysfunction. In: Peterson B (ed). The collected papers of Irwin M Korr. American Academy of Osteopathy, Colorado Springs, pp 200–207.

Korr I (1979) The collected papers of Irwin M Korr. American Academy of Osteopathy, Colorado Springs.

Kraus JF, Brown KA, McArthur DL, Peek-Asa C, Samaniego L, Kraus C, Zhou L 1996 Reduction of acute low back injuries by use of back supports. *International Journal of Occupation and Environmental Health*, **2**: 264–273.

Krause N, Ragland DR, Fisher JM, Syme SL (1998) Psychosocial job factors, physical workload and incidence of work related spinal injury: a 5-year prospective study of urban transit operators. *Spine*, **23**(23): 2507–2516.

Kroemer KHE, Grandjean E (1997) Fitting the task to the human, 5th edn. Taylor and Francis, London.

Kuhlman KA, Hennessy WJ (1997) Sensitivity and specificity of carpal tunnel syndrome signs. *American Journal of Physical Medicine and Rehabilitation*, **76**: 451–457.

Kumar S (1990) Cumulative load as a risk factor for back pain. *Spine*, **15**(12): 1311–1316.

Kumar S (1994) A conceptual model of over exertion, safety and risk of injury in occupational settings. *Human Factors*, **36**(2): 197–209.

Lancet (1875) A telegraphic malady – personation at examinations. April 24: 585.

Lander C, Korbon GA, DeGood DE, Rowlingson JC (1987) The Balons chair and its semi-kneeling position: an ergonomic comparison with the conventional sitting position. *Spine* **12**(3): 269–272.

Larsonn R, Cai H, Zhang Q, Oberg PA, Larsson SE (1998) Visualisation of chronic neck-shoulder pain: impaired microcirculation in the upper trapezius muscle in chronic cervico-brachial pain. *Occupational Medicine*, **48**(3): 189–194.

Laursen B, Jensen B, Sjogaard G (1998) Shoulder muscle EMG during repetitive work tasks with varying speeds and precision demands. In: Kumar S (ed) Advances in occupational ergonomics and safety. IOS Press, Amsterdam, pp 210–213.

Le Forestier N, Mouton P, Maisonobe T, Fournier E, Moulonguet A, Willer JC, Bouche P (2000) True neurological thoracic outlet syndrome. *Review Neurology* (Paris), **156**(1): 34–40.

Lee JH, Hoshino Y, Nakamura K, Kariya Y, Saita K, Ito K (1999) Trunk muscle weakness as a risk factor for low back pain. *Spine* **24**(1): 54–57.

Leino PI (1993) Does leisure time physical activity prevent low back disorders? *Spine* **18**(7): 863–871.

Lim SY (1995) Psychosocial and work stress perspectives on musculoskeletal discomfort. Premus 95 book of abstracts, 175–177.

Loisel P, Abenhaim L, Durand P, Esdaile J et al (1997) A population-based randomized clinical trial on back pain management. *Spine*, **22**(24): 2911–2918.

Lonn JH, Glomsrod B, Soukup MG, Bo K, Larsen S (1999) Active back school: prophylactic management for low back pain. *Spine*, **24**(9): 865–871.

Luoto S, Heliovaara M, Hurri H, Alaranta H (1995) Static back endurance and the risk of low-back pain. *Clinical Biomechanics*, **10**(6): 323–324.

McGill SM (1997) The biomechanics of low back injury: implications on current practice in industry and the clinic. *Journal of Biomechanics* **30**(5): 465–475.

McGill SM (1998) Low back exercise: evidence for improving exercises regimes. *Physical Therapy*, **78**(7): 754–765.

McGill SM (1999) Should industrial workers wear abdominal belts? Prescription based on the literature. *International Journal of Industrial Ergonomics*, **23**: 633–636.

McLean J, Tucker J, Latham J (1990) Radiographic appearances in lumbar disc prolapse. *Journal of Bone and Joint Surgery*, **72**B: 917–920.

McKenzie RA (1981) The lumbar spine. Mechanical diagnosis and therapy. Spinal Publications, Wellington, NZ.

Magnusson ML, Pope MH, Hansson T (1998) Does hyperextension have an unloading effect on the intervertebral disc? *Scandinavian Journal of Rehabilitative Medicine*, **27**: 5–9.

Mandal AC (1981) The seated work position. Theory and practice. *Applied Ergonomics*, **12**(1): 19–26.

Mandal AC (1985) The seated man. Homo sedens. Dafnia Publications, Denmark.

Marshall E, Mackey M, Adams R, Hunter S (1997) the effect of a supervised exercise programme on persons with a work-related low back injury. IEA 97 conference proceedings, Tampere, **4**: 306–308.

Martin B, Rempel D, Sudarsan P, Dennerlein J, Jacobson M, Gerard M, Armstrong T 1998 Reliability and sensitivity of methods to quantify muscle load during keyboard work. In: Kumar S (ed) Advances in occupational ergonomics and safety. IOS Press, Amsterdam, pp 495–498.

Massett DF, Piette AG, Malchaire JB (1998) Relationship between functional characteristics of the trunk and low back pain. *Spine*, **23**(3): 359–365.

Mathias AC, Salvendy G, Kuczek T (1998) Predictive models of carpal tunnel syndrome causation among VDT operators. *Ergonomics*, **41**(2): 213–226.

Mayer TG, Gatchel RJ, Mayer H, Kishino ND, Keeley J, Mooney V (1987) A prospective two-year study of functional restoration in industrial low back injury. *Journal of the American Medical Association*, **258**(13): 1763–1767.

Mealy K, Brennan H, Fenelon GCC (1986) Early mobilisation of acute whiplash injuries. *British Medical Journal*, **292**: 656–657.

Mercer SR, Jull GA (1996) Morphology of the cervical intervertebral disc: implications for McKenzie's model of the disc derangement syndrome. *Manual Therapy*, **2**: 76–81.

Millanvoye M (1998) Aging of the organism before sixty years of age. In: Marquie JC, Cau Bareille DP, Volkoff S (eds) Working with age. Taylor and Francis, London, pp 131–161.

Mital A (1991) Hand tools, injuries, illnesses, design and usage. In: Mital A, Karwowski W (eds) Workplace, equipment and tool design. Elsevier, Oxford, pp 218–256.

Mital A, Kilbom A (1992) Design, selection and use of hand tools to alleviate trauma at the upper extremities: part 1 – guidelines for the practitioner, and part 2 – the scientific basis (knowledge base) for the guide. *Journal of Industrial Ergonomics*, **10**: 1–21.

Miyamoto K, Linuma M, Maeda M, Wada E, Shimizu K (1999) Effects of abdominal belts on intra-abdominal pressure, intramuscular pressure in the erector spinae muscles and myoelectric activity of the trunk muscles. *Clinical Biomechanics*, **14**: 79–87.

Morrison DS, Frogameni AD, Woodworth P (1997) Non-operative treatment of subacromial impingement syndrome. *The Journal of Bone and Joint Surgery*, **79A**(5): 732–737.

Muto T, Sakurai H (1993) Relationship between exercise and absenteeism due to illness and injury in manufacturing companies in Japan. *Journal of Occupational Medicine*, **35**(10): 995–999.

Nicholas JJ (1999) Exercise prescription for the arthritic patient. In: Shanker K (ed) Exercise prescription. Hanley and Belfus, Philadelphia, pp 277–296.

Niere K, Robinson P (1997) Determination of treatment outcome in headache patients. *Manual Therapy*, **2**(4): 199–205.

NIOSH (1995) Annual survey of occupational injuries and illnesses. US Dept of Labor. National Institute of Occupational Safety and Health, Cincinatti.

NIOSH (1997a) Backbelts. NIOSH publication. June 1997. US Dept of Labor. National Institute of Occupational Safety and Health, Cincinatti.

NIOSH (1997b) Musculoskeletal disorders and workplace factors, Bernard BP (ed) US Department of Health and Human Services, National Institute of Occupational Safety and Health, Cincinatti.

Norman R, Wells R, Neumann P, Frank J, Shannon H, Kerr M (1998) A comparison of peak vs cumulative physical work exposure risk factors for the reporting of low back pain in the automotive industry. *Clinical Biomechanics*, **13**: 561–573.

Nykanen M (1995) Pulsed ultrasound treatment of the painful shoulder. *Scandinavian Journal of Rehabilitation Medicine*, **27**: 105–108.

O'Sullivan PB, Twomey LT, Allison GT (1997) Evaluation of specific stabilising exercise in the treatment of chronic low back pain with radiological diagnosis of spondylolysis or spondylolisthesis. *Spine*, **22**(24): 2959–2967.

Pfingsten M, Hildebrandt J, Leibing E, Franz C, Saur P (1997) Effectiveness of a multimodal programme for chronic low back pain. *Pain*, **73**: 77–85.

Pheasant S (1991) Ergonomics, work and health. Macmillan, London.

Pheasant S (1997) Bodyspace, 2nd edn. Taylor and Francis, London.

Pienimaki T, Tarvainen TK, Sirra P, Vanharanta H (1996) Progressive strengthening and stretching exercises and ultrasound for chronic lateral epicondylitis. *Physiotherapy*, **82**(9): 522–530.

Pienimaki T, Karinen P, Kemila T, Koivukangas P, Vanharanta H (1998) Long term follow up of conservatively treated chronic tennis elbow patients, a prospective and retrospective analysis. *Scandinavian Journal of Rehabilitation Medicine*, **30**: 159–166.

Porter J, Gyl D (1995) Low back trouble and driving. Premus 95 book of abstracts, 117–119.

Porterfield J, DeRosa C (1998) Mechanical low back pain, 2nd edn. WB Saunders, Philadelphia.

Punnett L, Fine L, Monroe Keyserling W, Herrin G, Chaffin D (1991) Back disorders and non-neutral trunk postures of automobile assembly workers. *Scandinavian Journal of Work Environment and Health*, **17**: 337–346.

Ramazzini B (1713) De Morbis Artificum. *Trans*: Wright WC (1940) Diseases of workers. University of Chicago, Chicago.

Randlov A, Ostergaard M, Maniche C, Kryger P, Jordan A, Heegard S, Holm B (1998) Intensive dynamic training for females with chronic neck/shoulder pain. A randomized controlled trial. *Clinical Rehabilitation*, **12**: 200–210.

Ranney D (ed) (1997) Chronic musculoskeletal injuries in the workplace. WB Saunders, Philadelphia, pp 145–168.

Ranney D, Wells R, Moore A (1995) upper limb musculoskeletal disorders in highly repetitive industries precise anatomical findings. *Ergonomics*, **38**(7): 1408–1423.

Rempel D (1996) Work related musculoskeletal disorders among computer users. Risk assessment for musculoskeletal disorders. Conference proceedings ICOH, Denmark, 39–41.

Rempel D, Keir P, Smutz WP, Hargens A (1997) Effects of static fingertip loading on carpal tunnel pressure. *Journal of Orthopaedic Research*, **15**: 422–426.

Rempel D, Bach JM, Gordon L, So Y (1998) Effects of forearm supination on carpal tunnel pressure. *The Journal of Hand Surgery*, **23A**: 38–42.

Richardson CA, Jull GA (1995) Muscle control – pain control. What exercises would you prescribe? *Manual Therapy*, **1**(1): 2–10.

Richardson C, Jull G, Hodges P, Hides J (1999) Therapeutic exercise for spinal segmental stabilization in low back pain. *Churchill Livingstone*, Edinburgh.

Riihimaki H (1997) Is sedentary work hazardous to the back – epidemiologic evidence. Proceedings of the 13th triennial congress of the International Ergonomics Association. IEA **974**: 102.

Rosenstock L (1997) Report of written testimony from National Institute for Occupational Safety and Health submitted to the subcommittee on workforce protection. May 21 1997. National Institute of Occupational Safety and Health, Cincinatti.

Royal College of General Practitioners (1996) Clinical guidelines for the management of acute low back pain. Royal College of General Practitioners, London.

Salminen J, Erkintalo M, Laine M, Pentti J (1995) Low back pain in the young. A prospective three-year follow-up study of subjects with and without low back pain. *Spine*, **20**(19): 2101–2107.

Scheer SJ, Radack KL, O'Brien DR (1995) Randomized controlled trials in industrial low back pain relating to return to work. Part 1 Acute interventions. *Archives of Physical Medicine and Rehabilitation*, **76**: 966–973.

Schoenen J, Sandor S (1999) Headache. In: Wall PD, Melzak R (eds) Textbook of pain. Churchill Livingstone, Edinburgh, **33**: 761–798.

Serina ER, Tal R, Remple D (1999) Wrist and forearm postures and motions during typing. *Ergonomics*, **42**(7): 938–951.

Shankar K, Nayak NN (1999) Effect of exercise on organ systems. In: Shankar K (ed) Exercise prescription. Hanley and Belfus, Philadelphia, pp 17–31.

Shekelle PG, Adams AH, Chassin MR, Hurwitz EL, Brook RH (1992) Spinal manipulation for low-back pain. *Annals of Internal Medicine*, **117**(7): 590–598.

Shephard RJ (1996) Financial aspects of employee fitness programmes. In: Kerr J, Griffiths A, Cox T (eds) Workplace health: employee fitness and exercise. Taylor and Francis, London, pp 29–54.

Sihvonen T, Lindgren KA, Airaksinen O, Manninen H (1997) Movement disturbances of the lumbar spine and abnormal electromyographic disturbances in recurrent low back pain. *Spine*, **22**(3): 289–295.

Silverstein B (1995) Work-related musculoskeletal disorders: primary prevention strategies. Premus 95 book of abstracts, 21–23.

Sjogaard G, Savard S, Juel C (1988) Muscle blood flow during isometric activity and its relation to muscle fatigue. *European Journal of Applied Physiology*, **57**: 327–335.

Skargren EI, Oberg BE, Calsson PG, Gade M (1997) Cost and effectiveness analysis of chiropractic and physiotherapy treatment for low back and neck pain. *Spine*, **22**(18): 2167–2177.

Smith MJ (1997) Psychosocial aspects of working with video display terminals and employee physical and mental health. *Ergonomics*, **40**(10): 1002–1015.

Smith MJ, Carayon P (1996) Work organisation, stress, and cumulative trauma disorders. In: Moon SD, Sauter SL (eds) Beyond biomechanics: psychosocial aspects of musculoskeletal disorders in office work. Taylor and Francis, London, pp 23–43.

Smith MJ, Karsh B, Conway FT et al (1998) Effects of a split keyboard design and wrist rest on performance, posture and comfort. *Human Factors*, **40**(2): 324–326.

Snyder-Mackler L, Epler M (1989) Effect of standard and aircast tennis elbow bands on integrated electromyography of forearm extensor musculature proximal to the bands. *The American Journal of Sports Medicine*, **17**(2): 278–281.

Solveborn S, Olerud C (1996) Radial epicondylalgia (tennis elbow): measurement of range of motion at the wrist and elbow. *Journal of Orthopaedic and Sports Physical Therapy*, **23**(43): 251–257.

Souza TA (1994) Sports injuries of the shoulder. Churchill Livingstone, New York.

Sporrong H, Palmerud G, Herberts P (1995) Influences of static hand muscle activity on muscle activity in human shoulder muscles. Premus 95 book of abstracts, 202–204.

Sporrong H, Palmerud G, Kaderfors R, Herberts P (1998) The effect of light manual precision work on shoulder muscles – an EMG analysis. *Journal of Electromyography and Kinesiology*, **8**: 177–184.

Stoddard A (1969) Manual of Osteopathic Practice. Hutchinson, London, pp 240–244.

Stoddard A, Osborne J (1978) Scheuermann's disease or spinal osteochondrosis: its frequency and relationship with spondylosis. *Journal of Bone and Joint Surgery*, **61B**: 56–58.

Straker L, Jones KJ, Miller J (1997) A comparison of the postures assumed when using laptop computers and desktop computers. *Applied Ergonomics*, **28**(4): 263–268.

Stromberg T, Darlin LB, Brun A, Lundborg G (1997) Structural nerve changes at wrist level in workers exposed to vibration. *Occupational and Environmental Medicine*, **54**: 307–311.

Swanson NG, Galinski TL, Cole LL, Pan CS, Sauter L (1997) The impact of keyboard design on comfort and productivity in a text-entry task. *Applied Ergonomics*, **28**(1): 9–16.

Taylor T, Marcucci M, Dimuria G, Stringa G (1989) The role of transitional vertebra in intervertebral disc degeneration and prolapse. *Journal of Bone and Joint Surgery*, **71B**: 164.

Theorell T (1996) Possible mechanisms behind the relationship between the demand-control-support model and disorders of the locomotor system. In: Moon SD, Sauter SL (eds) Beyond biomechanics psychosocial aspects of musculoskeletal disorders in office work. Taylor and Francis, London, pp 65–75.

Thirlaway K, Benton D (1996) Exercise and mental health: the role of activity and fitness. In: Kerr J, Griffiths A, Cox T (eds) Workplace health: employee fitness and exercise. Taylor and Francis, London, pp 69–82.

Thoumie P, Drape J, Aynrard C, Bedoiseau M (1998) Effect of a lumbar support on spine posture and motion assessed by an electrogoniometer and continuous recording. *Clinical Biomechanics*, **13**(1): 18–26.

Tittiranonda P, Burastero S (1995) Work posture and musculoskeletal disomfort among VDT users. Premus 95 book of abstracts, 526–527.

Tittiranonda P, Burastero S, Rempel D (1997) Six month keyboard intervention study in computer users with hand symptoms: typing performance and user preference. Proceedings of the 13th triennial congress of the International Ergonomics Association. IEA 97, **5**: 65–67.

Toohey J (1997) Osteopathic treatment of migraine: the patient's perspective. BSc(hons) thesis, British College of Naturopathy and Osteopathy, London.

Torstensen TA, Ljunggren AE, Meen HD, Odland E, Mowinckel P, Geijerstam S (1998) Efficiency and costs of medical exercise therapy, conventional physiotherapy and self-exercise in patients with chronic low back pain. *Spine*, 23(23): 2616–2624.

Travell JG, Simons DG (1983) Myofascial pain and dysfunction. The trigger point manual, vol 1, the upper extremities. Williams and Wilkins, Baltimore.

Travell JG, Simons DG (1992). Myofascial pain and dysfunction. The trigger point Manual, vol 2, the lower extremities. Williams and Wilkins, Baltimore.

Troup JDG, Videman T (1989) Inactivity and the aetiopathogenesis of musculoskeletal disorders. *Clinical Biomechanics* 4: 173–178.

Turner JA (1996) Does a successful outcome imply an effective treatment? In: Cohen MJM, Campbell JN Pain treatment centers at a crossroads; a practical and conceptual reappraisal. Progress in Pain Research and Management. IASP Press, Seattle, vol 7, pp 153–161.

Turner JA, Deyo RA, Loeser JD, Von Korff M, Fordyce WE (1994) The importance of placebo effects in pain, treatment and research. *Journal of American Medical Association*, 271(20): 1609–1614.

Turville KL, Psihogios JP, Ulmer TR, Mirka GA (1998) The effects of video display terminal height on the operator: a comparison of the 15 degree and 40 degree recommendations. *Applied Ergonomics*, 29(4): 239–246.

Udo H, Tajima T, Shinichi U, Yoshinaga F et al (1997) Low back load in two car seats. *Industrial Ergonomics*, 20: 215–222.

Van der Heijden GJMG, van der Windt DAWM, de Winter AF (1997) Physiotherapy for patients with soft tissue disorders: a systematic review of randomised clinical trials. *British Medical Journal*, 315: 25–30.

Veierstad KB (1998) Arm pain related to mechanical exposure of VDU use – a review of the epidemiology. In: Kumar S (ed) Advances in occupational ergonomics and safety. IOS Press, Amsterdam, pp 453–455.

Veierstad KB, Westgaard RH, Andersen P (1993) Electromyographic evaluation of muscular work pattern as a predictor of trapezius myalgia. *Scandinavian Journal of Work, Environment and Health*, 19: 284–290.

Vicenzino B, Wright A (1995) Effect of a novel manipulative physiotherapy technique on tennis elbow; a single case study. *Manual Therapy*, 1(1): 30–35.

Videman T, Markku N, Troup J (1990) Lumbar spine pathologyin cadaveric material in relation to history of back pain, occupation, and physical loading. *Spine*, 15(8): 728–740.

Viikari-Juntura E, Takala E, Riihimaki H, Malmivaara A, Martikainen R, Jappinen P (1998) Standardized physical examination protocol for low back disorders: feasibility of use and validity of symptoms and signs. *Journal of Clinical Epidemiology*, 51(3): 245–255.

Villanueva MBG, Jonai H, Sotoyama M, Hisanaga N, Takaeuchi Y, Saito S (1997) Sitting posture and neck and shoulder muscle activities at different screen height settings of the visual display terminals. *Industrial Health*, 35: 330–336.

Vollestad N, Roe C, Saugen E (1995) Effect of pain on activation of four shoulder and neck muscles. Premus 95 book of abstracts, 301–303.

Waddell G (1998) The back pain revolution. Churchill Livingstone, Edinburgh.

Weiss ND, Gordon L, Bloom T, So Y, Rempel D (1995) Position of the wrist associated with the lowest carpal tunnel pressure: implications for splint design. *The Journal of Bone and Joint Surgery*, 77A(11): 1695–1699.

Werner, RA, Franzblau A, Albers JW, Armstrong TJ (1997) Influence of body mass index and work activity on the prevalence of median mononeuropathy at the writst. *Occupational and Environmental Medicine* 54: 268–271.

Westgaard RH (1997) Limits to human performance: consideration of low-level work loads of long duration. Proceedings of the 13th triennial congress of the International Ergonomics Association. IEA 97, 4: 545–547.

Westgaard RH, De Luca CJ (1997) Motor unit substitution during sustained contractions: implications for ergonomics. Proceedings of the 13th triennial congress of the International Ergonomics Association. IEA 97, 4: 237–239.

Westgaard RH, Winkel J (1997) Ergonomic intervention research for improved musculoskeletal health: a critical review. *International Journal of Industrial Ergonomics*, 20: 463–500.

Willard F Neuroendocrine-immune network, nociceptive stress and the general immune response. Unpublished data.

Williams PL et al (eds) (1995) Gray's Anatomy. 38th edn. Churchill Livingstone, Edinburgh.

Williams RA, Pruitt SD, Doctor JN, Epping-Jordan JE (1998) The contribution of job satisfaction from acute to chronic LBP. *Archives of Physical and Medical Rehabilitation*, 79: 366–373.

Wilson A (1993) The incidence of spinal complaints in college students – a preliminary report. *Journal of the New Zealand Register of Osteopaths*, 6: 16–17.

Wilson A (1994) Are you sitting comfortably? Optima, London.

Wilson A (1996) The complete guide to good posture at work. Vermillion, London.

Wolfe F, Smythe HA, Yunus MB et al (1990) The American College of Rheumatology 1990 Criteria for the classification of fibromyalgia. Report of the Multicentre Criteria Committee. *Arthritis and Rheumatism*, 33: 160–172.

Wolstad JC, Sherman BR (1998) The effects of a back belt on posture, strength and spinal compressive force during static lift exertions. *International Journal of Industrial Ergonomics*, 22: 409–416.

Woolf CJ, Thompson SWN (1991) The induction and maintenance of central sensitization is dependent on N-methyl-D aspartic acid receptor activation; implications for the treatment of post-injury pain hypersensitivity states. *Pain* 44: 293–299.

Wright A (1999) Recent concepts in the neurophysiology of pain. *Manual Therapy*, 4(4): 196–202.

Yabuki S, Kikuchi S, Olmarker K, Myers RR (1998) Acute effects of nucleus pulposus on blood flow and endoneurial pressure in rat dorsal root ganglia. *Spine*, 23(23): 2517–2523.

Zecevic A, Miller DI, Harburn K (2000) An evaluation of the ergonomics of three computer keyboards. *Ergonomics* 43(1): 55–72.

Index